CENTRAL PAIN SYNDROME

Central Pain Syndrome (CPS) is a neurological condition caused by damage specifically to the central nervous system — brain, brainstem, or spinal cord. This is the only up-to-date book available on the clinical aspects (including diagnosis and therapy) of CPS management. The authors have developed a complete reference source on central pain, which includes background material, the pathophysiology of the syndrome, and diagnostic and therapeutic information. The syndrome has been a medical mystery for 100 years with no effective cure; this book turns the concept of incurability of central pain on its head, providing a rational approach to therapy based on a scientific theory.

Sergio Canavero set out to become a functional neurosurgeon after reading *Scientific American*'s special issue on the brain in September 1979. He graduated *magna cum laude* and went on to gain FMGEMS certification. Finding psychosurgery impossible to pursue in Italy, he moved on to the field of pain and movement disorders, introducing extradural cortical stimulation for Parkinson's disease and stroke rehabilitation. His lifetime focus is on the nature of consciousness. With Bonicalzi, he founded the Turin Advanced Neuromodulation Group, a think tank focusing on the advancement of neuromodulation. His secondary focus is on women, a subject he discussed in his book *Donne Scoperte* (*Women Unveiled*, 2005), which attracted media interest.

Vincenzo Bonicalzi graduated *magna cum laude* and took up a career in anesthesiology, pain therapy, and intensive care. He is a senior staff member at the Department of Neurosciences at the third-largest medical facility in Italy. He is an enthusiast for medical statistics and evidence-based medicine. With Canavero, he has explored the pitfalls of modern neurointensive care.

CENTRAL PAIN SYNDROME

PATHOPHYSIOLOGY, DIAGNOSIS AND MANAGEMENT

Sergio Canavero, MD (US FMGEMS)

Turin Advanced Neuromodulation Group (TANG), Turin, Italy

Vincenzo Bonicalzi, MD

Turin Advanced Neuromodulation Group (TANG), Turin, Italy

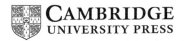

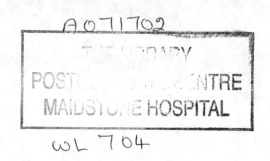
CAMBRIDGE UNIVERSITY PRESS
Cambridge, New York, Melbourne, Madrid, Cape Town, Singapore, São Paulo

Cambridge University Press
32 Avenue of the Americas, New York, NY 10013-2473, USA

www.cambridge.org
Information on this title: www.cambridge.org/9780521866927

First published 2007

Printed in the United States of America

A catalog record for this publication is available from the British Library.

Library of Congress Cataloging in Publication Data

Canavero, Sergio, 1964–
    Central pain syndrome : pathophysiology, diagnosis and
management / Sergio Canavero and Vincenzo Bonicalzi.
        p. ; cm.
    Includes bibliographical references and index.
    ISBN-13 978-0-521-86692-7 (hardback)
    ISBN-10 0-521-86692-8 (hardback)
    1. Central pain.   I. Bonicalzi, Vincenzo, 1956– . II. Title.
    [DNLM: 1. Pain–physiopathology.   2. Pain–therapy.   3. Central
Nervous System–injuries.   4. Central Nervous System Diseases
–physiopathology. WL 704 C213c 2006]
    RC368.C36 2006
    616'.0472—dc22
                                                                2006023246
ISBN 978-0-521-86692-7 (hardback)

To my parents, for their unfailing support
and
to Serena, Marco and Francesca, wishing them a world without pain

To my parents, source of my past
and
to Cecilia, path of my future

CONTENTS

LIST OF TABLES

PREFACE (OR, THE STORY OF AN IDEA)

"The man with a new idea is a crank — until the idea succeeds." (**Mark Twain**)

The story of this book goes back 15 enthusiastic years. At the end of 1991, S.C., at the time 26, was asked by C.A. Pagni, one of the past mavens of the field, to take up central pain. S.C. was back from a semester as an intern at Lyon (France) neurosurgical hospital. A dedicated bookworm, he often skipped the operating theater in favor of the local well-stocked library. In that year a paper was published by two US neurobiologists, espousing the idea of consciousness arising from corticothalamic reverberation: this paper drew his attention, as he was entertaining a different opinion as to how consciousness arises. At the beginning of 1992 he came across a paper written by two US neurologists, describing a case of central post-stroke pain abolished by a further stroke: the authors were at a loss to explain the reason.

Discoveries sometimes happen when two apparently distant facts suddenly fit together to explain a previously puzzling observation. And so it was. During a "girl-hunting" bike trip at Turin's best-known park, a sunny springtime afternoon, the realization came thundering in. Within a short time, a name was found and so the dynamic reverberation theory of central pain was born. It was first announced in a paper published in the February 1993 issue of *Neurosurgery* and then in *Medical Hypotheses* in 1994.

In May 1992 Pagni introduced Dr. Bonicalzi, a neuroanesthesiologist and pain therapist, to S.C. Over the following years, the combined effort led to further evidence in favor of the theory, in particular a neurochemical foundation based on the discovery that propofol, a recently introduced intravenous anesthetic, could quench central pain at nonanesthetic doses (September 1992). The idea of using propofol at such dosage came from reading a paper by Swiss authors describing its use in central pruritus. The similitude between central pain and pruritus, at the time not clearly delineated in the literature, was the driving reason. In 1988 Tsubokawa in Japan introduced cortical stimulation for central pain: it was truly ad hoc, as cortex plays a major role in the theory. Happily, since 1991, the cortex has gone through a renaissance in pain research, although neurosurgical work already pointed in that direction. We soon combined three lines of research — drug dissection, neuroimaging and cortical stimulation data — in our effort to tease out the mechanism subserving central pain.

Central pain as a scientific concept was the product of an inquisitive mind, that of Dr. L. Edinger, a neurologist working in Frankfurt-am-Main, Germany, at the end of the 1800s. Despite being recognized by early-twentieth-century neurologists as the initiator of the idea of "centrally arising pains," this recognition soon faded, shadowed by Dejerine and Roussy and their thalamic syndrome. At the beginning of the twenty-first century, due credit must go to the physician who deserved it in the first place, namely Dr. Edinger.

For a century, central pain has remained neglected among pain syndromes, both for a lack of pathophysiological understanding and a purported rarity thereof. Far from it! Recent estimates make it no rarer than Parkinson's disease, which, however, commands a huge literature. Worse yet, the treatment of central pain has only progressed over the past 15 years or so and much of the new acquisitions have not yet reached the pain therapist in a rational fashion.

As we set out to write this book, we decided to review the entire field and not only expound the dynamic reverberation theory, which, as we hope to show, may well represent "the end of central pain." It has truly been a "sweatshop work" as we perused hundreds of papers and dusted off local medical libraries in search of obscure and less obscure papers in many languages, as true detectives. We drew out single cases lost in a *mare magnum* of unrelated data and in the process gave new meaning to long-overlooked reports. We also realized that some bad science mars the field, and this is properly addressed.

The result is — hopefully — the most complete reference source on central pain in the past 70 years or so. The reader should finish the book with a sound understanding of what central pain is and how it should be treated. The majority of descriptive material has been tabulated, so that reading will flow easily. We hope this will be of help to the millions who suffer from central pain.

Special thanks go to the "unsung heroes" at the National Library of Medicine in Washington, DC, whose monumental efforts made our toil (and those of thousands of researchers around the world) less fatiguing. Thanks also to the guys behind Microsoft Word, which made the tabulations easy as pie. Also, due recognition must go to the Cambridge staff who have been supervising this project over the past two years, especially Nat Russo, Cathy Felgar, and Jennifer Percy and the people at Keyword, above all Andy Baxter and Andrew Bacon for the excellent editorial work.

Sergio Canavero, Vincenzo Bonicalzi
Turin, May 2006

"Frau R. Suicidium." (**Edinger 1891**)

DEFINITIONS

Ever since Dejerine and Roussy's description of central pain (CP) after thalamic stroke in 1906, *thalamic pain* (itself part of the *thalamic syndrome*) has remained the best-known form of CP and it has often − misleadingly − been used for all kinds of CP. Since CP is due to extrathalamic lesions in the majority of patients, this term should be discarded in favor of the terms central pain of brain−brainstem or cord origin (BCP and CCP). Other terms that are now obsolete and should be discarded include *pseudothalamic pain* (i.e., CP caused by extrathalamic lesions) and *anesthesia dolorosa*, when this refers to CP in an anesthetic region caused by neurosurgical lesions. If a stroke at whatever level is the cause of CP, the term central post-stroke pain (CPSP) is used. Even though some clinical features are similar, peripheral neuropathic pain (PNP) is not CP.

CP is akin to central dysesthesias/paresthesias (CD) and central neurogenic pruritus (CNP): actually, these are facets of a same disturbance of sensory processing following central nervous system (CNS) lesions. Dysesthesias and paresthesias differ from pain in their being abnormal unpleasant and non-unpleasant sensations with a nonpainful quality. While contributing to suffering, they can also be found in PNP. *Dysesthetic pain* used as a synonym of CP must also be abandoned.

Since 1978 there has been a tendency to combine CP and PNP under the general rubric of *deafferentation pain* on account of "shared clinical features," both being due to a decrease in afferent input into the CNS and consequent sensitization (see Tasker 2001). Deafferentation pain has never been included in the taxonomy published by the International Association for the Study of Pain (IASP) (Merksey and Bogduk 1994), and actually indiscriminate lumping of all neuropathic pains under this term has created much confusion and even contradictions, often hindering assessment of therapeutic strategies for single disease entities. The term *neural injury pain* should also be discarded. In 1990 a consensus group (Devor *et al.* 1991) concluded that: "The term 'deafferentation pain' as presently used is misleading and should perhaps be abandoned altogether for purposes of clinical diagnosis."

Virtually all kinds of slowly or rapidly developing disease processes affecting the spino- and quintothalamic pathways (STT/QST), i.e., the pathways that are most important for the sensibility of pain and temperature, at any level from the dorsal horn/sensory trigeminal nucleus to the parietal cortex, can lead to CP/CD/CNP. These do not depend on continuous receptor activation.

The IASP defines CP as "pain initiated or caused by a primary lesion or dysfunction of the central nervous system" (Merksey and Bogduk 1994), i.e., of the spinal cord, brainstem or cerebral hemispheres. This definition is too extensive, as it includes pain associated with motor disorders (Parkinson's disease and dystonia) and painful fits, which − although being CNS disorders − are not strictly CP: impairment of spinothalamocortical conduction, a cardinal finding of CP, is not seen in these conditions. However, there are cases of bona fide CP without clinical or electrophysiological signs of such impairment. We propose that CP/CD/CNP be considered only "spontaneous, constant and/or evoked pain, dysesthesia or pruritus initiated by a CNS lesion impinging on or interfering with the spinothalamoparietal path." Since CP appears to be the most frequent of these three conditions, we will generally refer to CP throughout the text. Parkinson's disease, epileptic pains and perhaps other diseases with a painful CP-like component should be classified as *central pain-allied conditions* (CPAC).

Once thought an uncommon neurological curiosity, CP is an important and underrecognized condition. CP produces immense suffering ("a great burden"), even when intensity is low: its generally very unpleasant and irritating, largely constant character makes it incomprehensible by almost all sufferers. Patients can be completely disabled and CP may be so devastating as to override any other disability in the chronic stage. By dominating the sensorium, interfering with the thought processes and undermining the morale, CP frequently alters mood, intellect and behavior with deterioration of personality, depression and neurotic tendencies, interfering with rehabilitation, and impairing daily activities and quality of life. Many patients with severe persistent pain undergo a progressive physical deterioration caused by disturbance of sleep and appetite, a restriction in physical and daily activities, and often become addicted to medications, all of which contribute to general fatigue, increased irritability and decreased libido and sexual activity. The social effects are equally devastating: many patients have progressively greater problems with their families and friends, reduce their social interactions and activities and are unable to work (Widar *et al.* 2004). There are hints that chronic pain may suppress the immune system and even alter insulin sensitivity. Some patients with severe persistent pain become so discouraged and desperate that they commit suicide, and usually not because of depression. Last, but not least, CP financially burdens both society and patients. Thus, it represents a true challenge.

HISTORY

"Those who cannot remember the past are condemned to repeat it." (**G. Santayana**)

Cases of CP following brain or cord damage have most certainly been observed since antiquity, but never understood as such. We have to wait until the nineteenth century for published descriptions of what we now understand to be CP (Table 1.1) in western medicine (there appear to be reports of what is most likely CP in ancient Chinese medicine, this being the result of a deficiency of the Qi and attendant blood stasis, in turn depriving the nourishing of meridians and tendons; see Kuong 1984).

TABLE 1.1. Historic highlights of central pain in the western literature (from Garcin 1937; DeAjuriaguerra 1937)*

Marcet (1811)	Describes pain after bulbar lesions
Fodera (1822)	Describes pain after spinal hemisection
Brown-Sequard (1850)	Describes the syndrome named after him; confirms previous description of hyperesthesia below lesion level on the plegic side
1860–70s	Descriptions of pain after spinal trauma during the U.S. Civil War
Marot (1875)	Further describes pain after bulbar lesions
Nothnagel (1879)	First precise description of constant pain following tumors of the pons Varolii (mentioned by other authors) and other sites
Page (1883)	Describes pain in spinal cord injury patients
Edinger (1891)	Birth of the concept of central pain
Hardford (1891)	Describes pain of cortical origin
Mann (1892)	Matches CP to infarctions of medulla at nucleus ambiguus level
Gilles de la Tourette (1889)	Describes syringomyelic pain
Wallenberg (1895)	Describes the syndrome named after him; insisted on facial pains; ascribed it to PICA embolism (verified autoptically in 1901)
Reichenberg (1897)	Describes CP as resulting from parietal stroke (autopsy confirmed)
Link (1899)	Describes CP as resulting from pontobulbar lesions
Dejerine and Roussy (1906)	Describe the syndrome named after them
Holmes (1919)	"Typical thalamic pain" observed in spinal cord injured patients (World War I soldiers)
Souques (1910), Guillain and Bertrand, Davison and Schick, Schuster, Wilson, Parker (1920s–30s)	Autoptic confirmation that CP may arise without thalamic involvement

* A great many authors described CP, but dates are not available through the two cited reviews: these authors include Halische, Joly, Duchek, Biernacki, Oppenheim, Bechterew (pre-1900), Barrè, Elsberg (cordonal pain), Foerster (dorsal horn pain), Vulpian, Gowers, Gerhardt (recognized CP in multiple sclerosis), Schlesinger, Lhermitte and DeMassary-Bonhomme (hematobulbia), Mills, Mattirolo, Hanser, and many others.

However, the possibility of *centrally arising* pains was simply dismissed by most authorities.

It was only in 1891 that Edinger, a German neurologist, challenging the prevailing opinion of the day, and *"avec une rare sagacité"* (with rare sagacity; Garcin 1937), introduced the concept of *centrally arising pains*. In his landmark paper *"Giebt es central entstehende Schmerzen? Mittheilung eines Falles von Haemorrhagie in den Nucleus externus Thalami optici und in das Pulvinar, dessen wesentliche Symptome in Hyperaesthesie und furchtbaren Schmerzen in der gekreuzten Seite, ausserdem in Hemiathetose und Hemianopsie bestanden haben"* (Are there centrally arising pains? Description of a case of bleeding in the nucleus externus thalami optici and in the pulvinar, whose essential symptom consisted in hyperesthesia and terrible pains in the contralateral side, besides hemiathetosis and hemianopsia), he remarked how only a few cases of pains associated with damage of the brain, brainstem and spinal cord were on record (*"Die Durchsicht der Literatur nach aehnlichen Beobachtungen hat nur wenig ergeben"* − A literature review of similar cases has borne little fruit), but that other reasons were adduced to explain them (generally peripheral nerve causes or muscle spasms). One of the few "well investigated" cases was that of Greiff (1883), concerning a 74-year-old woman who developed *"Hyperaesthesie und reissenden Schmerzen im linkem Arm, geringgradiger im linkem Beine"* (hyperesthesia and tearing pains in the left arm and of lesser intensity in the left leg) as a consequence of several strokes and which lasted for two months until death. At autopsy, two areas of thalamic softening were found, one of which was in what appears to be ventrocaudalis (Vc). Greiff commented on vasomotor disturbances as a possible cause of pain. According to Edinger *"Vielleicht giebt es auch corticale Schmerzen"* (perhaps there are also cortical pains), and he cited as evidence *". . . schmerzhaften Aura bei epileptischen, abnorme Sensationen bei Rindenherden und Reizerscheinungen im Bereich des Opticus bei Affectionen des Hinterhaupts-lappens"* (. . . painful aura in epileptics, abnormal sensations in cortical foci and signs of excitation in the territory of the opticus following diseases of the occipital lobe). Edinger reported on *"einen Krankheitsfall . . . in dem als Ursache ganz furchtbaren Schmerzen post mortem ein Herd gefunden wurde, der dicht an die sensorische Faserung grenzend im Thalamus lag. Der Fall erscheint dadurch besonders beweiskraftig fuer die Existenz 'centraler Schmerzen', weil die Hyperaesthesie und die Schmerzen sofort nach dem Insulte und monatelang vor einer spaeter auftretenden Hemichorea sich zeigten"* (a patient . . . in whom the origin of truly terrible pains was at autopsy a lesion that impinged on the fibers abutting the thalamus. This case is thus especially convincing evidence for the existence of "central pains," as the hyperesthesia and the pains showed immediately after the insult and months before a later arising hemichorea). The patient was *"Frau R."* (Mrs. R.), aged 48, who developed *"heftige Schmerzen und deutliche Hyperaesthesie in den gelaehmten Gliedern"* (violent pains and clear-cut hyperesthesia in the paretic limbs: right arm and leg); *"Wegen der furchtbaren Schmerzen Suicidium 1888"* (due to the terrible pains, suicide 1888). This woman developed an intense tactile allodynia for all stimuli bar minimal, which hindered all home and personal activities (e.g., dressing) and made her cry; also *"Laues wasser wurde als sehr heiss, kaltes als unertraeglich schmerzend"* (lukewarm water was felt as very hot, and cold water as intolerably painful) in both limbs. Very high doses of "*Morphium*" were basically ineffective. This patient's pain reached intolerable peaks, but sometimes could be tolerated for a few hours or at most half a day before shooting up again. In this patient, "*Vasomotorische Stoerungen, wie sie in dem Lauenstein (D.Arch.f.klin.Med. Bd.XX.u.A.)'schen... Falle bestanden haben, sind nicht zur Beobachtung gekommen*" (vasomotor disturbances, as present in Lauenstein's case, were nowhere to be observed). At autopsy, "*Der Herd im Gehirn nimmt also den dorsalen Theil des Nucleus externus thalami und einen Theil des Pulvinar ein, er erstreckt sich lateral vom Pulvinar fuer 1 mm in den hintersten Theil der inneren Kapsel hinein. Der Faserausfall, der dort in Betracht kommt, ist sehr gering.*" (The brain lesion involved the dorsal portion of the nucleus externus thalami and a portion of the pulvinar, extending laterally from pulvinar for 1 mm into the most posterior part of the inner capsule. The loss of fibers, that can be observed at this point, is minimal.) Thus, in Greiff's and Edinger's patients lesions were respectively found at autopsy in right thalamic nucleus internus and ventral thalamus and in thalamic nucleus externus and pulvinar.

Edinger should be given the credit as the one who introduced the concept of CP to neurology, as he wrote: "*Man kommt zum Schlusse, dass hier wahrscheinlich durch directen Contact der sensorischen Kapselbahn mit erkranktem Gewebe die Hyperaesthesie und die Schmerzen in der gekreuzten Koerperhaelfte erzeugt worden sind*" (one concludes that here both the hyperesthesia and the pains in the crossed half of the body have been likely caused by direct contact of injured tissue with the sensory path coursing in the internal capsule), actually being the first to propose an irritative theory of CP. Incidentally, he stressed the importance of the internal capsule, a forerunner of our theory (Canavero 1994).

One year later, Mann (1892), another German neurologist, concluded, in Edinger's wake, that CP can be also observed outside the thalamus, namely in the medulla oblongata, thus antedating Wallenberg's classic description (autopsy of this patient performed in 1912 confirmed Mann's clinical diagnosis and the involvement of the spinothalamic tract). Thereafter, an explosion of reports ensued. In the first decade of the twentieth century, Dejerine and Roussy (1906) described six cases of what they called "*Syndrome thalamique*," whose signs and symptoms were summarized by Roussy (1906) in his thesis:

1) slight hemiparesis usually without contracture and rapidly regressive;
2) persistent superficial hemianesthesia of an organic character which can in some cases be replaced by cutaneous hyperesthesia, but always accompanied by marked and persistent disturbances of deep sensations;
3) mild hemiataxia and more or less complete astereognosis.

To these principal and constant symptoms are "*ordinairement*" (ordinarily) added:

1) severe, persistent, paroxysmal, often intolerable pain on the hemiparetic side unyielding to any analgesic treatment;
2) choreoathetotic movements in the limbs on the paralyzed side.

On the basis of an autopsy study of three cases, they concluded that the lesion is localized to the external, posterior and inferior region of the thalamus (thus including the main sensory nucleus Ventrocaudalis, or Vc), impinges on the median nuclei and, to a lesser extent, involves a part of the posterior limb of the internal capsule. Certainly, the complete syndrome is very rare. In their original paper on the *syndrome thalamique*, Dejerine and Roussy evaluated microscopically the thalamic lesion responsible for the syndrome. In their first case they noted a lesion in the posterior thalamus, involving both external and internal nuclei and the internal capsule. The lesion impinged more diffusely on the external thalamic nucleus. In their second case the lesion again impinged more on the external thalamic nucleus, but they also noted the lesion of the internal and median nuclei, internal capsule and pulvinar. The lesion also impinged on the posterior pulvinar. In their third case a less extended lesion was noted, impinging on the posterior part of the thalamic external nucleus, the internal and median nuclei, the posterior part of the internal capsule and part of the lenticular nucleus. They concluded that the thalamic syndrome follows a lesion of the postero-external part of the external thalamic nucleus, impinging also on part of median and internal thalamic nuclei and on the near part of the internal capsule.

A few years later, Head and Holmes (1911), on the basis of personal and literature autoptic evidence, concluded that thalamic pain depends on the destruction of the posterior part of the external thalamic nucleus. In their book-size article, they provide the best and first quantitative description ever of somatosensory alterations in CP patients (Chapter 2).

During World War I several observations on "thalamic pains" associated with spinal cord war lesions were published, as previously done – but only descriptively – during the U.S. Civil War in the 1860s.

The term central pain was first used in the English literature by Behan (1914). In 1933 Hoffman reported a tiny lesion in the most basal part of the Vc, where spinothalamic fibers end (Hassler's Vcpc). This is probably the smallest reported lesion causing CP.

In the 1930s three major reviews on CP were published (De Ajuriaguerra 1937; Garcin 1937; Riddoch 1938). Here, the interested reader will find an unparalleled review of the literature of the nineteenth and early twentieth centuries, plus unsurpassed descriptions of CP, whose ignorant neglect (admittedly also out of language barriers) on the part of modern investigators is responsible for several "re-discoveries." Nothing new has been basically added to the clinical literature since.

Riddoch gave this definition: "By central pain is meant spontaneous pain and painful overreaction to objective stimulation resulting from lesions confined to the substance of the central nervous system including dysaesthesiae of a disagreeable kind."

It was clear how "thalamic pains" could follow a lesion of the lateral thalamic area, in the territories of the lenticulo-optic, thalamo-geniculate and thalamo-perforating arteries, but also of the cortex (rarely), internal capsule, medulla oblongata and less frequently the pons (no mesencephalic lesions were on record) and the spinal cord (not infrequently; particularly following injury and syringomyelia). Thermoalgesic sensory loss and somatotopographical constraints were clearly delineated. However, De Ajuriaguerra, based on a patient with a thalamic lesion and CP without sensory derangement described by Lhermitte, concluded against a role of the sensory relay nuclei in the genesis of CP (actually that patient had minimal sensory loss and loss of cells and fibers also included Vc).

The most frequent cause of CP appeared to be vascular at all levels, except the brainstem, where tumors, tuberculomas, multiple sclerosis, syringobulbia and hematobulbia contributed; Mills's 1908 patient suffered mostly central paresthesias. Epileptic pains were also considered CP.

Unfortunately, over the years, despite ample evidence that other lesions can cause CP as well, the term *thalamic syndrome* became synonymous with CP, despite it being clear to many that it was not so.

In 1969 Cassinari and Pagni, in their monograph *Central Pain: A Neurosurgical Survey*, wrote: "the conclusions of the various workers who have tried ... to identify the structure in which lesions are responsible for the onset of central pain sometimes conflict. The divergence of opinion is fairly easily explained by the fact that spontaneous lesions are usually extensive, difficult to define, often plurifocal, and affect several systems with different functions." By studying iatrogenic "pure" lesions (which they equated to "experimental lesions") giving rise to CP, they reached the conclusion that the essential lesion was damage to the pain-conveying spinothalamocortical tract. Also, they observed how operations that interrupt the central pain pathways in order to allay pain may themselves originate CP (sometimes more severe than the pain that led to the operation), an occurrence practically impossible to foresee. However, the genesis of CP remained an enigma.

Thereafter, the subject received little additional attention (the "hidden disorder": Schott 1996). CP remained a neglected field among most medical educators and also among neurologists and neurosurgeons at large. Bonica (1991) found that, of 26,281 pages of text in 14 textbooks of neurology, neurosurgery, medicine and surgery, only 6.5 (0.025%) dealt specifically with CP, a situation that persists almost unchanged to this day. Consequently, most physicians in practice have little or no awareness of the subject.

Until the mid 1980s, little or no research on the clinical characteristics as well as the basic mechanisms and pathophysiology of CP was done, with only a handful of basic and clinical scientists devoting efforts to these objectives. Not even the establishment of the IASP in 1973 and of the journal *Pain* in 1975 changed this dismaying panorama. At the end of the 1990 Ann Arbor symposium on central pain syndromes (Casey 1991), Lindblom epitomized the problem: "The pain mechanisms of central pain syndromes are virtually unknown and specific analgesic measures are lacking for the vast majority of patients": CP remained a "puzzling mystery" (Pagni 1989).

The extent of the "puzzle" is given by the bewildering array of theories proposed over 100 years, several directly contradicting one another:

1) Irritation of cells and fibers of spinothalamic and lemniscal systems.
2) Irritation of the sympathetic system, outside the CNS, central cerebrospinal sensory pathways being destroyed.
3) Diversion of pain impulses to the hypothalamus.
4) Summation and wrong integration of pain impulses on a few spared nociceptive neurons.
5) Loss of inhibitory pain mechanisms exerted by thalamus, cerebral cortex, striopallidum, medial lemniscus, brainstem.

6) Activation of alternative secondary pathways, not usually opened and not used when conduction via the spinothalamic complex is available.

7) Abnormal spontaneous or provoked activity in deafferented central sensory neuronal pools which may act as spontaneous dysesthesia and pain-generating mechanisms.

8) Hypersensitivity of deafferented medial midbrain tegmentum, posterior thalamus, thalamic radiations and somatosensory cortex.

9) Activation of nonspecific polysynaptic pathways (paleospinothalamic system), i.e., the neospinothalamic complex and lemniscal system being damaged, nociceptive stimuli are conveyed to the conscious level on this diffuse network of short neurons.

Much has changed over the past 15 years, with several groups applying modern neuroimaging and neurophysiologic techniques to the study of CP. In particular, it is our contention that an explanation and a cure for this "enigma" can now be offered.

2 CENTRAL PAIN OF BRAIN ORIGIN

EPIDEMIOLOGY AND CLINICAL FEATURES

1. Lesions causing CP and location (Table 2.1a,b)

BCP has been caused by all kinds of lesions at any level along the spinothalamo-parietal path, from brainstem to cortex, a fact already appreciated in the 1930s (Garcin 1937; DeAjuraguerra 1937; Riddoch 1938). These include rapidly or slowly developing processes, apparently without differences in probability of triggering CP (but systematic studies have not been conducted), compressive or disruptive/distractive (these latter perhaps being more often associated with CP).

Stroke, either hemorrhagic or ischemic, is the commonest cause of BCP (without differences between the two); dismayingly, iatrogenic CP is not rare. In agreement with their known incidence, in all studies, infarcts are more common than hemorrhages (roughly 4:1).

When the lesion is thalamic, Vc is always involved (the case of Gonzales *et al.* [1992] had signs of capsular involvement). Contrary to previous belief, one third or even less of BCP cases are purely thalamic (e.g., Hirato *et al.* 1993; Andersen *et al.* 1995; Tasker 2001b; Widar *et al.* 2002; Oliveira *et al.* 2002; see also Schmahmann 2003) and complete thalamic syndromes are exceptional. CP does not arise following thalamic lesions only damaging the kinesthetic afferent pathway and probably the spindle afferent pathway as well (Ohye 1998). In all other cases, lesions are cortico-subcortical, in the brainstem, capsulothalamic or lenticulocapsular, or diffuse. Most CPSP is supratentorial (roughly 80%; Tasker 2001).

All cortical lesions responsible for CP involve, exclusively or in combination, the parietal lobe, and specifically SI (and also SII) (e.g., Bassetti *et al.* 1993). Pain occurring acutely immediately after traumatic cortical injury (e.g., penetrating head injuries) – a lancinating pain felt by the patient at the very moment of injury – has been considered CP of cortical origin (Garcin 1937): it fades away rather quickly (hours to days).

The most common site of brainstem lesions (either stroke or hematobulbia, syringobulbia, tumors and MS) is the medulla oblongata, with few cases of pontine and no pure midbrain spontaneous CP having been reported. However, this may actually be an underestimation, as a brainstem lesion was found in 70% of stroke patients in whom MRI was performed (Vestergaard *et al.* 1995). CP of bulbar origin is generally due to thrombosis of the posteroinferior cerebellar artery (PICA) giving rise to Wallenberg's syndrome, in which a lesion impinges on the spinothalamic

TABLE 2.1. Lesions causing CP and their location

a: Lesions causing BCP

(1) Vascular lesion (ischemia/infarct*; hemorrhage, including intracerebral[†] and subarachnoid (independent of surgery, due to spasm and infarction or direct brain injury), vascular malformations (AVM through compression, theft ischemia or hemorrhage, cavernomas through hemorrhage and perhaps compression, compressing nonhemorrhagic saccular aneurysm, venous angioma), migraine-induced vasospasm). [est. 85%]

(2) Penetrating trauma [est. 1–2%]

(3) Inflammation: MS, etc.

(4) Infection: abscess (e.g., toxoplasma), gumma, tuberculoma, encephalitis, etc. [est. 4%]

(5) Tumor (glioma, meningioma, etc., including intratumoral hemorrhage) [est. 1–2%]

(6) Epilepsy

(7) Iatrogenic[‡]

---

* There appears to be no difference between hemorrhages and infarcts as regards the tendency to induce CP, but infarcts being more frequent (85% vs. 15%) are more commonly cause of CPSP. Likewise, about 80% of all infarcts occur in the carotid territory and engage the thalamus (thalamogeniculate and thalamostriate arteries), while PICA strokes engage the lower brainstem. Ischemic lesions may be multiple, often small infarcts especially in the corona radiata and brainstem.

† Intracerebral hemorrhages may act like tumors and provoke CP by compression.

‡ Also includes one patient with a thalamic DBS apparatus for motor control who developed CP after cardioversion, patients with resected vestibular schwannomas and cerebellar tumors.

b: Site of lesions causing brain central pain

Kameyama (1976)

Anatomopathological study on 87 patients with thalamic lesions mainly involving the Vc nucleus.

Author's conclusion: Thalamic pain is more common in right-sided lesions. Thalamic pain is more frequent in lesions confined to Vc (16% out of 38 cases) or involving Vc nucleus and extending to internal capsule (13% out of 31 cases). Patients with combined Vc and pulvinar lesions (19 cases) developed thalamic pain in 11% of cases. Vc lesions extending to nucleus centrum medianum (11 cases) were never associated with the development of CP. This group of patients, however, suffered from more frequent disturbances of deep sensation. As individual variations are common in this area, even very similar lesions do not necessarily produce the same syndrome.

Graff-Radford et al. (1985)

CT study of 25 patients with non-hemorrhagic thalamic infarction. The location of the lesion was determined by CT slices plotted on appropriate templates of human brain. Blinded assessment. Patients were divided into 4 groups with different clinical hallmarks:

(1) posterolateral thalamic infarcts (9 cases, geniculothalamic artery infarct): sensory loss in all primary modality, without major cognitive deficits or aphasia; dysesthesia, hemiparesis, hemianopia and choreiform movements may be associated

(2) anterolateral thalamic infarcts (5 cases, tuberothalamic artery [paramedian thalamic artery, anterior internal optic artery or premamillary pedicle] infarct): normal sensory findings or transient proprioceptive loss

(3) medial thalamic infarcts (3 cases, deep interpeduncular profunda artery [paramedian thalamic artery, posterior internal optic artery or thalamoperforating pedicle] infarct): normal sensory findings or transient proprioceptive loss

(4) lateral thalamus and posterior internal capsule lesions (depending on the partial or whole involvement of the anterior choroidal territory): diminished pinprick in 4/8 pts

Authors' conclusion: Geniculothalamic (posterolateral) infarction may cause Dejerine–Roussy syndrome. Dysesthesia developed in 4/9 pts. A geniculothalamic lacune in primary sensory nuclei (Vc) causes a "pure sensory loss." Complete geniculothalamic infarction causes a contralateral loss of both proprioception and pain sensation. A partial lesion (lacune) in the same territory causes impaired pain and light touch sensation but preserved proprioception or vibratory sensibility.

Kawahara et al. (1986)

37 patients with small (less than 2 cm) thalamic hemorrhage recognized on CT scans. The precise location of each hematoma determined from a stereotactic atlas.

Hematomas classification: (1) anterolateral type, (2) posterolateral type, (3) medial type, (4) dorsal type

Posterolateral hematomas (thalamogeniculate and thalamoperforate arteries hemorrhages) accounted for 76% of cases (28/35 patients). In 9 cases, the posterior third of the internal capsule was spared, but in 19 cases the hematoma traversed it and in some cases ruptured into the third ventricle. Severe hemiparesis and hemihypesthesia/anesthesia were noted only with posterolateral lesions. Six patients complained of paresthesia. Patients with posterolateral lesions also had the poorest prognosis

Authors' conclusion: Sensory loss is due to the (probable) lesion of the ventral posterolateral and posteromedial nuclei and dysesthesia to a lateral thalamic lesion.

Schott et al. (1986)

Study of 35 patients with thalamic or thalamocapsular lesions (with or without CPSP) and of 8 patients with pseudothalamic syndrome and CP following cortical or subcortical lesions. Site of the lesion was determined on CT slices superimposed to a stereotactic atlas in 42 patients and on scintigraphic scan in 1 case. SSEP in all pts. CPSP present in 20 pts

Thalamic lesions and clinical finding in 20 CPSP pts:
geniculothalamic infarct: 5 pts; spontaneous pain absent in 2/5 pts
posterior choroidal infarct: 4 pts; spontaneous pain absent in 1/4 pts
hemorrhagic lesion of the posterior, external, posteromedial, medial and subthalamic nuclei: 1 pt each (=4)
thalamo-capsular hemorrhagic stroke: 7 pts (among these, posterior nuclei were involved in 3 cases, posterolateral nuclei in 1 case and geniculothalamic territory in 1 case); spontaneous pain absent in 7/7 pts

The authors state that 5 out of 20 patients with thalamic or thalamocapsular lesion complained of mild pain; yet a review of data shows that 15 cases complained of spontaneous pain and that 5 pts had only tactile allodynia and/or hyperpathia

Data in text and in tables are not in agreement.

Thalamic lesions and clinical finding in 15 pts without CP:
thalamo-capsular stroke: 9 pts (large thalamic stroke involving the territories of the thalamogeniculate and posterior cerebral arteries in 6 pts; stroke affecting the posterior, posterolateral and median thalamus, and posterior thalamus and capsule in 3 pts)
lesion of the median thalamus: 6 pts

Authors' conclusion: CPSP do not develop after median thalamic lesions or complete deafferentation of the ventrolateral nuclei.

Mauguière and Desmet (1988)

Some or many pts already described in Schott et al. (1986)

Study on 30 pts (with or without CPSP) with thalamic vascular lesions. SEPs assisted identification of 4 subgroups of thalamic pain syndrome. CT evidence of a single thalamic lesion:

10 patients with CPSP:
posterolateral thalamic focal infarct (territory of the geniculothalamic artery): 6 cases
posterior thalamic hemorrhagic lesion: 3 cases
residual hypodense capsulothalamic area (residual scar of a hematoma?): 1 case

6 patients with painful paresthesia and hyperpathia:
ischemic lesion in the geniculothalamic artery territory similar to that previously described: 4 cases (in one case associated to posterior cerebral artery infarct)
capsulothalamic hemorrhage: 2 cases

8 patients without spontaneous pain but with hyperpathia: small ischemic or hemorrhagic lesion involving:
anterolateral thalamus: 2 cases

(continued)

TABLE 2.1. Lesions causing CP and their location

b: Site of lesions causing brain central pain *(cont.)*

caudal pole of the posterior thalamus: 1 case
posterolateral thalamus: 5 cases

6 patients without CPSP:
posterolateral thalamic infarction: 6 cases (in 5 cases with concomitant occipital infarction)
Posterolateral thalamic lesions (territory of the geniculothalamic artery, supplying the somatosensory nuclei) in pts with CPSP were similar to that of patients without pain

---

Bogousslavsky *et al.* (1988)

Prospective study. Long-term follow-up. 40 pts. CT-proven pure thalamic infarct, without involvement of the superficial territory of the posterior cerebral artery. Topographic diagnosis of thalamic infarction determined by means of reported templates

Vascular territories analyzed according to studies delineating 4 main arterial territories:
(1) inferolateral territory (supplied by the inferolateral arteries or thalamogeniculate pedicle – also named infero-external optic artery – supplying mainly **Vc**)
(2) tuberothalamic territory (supplied by the tuberothalamic artery, also named polar artery or anterior optic arteries or premamillary pedicle, supplying mainly the anterior thalamic region, including VA and part of VL)
(3) posterior choroidal territory (supplied by the posterior choroidal arteries, also named posteromedial and postero- lateral systems, supplying also part of the CGL)
(4) paramedian territory (supplied by the retromamillary or thalamoperforate pedicle – also named posterior thalamo- subthalamic paramedian artery – which supplies the paramedian part of the upper midbrain and thalamus, including the intralaminar nuclei and most of the dorsomedial nucleus). In some cases, the thalamoperforate pedicle may supply the paramedian territory of both sides and the corresponding infarct may be bilateral

All the thalamic vascular territories are supplied by the vertebrobasilar system (PCA) with the exception of the tuberothalamic artery, which usually originates from the posterior communicating artery and may be supplied either by the vertebrobasilar or the carotid system. In cases where this artery is absent, the corresponding territory is supplied by the paramedian branches

Site of thalamic infarcts:
inferolateral (geniculothalamic) territory: 18/40 cases (45%). **CPSP in 3/18 pts (16.6%)**
tuberothalamic territory: 5/40 cases (12.5%)
posterior choroidal territory: 3/40 cases (7.5%)
paramedian territory: 14/40 cases (35%). Paramedian infarcts bilateral in 5 cases

CPSP developed in 3/27 pts (7.5%) with sensory dysfunctions, but only in pts with inferolateral (geniculothalamic) infarct. All these patients had a lesion of the thalamic Vc region and no thalamic pain was observed in patients with infarcts outside of it

---

Leijon *et al.* (1989) and Boivie *et al.* (1989)

2 studies on the same 27 selected CPSP pts

Site of the stroke (CVL):
brainstem (BS): 8 pts
thalamus (TH): 9 pts (CT-verified lesion restricted to the thalamus only in 2 pts, the other 7 CVL being large lesions (in most cases larger than 50 mL) extending into the thalamus, but affecting internal capsule, basal ganglia and other structures)
supratentorial extrathalamic (SE): 6 pts (CT-verified: 4 pts; 2 of the lesions located close to the thalamus involved the anterior limb of the internal capsule, but spared the posterior limb and the thalamus. One of the lesions included the basal ganglia. In 2 pts no lesions on CT)

Impossible CT localization of the relevant lesions (UI): 4 pts (bilateral supratentorial lesions).
A lesion of the internal capsule/basal ganglia was present in 1/8 BS pts, 7/9 TH pts, 3/6 SE pts and 1/4 UI pts.
A cortical/subcortical lesion was present in 1/8 BS pts, 5/9 TH pts, 3/6 SE pts and 4/4 UI pts.
It was impossible to localize the relevant CVL with CT criteria in 4/8 BS pts, 2/6 SE pts and 4/4 UI pts.

Authors' statement: In thalamic stroke, the lesion of the ventroposterior thalamic region, including the somatosensory nuclei, was likely, but could not be determined with certainty. In 4 of these pts the lesion extended to the cortex.

Michel *et al.* (1990)

12 cases of cortical CP due to ischemia (11) or hemorrhage (1) sparing the thalamus (on MRI or CT), but involving SI or extending to the thalamoparietal radiations. In 3 cases SI was spared and the cortex involved was prerolandic or posterior parietal. In this series, painful paroxysms resembled painful fits with a jacksonian march in 3 cases (pts 7, 8, 11)

	Hand*	Pain site	Sensibility			Cortical lesion site and type (CT scan)	Notes
			Pin	Ther	Tact		
1	R	L Hemibody (+ head)	I	I	Lo	R parietal (postcentral gyrus, supramarginalis gyrus) ischemic infarct	Cigarette smoking induced severe pain over the trunk. Spontaneous very slow (yrs) pain improvement (dysesthesia with smoke). No allodynia Max. pain site: face
2	R	L Hand	I	N	I	R parietal (postcentral gyrus, gyrus angularis) – occipital ischemic infarct	Pain disappearance after a 2nd infarct. No allodynia
3	R	L Hemibody	Lo	Lo	Lo	R perisylvian (postcentral gyrus, SII, supramarginalis gyrus) ischemic infarct	Hemianesthesia (all modalities). Mechanical allodynia. Hyperpathia. Max. pain site: lower limb
4	R	L Hemibody (+ head)	I	I	I	Massive R sylvian (MCA) ischemic infarct sparing the thalamus (RMI confirmed)	Hemihypoesthesia (all modalities). No allodynia. Patchy max. pain (more intense over joints)
5	R	R Hemibody (+ head)	I	I	I	L fronto-insular (prerolandic) ischemic infarct. Postcentral gyrus spared (?)	No allodynia. Max. pain: calf/ankle
6	R	L Hand/wrist	I	I	I	R parietal (postcentral gyrus, supramarginalis gyrus, gyrus angularis) ischemic infarct	Hypoesthesia (all modalities). Allodynia (mechanical, cold). Hyperalgesia
7	R	L Hemibody	I	I	I	Massive R sylvian (MCA) ischemic infarct sparing the thalamus (RMI confirmed)	No allodynia. Patchy max. pain (joints). CPSP appearance 2 yrs after the infarct. Lancinating radiating pains. 50% pain improvement with TENS
8	R	L Face and forearm/hand	I	I	I	R rolandic-parietal (postcentral gyrus, SII, supramarginalis gyrus) ischemic infarct (RMI confirmed)	Lancinating radiating pains. No allodynia
9	R	L Leg (distal half/foot)	I	I	I	R RMI confirmed small infarct of the ascending frontal convolution (precentral gyrus) (not showed by CT scan). Postcentral gyrus spared(?)	Allodynia

(continued)

TABLE 2.1. Lesions causing CP and their location

b: Site of lesions causing brain central pain *(cont.)*

	Hand*	Pain site	Sensibility			Cortical lesion site and type (CT scan)	Notes
			Pin	Ther	Tact		
10	R	L Leg/foot	I	I	N	R parietal prerolandic ischemic infarct (or hematoma?). Postcentral gyrus spared (?)	Tactile allodynia. Lesion described as ischemic in Table 1, but as hematoma in text
11	R	L Face, hand, stump	N	(Lo)	N	R frontal-rolandic (postcentral gyrus) hematoma	Previous (3 yrs) L leg amputation (ischemic disease). Phantom limb without phantom pain Patchy pain. No allodynia Warm hypoesthesia over the L hand, with cold and pinprick sensibility spared. Epileptic painful fits (showing a jacksonian march from hand to face and involving the phantom foot), phenytoin responsive (disappearance of fits and pain). Pain relief from cold bath
12	R	L Forearm/ hand	N	I	N	R sylvian (postcentral gyrus, SII, supramarginalis gyrus)	Tactile (and cold?) allodynia

* Hand: handedness; R: right; L: left; Pin: pinprick; Ther: thermal; Tact: tactile; I: impaired (reduced); Lo: lost; N: normal.

Authors' conclusion: Cortical areas generally involved in cortical CP: postcentral gyrus (particularly operculus parietalis, SII and insula) with extension to gyrus supramarginalis; Brodmann's area 7 and SI. If parietal areas are spared, the thalamoparietal radiations are involved.

Masson et al. (1991)

One pt with a pseudothalamic cortical syndrome, associated with pain asymbolia; MRI confirmed right infarction restricted to the posterior insula, superior margin of T1, the parietal operculum and the supramarginal gyrus (SI, thalamus, posterior parietal cortex and MI were spared)

Left hemibody (head included): complete hemianalgesia, no response to pinprick and pressure pain. Impaired thermal, tactile, vibratory and position sensibilities. Right hemibody: pain sensibility completely lost. Normal pinprick, tactile, thermal vibratory and position sensibilities

Asymbolia was imputed to a disconnection between SII at insula level and the limbic system.

Tasker et al. (1991)

Lesion localization possible in 40/73 pts (CT, autopsy, clinical examination). 11 pts with CPSP from thalamic lesion. Small lesion restricted to thalamus in 2 cases (1 R, 1 L), large thalamic lesion in 4 cases (3 R, 1 L) and right thalamo-suprathalamic lesion in 5 cases

Other lesion sites: brainstem (infratentorial): 14, suprathalamic only sparing thalamus: 11, diffuse: 1, no lesions on CT scan: 2 cases

Schmahmann and Leifer (1992)

Parietal CP. 6 pts

Cortical lesion site and type (CT scan)	Notes
White matter deep to the inferior aspect of the postcentral and supramarginal gyri; cortex and white matter of the superior aspect of the L postcentral gyrus and posterior parietal region; caudal superior temporal gyrus	Resection of L-sided parietal meningioma. Four mos later discomfort in the R hand. Seven yrs later traumatic hemorrhage in the inferior aspect of the L postcentral gyrus and rostral part of the L posterior parietal cortex (within the surgical scar). Max. pain: R hand
White matter deep to the L postcentral and supramarginal gyri; some involvement of the cortex of the postcentral gyrus; white matter deep to the middle and inferior frontal gyri (small lesion)	Embolic L stroke. CPSP 1 yr later
White matter deep of the postcentral and supramarginal gyri; posterior aspect of the insular cortex	L posttraumatic temporoparietal hematoma. CP 1 wk later
Caudal part of the insula; cortex and underlying white matter of the R angular and supramarginal gyri and superior temporal gyrus	R temporoparietal infarct (recurrent). Carotid endarterectomy. CP 4 yrs later. Pain exacerbated by cold and damp weather
Pericentral regions, posterior parietal cortex, superior temporal gyrus; caudate nucleus and basal ganglia atrophy	Carotid occlusive disease. Incomplete L MCA territory infarction
L sylvian fissure, extending upward into the white matter beneath the postcentral guys and the rostral inferior parietal lobule	Embolic cerebral infarction. Acute hemianesthesia and hemiparesthesias. Touch-provoked dysesthesias. Max. pain: distal arm and hand (overlapping max. sensory impairment area)

Authors' conclusion: In all cases the thalamus was spared and a common lesioned area was identified in the parietal lobe, located in the white matter deep to the caudal insula and deep to the opercular region of the rostral posterior parietal cortex. Cerebral cortex lesions were also noted, but the area of overlap was in the white matter. The cortex overlying this common white matter injury zone includes the rostral inferior parietal lobule and SII.

Gonzales *et al.* (1992)

2 pts with AIDS. CP due to toxoplasma abscesses in the thalamic region.

Postmortem examination (1st case): left-sided lesion in the posterior limb of the internal capsule. Histologic examination: area of necrosis and macrophage infiltration in the left thalamic reticular nucleus. Vc was spared, but a focus of myelin degeneration was noted in the suprathalamic white matter tracts and sections of the spinal cord revealed wallerian degeneration in the right corticospinal tract.

Authors' conclusion: Involvement of the Vc by flogosis and edema not seen pathologically might have contributed early to the initiation of the thalamic syndrome, but "it is possible that injury to the shell-like reticular nucleus may be the important element in the development or modulation of central pain in this case."

CT study (2nd case): single ring enhancing lesion in the left lateral thalamus and adjacent posterior limb of the internal capsule. In this pt **pain disappeared** after anti-toxoplasmosis therapy and 6-months treatment with amitriptyline.

Diaz and Slagle (1992)

Multiple MRI-confirmed toxoplasma abscesses affecting right lenticular nucleus and right and left thalamus. Right lesion affecting medial posterior thalamus, but involving the lateral thalamic structures. CP amitriptyline responsive

Samuelsson *et al.* (1994)

39 pts with lacunar infarct syndromes. CPSP in 3/39 pts. Thalamic lesion site:
pure sensory stroke (PSS) (9/10 pts with identified lesion): posterolateral part of the thalamus (in 1 case involving the posterior part of the internal capsule). CPSP in 3 pts

(continued)

TABLE 2.1. Lesions causing CP and their location

b: Site of lesions causing brain central pain *(cont.)*

Sensorimotor stroke (SMS) (9/12 pts with identified lesion): 8 infarcts in the posterior part of the internal capsule (often involving the putamen; in 2 cases involving the lateral thalamus), 1 infarct of the centrum ovale. No CPSP

Pure motor stroke (PMS) (14/17 pts with identified lesion): 9 infarcts in the posterior part of the internal capsule (often involving the putamen), 4 pontine infarcts, 1 infarct of the centrum ovale. In 4 cases, extension into the corona radiata and periventricular gray matter. No CPSP

Involvement of the thalamus was characteristic for pts with PSS, whereas sites of the infarcts in pts with SMS and PMS were largely similar. Thalamic infarcts predominated among the pts with the most pronounced sensory (QTT) abnormalities

Wessel *et al.* (1994)

Single CT-documented ischemic thalamic lesion. 18 pts with somatosensory disturbances. CP in the opposite hemibody in 10/18. Infarction classification on the CT scans, according to the vascular territory of the different arteries supplying the thalamus

CT-verified lesions among 10 pts with CPSP (classic or pure algetic thalamic syndrome):
anterolateral (tuberothalamic artery): 2/10 pts
posterolateral (geniculothalamic artery, supplying the major somatosensory relay region): 4/10 pts
paramedian (interpeduncular profunda artery or posterior thalamo-subthalamic arteries): 2/10 pts (unilateral infarct)
capsulothalamic lesions (grouping impossible according to these arterial territories): 2/10 pts

CT-verified lesions among 8 pts with severe somatosensory deficits, but without CPSP 1 yr after the stroke (analgetic thalamic syndrome):
posterolateral: 6/8 pts
capsulothalamic: 2/8 pts

Authors' conclusion: A paramedian or an anterolateral thalamic lesion (showed only in pts with CPSP) may be an indicator for the development of CP.

Kumral *et al.* (1995)

Prospective study. Thalamic hemorrhage. 100 pts. CT scan performed between 1 and 5 days after the stroke. Clinicotopographic analysis. Precise location of each hemorrhage determined by a stereotactic atlas

Types of thalamic hemorrhage determined:
anterolateral (including ventroanterior and ventrolateral nuclei): 21 pts
posterolateral (including posteroventrolateral and pulvinar nuclei): 55 pts
medial (including dorsomedial and intralaminar nuclei): 15 pts
dorsal (including mainly dorsomedial nucleus): 9 pts

Small thalamic hemorrhage (<2 cm in diameter or 4 mL in volume): 33 pts
anterolateral: 7
posterolateral: 16
medial: 8
dorsal: 2

Large thalamic hemorrhage (>2 cm in diameter or 4 mL in volume): 67 pts
anterolateral: 14
posterolateral: 39
medial: 7
dorsal: 7

All pts with posterolateral thalamic hemorrhage had sensorimotor deficits, as the adjacent internal capsule was presumably involved in the lesion. Sensory deficits could be detected in 66 pts, but no pts had acute thalamic pain

CPSP (thalamic pain) 1 month after the stroke: 9 pts:

Site of the lesion:
large anterolateral: 1 pt
large medial: 1 pts
large dorsal: 1 pt
posterolateral (1 small and 5 large): 6 pts

A classic syndrome of Dejerine–Roussy developed only in 6 pts, 5 of them with posterolateral lesion and 1 with medial large lesion. All 6 with chorea/ataxia

CPSP in pts with large dorsal and medial hemorrhages explained by the effect of the size of hemorrhage

Mori *et al.* (1995)

104 pts with thalamic hematoma. 86 survivors at 6 mos (52/63 men, 34/41 women)

Extent of hematoma	No. of pts (%)		
		Deaths	Thalamic pain
Localized within the thalamus	21 (20.2)	0	2 (9.5)
	VP: 7	VP: 0	
Extending to the internal capsule	52 (50)	5	3 (5.7)
	VP: 24	VP: 4	
Extending to the midbrain or putamen	31 (29.8)	13	1 (3.2)
	VP: 15	VP: 7	
Total	104	18	6 (5.7)

VP: ventricular penetration.

Chung *et al.* (1996)

Retrospective analysis. Thalamic hemorrhage. 175 consecutive pts admitted at three hospitals. Investigation on the impact of hematoma location (vascular territory) on the clinical symptoms and signs. Thalamic hematomas classification (4 regional type and 1 global type) based on CT and/or MRI findings. Extrathalamic extension of hematomas, including the involvement of the limb of the internal capsule, the lentiform nuclei, the head of caudate nucleus and adjacent subcortical white matter also evaluated.

Hematoma type, frequency and clinical data (pain not explicitly mentioned as part of the Dejerine–Roussy syndrome):

anterior type, mainly located in the region supplied by the polar or tuberothalamic artery (anterior thalamic region): 11/175 cases (6.3%). This type had the smallest size. Occasional involvement of the anterior limb of the internal capsule or of the caudate nucleus. Ventral lateral nucleus (important motor relay structure) often reached. No CP

posteromedial type, mainly located in the region supplied by the thalamic-subthalamic paramedian artery (medial thalamic region): 24/175 cases (13.7%). These hematomas involve mainly the dorsomedial and centromedian nuclei and frequently rupture into the third ventricle or extended mediocaudally in the midbrain (19/24 pts, "thalamomesencephalic hemorrhage"). 13/19 pts with midbrain involvement died. 33% of pts (8/24) had **hypesthesia** and 25% (6/24) developed **Dejerine–Roussy syndrome** (judging by data in Fig. 8B)

posterolateral type, mainly located in the region supplied by the thalamogeniculate artery: 77/175 pts (44%): This was the commonest type of thalamic hematomas in this series and was usually large. It ruptured into the ventricles in 58/77 pts and it extended to the posterior limb of the internal capsule in 61/77 pts (79.2%). The lentiform nucleus was involved in 30/77 cases (38.9%) and in 10 pts (12.9%) the hematoma extended deep into the adjacent white matter. The midbrain was involved in 6/77 cases (7.8%). **Sensory symptoms and signs** were frequent in pts with this type of hematoma: the authors stated in text that 31/77 cases (40.2%) had paresthesias at onset and decreased touch and pain sensation on examination. Judging by their Fig. 8B, 16/77 (21%) had paresthesias at onset and 50/77 (65%) had hypesthesia. Neurologic sequelae were frequent and 23/77 pts died. 32% of pts (25/77) developed **Dejerine–Roussy syndrome** between 3 and 15 days after the onset

(continued)

TABLE 2.1. Lesions causing CP and their location

b: Site of lesions causing brain central pain *(cont.)*

dorsal type, mainly located in the dorsal aspect of the thalamus (i.e. at a higher level of CT scans): 32/175 pts (18.2%). In 14 pts (43.7%) the hematoma extended posterolaterally into the corona radiata or centrum semiovale, thereby causing motor and sensory deficits. Disruption of the distal branches of the lateral posterior choroidal artery causes a pure dorsal thalamic hematoma, not involving the pulvinar, usually presenting as sensorimotor stroke. This type of stroke is mild and reversible. 11 pts (34.3%) had paresthesias at onset and, judging by Fig. 8B, 23 pts (71.8%) had hypesthesia. **Thalamic syndrome** of Dejerine–Roussy developed in 8 pts (32%)

global type, large hematomas occupying the whole thalamus. In these hematomas the bleeding focus was difficult to assess on brain images: 31/175 pts (17.7%). These hematomas were large enough to occupy the entire area of the thalamus and often extended into the internal capsule and putamen. In most cases the clinical and radiological char- acteristics were very similar to those of the **posterolateral type,** except that the hematomas were too large to define the bleeding focus. The majority of them were probably caused by lesion of thalamogeniculate arteries. **Hypesthesia** was present (Fig. 8B) in 17 pts (54.8%). 24 pts (77.4%) died, but the authors did not report any case of Dejerine–Roussy syndrome

Nasreddine and Saver (1997)

Systematic review of thalamic CPSP. Lesions were confined to the thalamus in approximately half the cases (45/87, 51.7%). An additional 21% extended into the internal capsule and in the remaining one-third there were additional lesions, most often (13%) in the occipital lobe, reflecting concomitant infarction in the territory of the posterior cerebral artery

In 117 cases it was possible to localize the lesion within the thalamus: the **ventral posterior thalamus** was affected in 73% of cases and possibly in another 10%. Ischemic stroke generally affected the **geniculothalamic artery territory.** In one case each, the lesion affected the anterior, paramedial, lateral superior, medial posterior, posterior superior and central thalamus. The lateral thalamus was affected in 6 cases and the anterolateral thalamus in 4 cases. Infarcts were located in the territory of the posterolateral choroidal artery in 3 cases

These authors noted that all pain cases in 4 series of pts with thalamic stroke occurred with lesions in the geniculothalamic territory

Paciaroni and Bogousslasky (1998)

Pure sensory thalamic stroke 25 pts. Topographic diagnosis of thalamic lesion made on reported templates by means of CT or MRI scans and MR angiography. The only clinical manifestation of stroke was sensory dysfunction. The infero- lateral region (thalamogeniculate arteries) was involved in all of the pts

Symptoms during the stroke:
pain and/or dysesthesia: 6 pts (involvement of the n. ventrocaudalis in 5 of them; in 3 associated with lesion of the n. ventro-oralis intermedius and in 1 of the pulvinar)
contralateral paresthesias: 18 pts (involvement of the n. ventrocaudalis in 16 of them; associated with lesion of the n. ventro-oralis intermedius in 4 cases, of the n. ventro-oralis intermedius plus n. ventro-oralis externus in 1 case and of the n. parvocellularis and pulvinar in 1 case)

Delayed pain and/or dysesthesia (CPSP): 4/25 pts (16%). Pts with CPSP had a median involvement of 1 nucleus (range 1–3). Thalamic infarcts were very small. The thalamic nuclei involved by the lesion in these pts were the nucleus ventrocaudalis in 3/4 cases and nucleus ventrocaudalis, nucleus parvocellularis and pulvinar in 1/4 cases

Pts without CPSP: Pts without CPSP had a median involvement of 2 nuclei (range 1–5). An isolated lesion of the n. ventrocaudal was however present in 7 pts

Authors' conclusion: Sensory dysfunction and delayed thalamic pain are more commonly found in lesions involving the nucleus ventrocaudalis and n. ventro-oralis intermedius.

Bowsher *et al.* (1998)

Aim of the study: to correlate the pain characteristics and quantitative sensory findings with the location of lesions revealed on MRI. 73 CPSP pts (65 post-stroke, 8 post-SAH). Post-stroke sensory deficit without pain in 13 pts (control).

Multiple lesions in most pts

*Location of all identified **brainstem** and **contralateral supratentorial** lesions in all CPSP pts (n = 73) and controls (n = 13) undergoing MRI:*
brainstem w/ crossed signs: 5 pts (2 controls)
brainstem w/ uncrossed signs: 20 pts (1 control)
ventroposterior thalamic n.: 49 (43?) pts (7 controls)
other thalamus: 29 pts (3 controls)
internal capsule: 35 pts (7 controls)
basal ganglia: 33 pts (6 controls)
insula: 22 pts (3 controls)
parietal cortex: 13 pts (4 controls)
no detectable abnormalities: 3 pts

*Location of identified **homolateral** to the symptomless side **supratentorial** lesions in 16 CPSP pts and 2 controls (total: 18 pts):*
ventroposterior thalamic n. alone: 2 pts
ventroposterior thalamic n. plus internal capsule: 4 pts
internal capsule alone: 8 pts (2 controls)
parietal cortex alone: 1 pt
parietal cortex plus internal capsule: 1 pt

Pts subgroups according to lesion site (70 pts):
Purely infratentorial: 9 pts + 3 pts with additional supratentorial lesions but crossed sign/symptoms (2 (3?) controls). "A number of cases had single lesions extending from the upper brainstem ... into the VPL, and ... into the IC as well"
Thalamic (± internal capsule): 27 pts (including 2 purely capsular) (4 controls). VPL involved in 43 pts (without infratentorial or cortical lesion in 23, w/ additional parietal/insular and/or brainstem lesions in 20). VPL + IC lesions in 22 VPL pts. VPL lesions in 61% of all cases w/ MRI-detected lesions (43 pts) and in 7/13 controls
Supratentorial (thalamic ± internal capsule + parietal cortex ± insula): 18 pts (including 2 purely capsular) (6 controls). Circumscribed supratentorial lesions only in 8 pts. Purely supratentorial lesion not involving VPL in 9 pts (central thalamus: 2, IC: 2, parietal cortex) and 4 controls (IC: 2, cortex: 2). Basal ganglia involvement in 33 pts and 6 controls. Basal ganglia + VPL in 14 pts. Basal ganglia involved but VPL spared: 2 pts
Infra- and supratentorial + cortical: 6 pts (no control). Many pts had periventricular spots. Cortical lesions (involving parietal cortex ± insular/retroinsular regions) in 17 pts and 5 controls. Basal ganglia + infra-/supratentorial lesions: 11 pts. Gray matter lesion: 19 pts. White matter lesion: 12 pts. Gray + white matter lesion: 39 pts
Infra- and supratentorial only: 7 pts (1 control)
No detectable abnormalities: 3 pts
Lesions in symptomless hemispheres: 16/70 pts, 2/13 controls. Infratentorial: 3/11; thalamus (± IC): 13/27 pts (3 basal ganglia only); supratentorial: 2/18 pts; infra- and supratentorial: 1/6 pts; infra- and supratentorial only: 2/7 pts (basal ganglia only: 1)

Authors' conclusion: Under these circumstances "it would be extremely difficult to draw outlines that would have any real claim to 'illustrate' the lesion."

Kim (1998)

6 pts with early-onset CPSP contralateral to the ischemic lesion followed by delayed ipsilateral sensory symptoms with onset of mild ipsilateral pain mirroring the site of the most severe CPSP (without objective sensory deficits). No new ischemic lesions.

2 medial medullary infarct (MMI) pts with CPSP

(continued)

TABLE 2.1. Lesions causing CP and their location

b: Site of lesions causing brain central pain *(cont.)*

	Pain site (early CPSP)	Sensibility	Cortical lesion site and type (MRI or CT scan)	Notes
1	L perioral area, hard palate, palm/fingers, toes except the fifth	Decreased (all modalities)	R thalamic infarct (MRI)	Delayed symptoms 16 mos after stroke (first 2 fingers, toes). Aggravating factors (both sides): movements, fatigue, cold water. Follow-up: 60 mos
2	L shoulder, trunk, leg	Decreased (all modalities)	R thalamic infarct (MRI)	Delayed symptoms 6 mos after stroke (shoulder, thigh). Follow-up: 24 mos
3	R hemibody + face	Decreased (all modalities)	L lenticulocapsular hemorrhage (CT)	Delayed symptoms 24 mos after stroke (lower leg). Aggravating factors (both sides): movements, fatigue. Follow-up: 27 mos
4	L hemibody + face	Unchanged	R pontine infarct (MRI)	Delayed symptoms 24 mos after stroke (foot, fingers). Follow-up: 36 mos
5	L hemibody + face	Unchanged	R medial medullary infarct (MRI)	Delayed symptoms 9 mos after stroke (hand). Aggravating factors (both sides): movements, fatigue, humid weather. Follow-up: 23 mos
6	L hemibody + face	Decreased (all modalities)	R medial medullary infarct (MRI)	Delayed symptoms 15 mos after stroke (hand, foot). Aggravating factors (both sides): cold weather. Follow-up: 31 mos

Clinical sensory examination: pinprick, temperature, vibration, light touch, position.

Author's conclusion: Pts with MMI often develop CPSP.

Kumral et al. (2001)

16 consecutive pts. MRI-confirmed **bilateral** thalamic infarction. MR angiography of posterior cerebral, basilar and vertebral arteries in all pts. Vascular territories according to templates of Bogousslavsky *et al.* (1988) (polar artery, paramedian [thalamo-subthalamic] artery, thalamogeniculate artery and posterior choroidal artery). Bilateral infarct site:

thalamic paramedian artery territory: 8 pts
paramedian and contralateral thalamogeniculate arteries territory (2 infarcts): 3 pts
polar and contralateral thalamogeniculate arteries territories (2 infarcts): 2 pts
thalamogeniculate artery territory: 3 pts

CPSP (thalamic pain): 1 pt (bilateral thalamogeniculate infarct)

Oliveira et al. (2002)

40 pts. Lesion CT/MRI confirmed

Lesion site:
supratentorial extrathalamic: 15 pts
thalamic: 8 pts
thalamocapsular: 5 pts
brainstem: 8 pts
undetermined: 4 pts

21 pts had multiple lesions

Ischemic stroke in 87.5% of pts; hemorrhagic stroke in 12.5% of pts

Kim (2003)

20 pts with CPSP or paresthesia after lenticulocapsular hemorrhage – LCH

The lesions involved the dorsal part of the posterior limb of the internal capsule, probably damaging the thalamocortical sensory pathway. The CPSP usually developed some time after the onset, tended to persist, and partially responded to medications. These characteristics are consistent with CPSP that developed in pts with stroke occurring in other regions. Thus, LCH should be considered one of the causes of CPSP

The LCHs involved the posterior portion of the putamen and the dorsal part of the posterior limb of the internal capsule just adjacent to the thalamus, where ascending sensory tracts are believed to be prominently located. Follow-up imaging results also showed that the lesions involved the posterior limb of the internal capsule (pts 8, 10, 12, 15 and 20). However, a part of the posterolateral part of the thalamus may have been involved as well in some pts (pts 2, 5, 6, 9 and 19). The mildness of limb weakness may be explained by the partial involvement of the descending pyramidal fibers at the dorsal part of the posterior limb of the internal capsule

Interestingly, **the CPSP was distinctly more severe in the leg than in the arm or face in the majority of the pts.** Considering the neuroradiologic data of the pts, the lesions may have involved the sensory tracts originating from the most dorsolateral portion of the ventral posterior nucleus, which would explain the leg-dominant sensory symptoms

Greenspan et al. (2004)

13 consecutive CPSP pts. MRI confirmed lesion. Stroke type:

BS (LMI)	TH	SE	UI
2	4	6	1
	L thalamus + corona radiata + IC	R basal ganglia + IC	
	R ventrocaudal thalamus (2 pts)	L parietal cortico-subcortical	
	L posterior thalamus	R insula (2 pts)	
		L insula	

BS: brainstem; LMI: lateral medullary infarction; TH: thalamic; SE: supratentorial extrathalamic; UI: unidentified; IC internal capsule.

Bowsher et al. (2004)

4 pts with small restricted cerebral cortical infarcts, sparing in all case SI (postcentral gyrus)

Pt 1: lesion confined to the parietal operculum (SII)

Pt 2: SII lesion also encroaching on the posterior insula

Pt 3: lesion involving both banks of the sylvian fissure and the dorsal insula

Pt 4: lesion involving the upper bank of the sylvian fissure

Cahana et al. (2004)

1 pt with Wallenberg syndrome (?) from *Listeria rhomboencephalitis* (MRI findings: left pontine tegmentum lesion involving the spinal-trigeminal tract and nucleus)

Hansson (2004)

43 pts with evidence of unequivocal stroke, CPSP pain lasting > 6 mos
(Data from Widar et al. 2002; Andersen et al. 1995; Leijon et al. 1989)

Location of stroke:
brain stem 5
thalamus 5
supratentorial/extrathalamic 27
not located 6

Author's conclusion: In most cases of CPSP, stroke lesions are extrathalamic.

Willoch et al. (2004)

5 CPSP pts

Pt 1: R Ischemic stroke (PCA, small lacunar lesion of VP thalamus + mediobasal part of occipital lobe)

(continued)

TABLE 2.1. Lesions causing CP and their location

b: Site of lesions causing brain central pain *(cont.)*
Pt 2: R ischemic stroke (posterior thalamus + mesial temporal lobe)
Pt 3: L ischemic stroke (posterior thalamus + border zones of PCA bilaterally)
Pt 4: L postoperative hemorrhage (hemangioma in the L inferior parietal lobe, bordering occipital and temporal lobes)
Pt 5: R hemorrhagic stroke (R midbrain, affecting medial lemniscus, spino-trigemino-thalamic tract and reticular formation)

Kong *et al.* (2004)

Stroke site in 13 CPSP pts out of 107 selected post-stroke pts:
thalamic: 7 (54%)
middle cerebral artery: 4 (31%)
basal ganglia: 2 (15%)

Seghier *et al.* (2005)

Structural MRI: small residual cavity confined to the right thalamic VPL nucleus and the adjacent posterior third of the posterior arm of the internal capsule

Montes *et al.* (2005)

Authors' conclusion: After projection of 3D MRI images onto a human thalamic atlas: well localized left thalamic infarct centered on the VP, involving the anterior 2/3 of the VPL nucleus and, to a lesser extent, VPM (VPMpc), VL (VLp) and VPI nuclei. The lesion spared the posterior thalamic nuclear group and did not extend posterior and ventral enough to concern the putative location of the spinothalamic-afferented nucleus VMpo.

tract and on the nucleus and/or the descending root of the trigeminal nerve on the same side.

2. Incidence and prevalence (Table 2.2)

For more than a century, BCP has been considered rare, based on sheer opinion (1 out of 1500 strokes according to Davis and Stokes 1966), a concept upheld by the "rapid retrospective survey" on 400 stroke patients (with unclear definition of source population under consideration) performed by Bowsher (1993), 2% of whom (out of 25% with somatosensory deficits) developed CP. Several studies dealing with this question have been published; unfortunately, the vast majority has a strong selection bias, being retrospective in nature or drawing from hospitalized patients in single neurology departments (i.e., not mirroring the true prevalence in the general population). One confounding factor has also been the delayed onset in several patients (up to years; Table 2.5), leading to underestimations.

Luckily, prospective studies conducted over the past decade overturned this misconception. Today, we know that no less than 8% of all strokes (brain and brainstem, ischemic and hemorrhagic) originate CP/CD/CNP; this figure rises to roughly 20% if somatosensory signs are present.

Almost 5 million Americans (2.4% of adults) had a stroke, with almost 600 000 new survivors each year. Stroke prevalence in the EU is about 1100/100 000. An estimated 15 million people worldwide survive a minor stroke each year (WHO estimate 2002). As stroke attacks seems to be lower in Western than in Eastern Europe or China for both men and women and blacks have a higher incidence of

TABLE 2.2. Incidence and prevalence (only best evidence studies included; excluded ones can be found in bibliographies attached to cited papers)

Author	Pathology	No. of pts	Pts with CP
Kameyama (1977)	Vc vascular lesions	87	Clinicopathological study. Cases selected at random from a routine autopsy series Thalamic spontaneous pain present in 12 pts (14%) "Dysesthesia" in 25 pts (29%)
Graff-Radford et al. (1985)	Nonhemorrhagic thalamic infarction	25	"Dysesthesia" in 4/25 pts (16%). Dysesthesias present only in a subgroup of pts with posterolateral (geniculothalamic) infarction in whom the incidence raised to 44.4% (4/9 pts)
Kawahara (1986)	Small thalamic hemorrhage	37	"Paresthesia and/or dysesthesia" in 6/37 pts (16.2%). Symptoms present only in pts with posterolateral thalamic lesions (6/28 pts (21.4%))
Bogousslavsky et al. (1988)	Thalamic infarct	40	Prospective study (all pts with a thalamic infarct admitted to the neurology department between 1978 and 1986) reporting clinical findings and long-term follow-up of 40 pts with a CT-proven "pure" thalamic infarct. Delayed onset (1 week, 2 months and 3 months) severe (2 cases) or moderate (1 case) CP in 2 women and 1 man out of 27 pts with sensory dysfunctions *Pain incidence:* whole group: 3/40 pts (7.5%) pts with sensory impairment: 3/27 (11%) pts with inferolateral territory infarct and lesion of the thalamic Vc region: 3/19 (17%) pts with infarcts outside the Vc region: no thalamic pain observed
Samuelsson et al. (1994)	Lacunar infarct syndromes	39	Pts collected from a series of 100 consecutive pts. Pure sensory stroke (thalamic) in 10 cases *Pain incidence:* whole group: 3/39 (7.7%) (severe in 2) (5.1%) PSS: 3/10 (30%) (severe in 2) (20%)
Kumral et al. (1995)	Thalamic hemorrhage	100	Consecutive pts affected by thalamic hemorrhage and admitted to a single neurology department between 1988 and 1993 Sensory deficits: 66/100 pts Acute thalamic pain: 0/100 pts Delayed (1 month) thalamic pain: 3 pts (large anterolateral, posterolateral and dorsal thalamic hemorrhage, respectively) Delayed (1 month) thalamic pain plus chorea plus ataxia (thalamic syndrome): 6 pts (small posterolateral hemorrhage [1 case], large posterolateral hemorrhage [4 cases], large medial hemorrhage [1 case]) CPSP incidence in the whole group: 9% (not reported if CPSP arose only in pts with somatosensory deficits)
Andersen et al. (1995)	Unselected stroke population	267	Study evaluating the incidence of CPSP in 207 (out of 267) pts (age < 81 yrs) surviving at least 6 mos after a stroke and who were able to communicate reliably. Sampling bias reduced by

(continued)

TABLE 2.2 *(continued)*

Author	Pathology	No. of pts	Pts with CP
			also examining 1/3 of the 10% non-hospitalized pts. 60 pts (23%) died in the first 6 mos after stroke and were not examined. Exclusion criteria: pts with SAH, Binswanger's disease, degenerative or expansive neurological diseases. Characterization of the site and extension of the lesions by means of a CT scan. Neuropsychiatric examinations and detailed sensory test made in the first week, at 1, 6 and 12 mos after the stroke. Pts lost to follow-up: <5%. **Incidence of CPSP at follow-up (% of pts):** 1 mo: 4.8% 6 mos: 6.5% 1 yr: 8.4% (16/191 pts) (moderate or severe in 5%). Evoked dysesthesia or allodynia in all but 1 pt. One further pt had persistent evoked non-painful dysesthesia. **In 2 additional pts pain disappeared spontaneously;** 1 pt had evoked dysethesia and shoulder pain at 1 month and another (lower brainstem infarction), complained of ocular pain with a Horner syndrome. **Incidence of CPSP in pts with some somatosensory deficits: 18%.** *Authors' conclusion:* 8% CPSP incidence may be a minimum figure. CP is not associated with age, sex and previous stroke.
Naver *et al.* (1995)	Stroke	37	Consecutive pts with acute monofocal stroke. Hemispheric lesion in 26 pts, brainstem stroke in 11 pts. Pain contralateral to the lesion side in 6 pts (16.2%), most of them with impaired temperature sensibility
Mori *et al.* (1995)	Thalamic hematoma	104	104 pts with thalamic hematoma. 86 survivors at 6 mos (52/63 men, 34/41 women)

Extent of hematoma		Thalamic pain
Localized within the thalamus	21 (20.2%)	2 (9.5%)
Extending to the internal capsule	52 (50%)	3 (5.7%)
Extending to the midbrain or putamen	31 (29.8%)	1 (3.2%)
Total	104	6 (5.7%)

Author	Pathology	No. of pts	Pts with CP
Chung *et al.* (1996)	Thalamic hemorrhage	175	Retrospective survey of 175 consecutive pts with thalamic hemorrhage Paresthesia and decreased touch and pain sensation at onset in 31/77 pts (40%) with posterolateral lesions. "About one third of them developed Dejerine-Roussy thalamic syndrome between 3 and 15 days after the onset" Paresthesia at onset also noted in 34% of pts with dorsal thalamic lesions Incidence of thalamic syndrome: 25% of pts with posteromedial hemorrhage (6 cases) 32% of pts with posterolateral hemorrhage (25 cases?) 25% of pts with dorsal hemorrhage (8 cases) Data from text and figure (Fig. 8) are not in agreement as far as posterolateral lesions are concerned. The presence of pain in thalamic syndrome is not specifically noted. No follow-up reported

Author	Pathology	No. of pts	Pts with CP
Kim and Bae (1997)	Brainstem stroke	17	Pure or predominant sensory stroke. MRI or CT confirmed lesions. Follow-up: 1 mo–3 yrs Paresthesia was the initial and main complaint in all pts. Sensory symptoms (almost) completely resolved in 5 pts. Paresthesia usually persisted in the others **CPSP:** in 2 pts (12%) paresthesia worsened, became painful and was often exacerbated by cold weather or fatigue, mimicking the so-called "thalamic pain syndrome" (follow-up: 18 mos, 3 yrs)
Nasreddine and Saver (1997)	Thalamic stroke	180	Systematic review on pain after thalamic stroke Frequency of CP after any thalamic stroke: 11% (range 8–16%). Frequency of CP after geniculothalamic artery stroke: 24% (range 13–59%)
McGowan et al. (1997)	LMI: lateral medullary infarction (Wallenberg's syndrome)	63	Mainly retrospective analysis. LMI diagnosis confirmed by MRI. Frequency of CP: 25.4% of pts (16/63). Loss of some pts to follow-up Rare (less than twice monthly) non-painful dysesthesias in a limb or cheek in 11 additional pts. **Two pts with crossed sensory deficits without pain suffered from a compulsive urge to scratch and pick their painless cheek** and developed excoriated ulcers No CP after medial medullary stroke in Bassetti et al. (1997)
Paciaroni and Bogousslasky (1998)	Pure thalamic sensory stroke	3628	Isolated sensory dysfunction with confirmed thalamic lesion in 25 pts among 3628 included in the Lausanne Stroke Registry. Clinical symptoms strongly suggestive of pure thalamic sensory stroke with normal findings on CT or MRI scans in other 34 pts *Symptoms during the stroke:* pain and/or dysesthesias in 4/25 pts (transient in all 4) contralateral paresthesia in 18/25 delayed pain and/or dysesthesias: 4/25 pts (16%)
Kim and Choi-Kwon (1999)	Lateral medullary infarction (LMI) (Wallenberg's syndrome) Medial medullary infarction (MMI)	41 14	Group of 55 (out of 64 consecutive pts) with a single episode of a MRI identified medullary infarction *Subjective residual sensory symptom 6 to 40 (mean 21) mos after the stroke onset:* on the face: LMI: 56% of pts; MMI: 7% of pts on the body/limbs: LMI: 83% of pts; MMI 71% of pts CPSP incidence: about 25% (according to the authors' statement that "pain" was defined as sensory symptoms more severe than grade 5 or 6 on a 10-point visual analog scale) However, symptoms were not described as "pain" by the majority of these pts, so the terms "central post-stroke paresthesia" describe more appropriately their sensory sequelae **LMI:** predominantly burning or cold sensations (VAS $\geq$ 5) on the face in 6 pts (14.6%) and/or on the body/limbs in 10 (24.3%). Severe lancinating sensations on the face in 1 pt. Severe paresthesias in 14 pts (34.1%)

(continued)

TABLE 2.2 *(continued)*

Author	Pathology	No. of pts	Pts with CP
			MMI: Severe burning or cold body/limbs sensations in 1 pt (7.1%) and severe squeezing/numbness sensations in 4 pts (28.5%)
Mukherjee et al. (1999)	Stroke	17 000	Door-to-door survey of 4600 families in Calcutta. 37 of 17 000 subjects suffered a stroke. CPSP in 17(12 F, 5 M)/37 pts (46%)
Kumral et al. (2001)	Bilateral thalamic infarction	16	1/16 pts (6.25%) developed CPSP with burning pain. Another pt reported Dejerine–Roussy syndrome. CPSP among thalamogeniculate infarct pts: 1/3 pts (33.3%)
Bowsher (2001)	Stroke	1071	Elderly post-stroke population. Survey about stroke in 1071 elderly (median age: 80 yrs, range 69–102) subjects. Completed stroke in 72/1071 (6.7%) CPSP observed in 8/72 (5 men) pts (11%) Shoulder pain excluded
Lampl et al. (2002)	Ventroposterior thalamic stroke	39	Prospective study aimed at investigating the incidence of CPSP in thalamic stroke pts either under prophylactic treatment (1 yr) with amitriptyline or assuming placebo *CPSP incidence*: whole group: 18% amitriptyline group: 17% placebo group: 21%
Weimar et al. (2002)	Ischemic/ hemorrhagic stroke	119	11 (9.2%). CPSP probable in 6 pts, confirmed in 5 pts. 1 pt with recurrent pain in the right extremities from recurrent focal seizures Frequency of (assumed) CPSP after hemorrhagic stroke: 4/13 pts (31%)
Widar et al. (2002, 2004)	Ischemic-hemorrhagic strokes	43	Neurological clinic inpatients with CT-confirmed stroke and long-term pain CPSP (2 yrs after stroke) in 15/43 pts (35%). Nociceptive (shoulder) pain in 18/43
Kim (2003)	Lenticulocapsular hemorrhage (LCH)	20	20 pts with CPSP or paresthesia after LCH. Not all pts were evaluated so no data on general prevalence of CPSP among pts with LCH can be extrapolated.
Gonzales et al. (2003)	Cancer-associated CP		Retrospective review of medical records of pts evaluated by 2 different services: the Pain Service and the Neurology Service, at Memorial Sloan-Kettering Cancer Center CP prevalence: **4% and 2%**, respectively. Primary and metastatic tumors and their therapy, including surgery, radiation and chemotherapy, were all potential causes of CP CP in pts with primary CNS tumors higher in pts with spinal cord tumors compared to pts with brain tumors ($P < 0.0001$)
Solaro et al. (2004)	Multiple sclerosis	1672	Multicenter (26 centers) cross-sectional study with a structured face-to-face questionnaire compiled by a neurologist; compared with 220 prospectively acquired pts. Only exclusion criterion: relapse in the last month before study beginning. Of 2077 questionnaires collected, 405 excluded from analysis due to incomplete data Females: 69%, males: 31%. Mean age 40 years (median 40, range: 14–75). Mean disease duration: 10.5 years (median 8, range 0–47). RR 74%, SP 20.5%, PP 5.5%.

Author	Pathology	No. of pts	Pts with CP
			Mean EDSS 2.9 (median 2.5, range 0–7). 717 (42.9%) had pain: these were significantly older (41.7 vs. 37.6), had a higher EDSS score (3.5 vs. 2.5) and a longer mean disease duration (14.4 vs. 9.2), were more likely SP/PP. Sex differences were not significant (A) Neuropathic pain: Dysesthetic pain (CP): 18.1%, Lhermitte's sign: 9%, trigeminal neuralgia: 2% (B) Nociceptive pain: Back pain: 16.4%, visceral pain 2.9%, painful tonic spasms: 11% 550 subjects reported one painful symptom, 167 more than one. 157 (9.4%) were on pain medication CP: 303 pts (18.1%); 71.6% females (not significant), mean age (43.6 yrs), mean EDSS (3.8), mean disease duration (11.9 yrs), RR/SP/PP percentages (59.6%, 30.1%, 10.3%) highly significant ($p < 0.001$) compared to no pain Trigeminal neuralgia (2.2%), 80.8% females with mean age 48.5, mean EDSS 4.4, mean disease duration 15.3, almost similar proportions between RR and SP Lhermitte's sign (9.1%), 64% females with mean age 39.2 yrs, mean EDSS 3.1, mean disease duration 10.2, three quarters in RR
Kameda et al. (2004)	MRI-confirmed medullary infarction (LMI and MMI)	214	157 LMI pts with information of sensory function. CP (thermal hypesthesia with touch and thermal allodynia) in 40 pts (25%). No correlation with a specific topographical subgroup
Kong et al. (2004)	Ischemic/hemorrhagic stroke	107	107 out of 475 pts attending the outpatient clinic of a rehabilitation center, without significant cognitive and/or language deficits, post-stroke duration more than 6 mos. CPSP in 13 pts (12.1%)
Nakazato et al. (2004)	Wallenberg's syndrome	32	CPSP in 14/32 pts (44%)
Widar et al. (2004)	Stroke	356 (?)	Pts with cerebral infarct or hemorrhage registered in an inpatient register at a neurological clinic in a university hospital in Sweden. 356 people contacted, 65 non-responders, 245 no pain or other pain conditions. 15 CPSP pts. CPSP incidence in the whole group: 4–5% (15/356 or 291 pts)
Svendsen et al. (2005)	Multiple sclerosis	50	50 MS pts with pain. CP in 29 pts (58%) (CP = pain in a body territory with decreased or increased sensation to touch, pinprick, warm or cold, without evidence of nociceptive, visceral or peripheral neuropathic pain)

stroke than whites (at least in the United States and the UK), the worldwide prevalence of CPSP alone may amount to several million patients.

As regards other causes of brain lesions, trauma, particularly penetrating head injury, is said to be rarely associated with CP (2 of 11 patients with somatosensory abnormalities in a 1000 patient series; Marshall 1951). No prospective study exists, although clinical experience would suggest that CP in such cases is indeed rare. CP arises only after disruptive or compressive lesions along the spinothalamoparietal axis; contusions mainly involve basal frontal and temporal areas and hematomas (extradural and subdural) rarely impinge on the parietal lobe to such extent to disrupt it. Moreover, half of patients with severe head injury go on to die within days or weeks of trauma or develop severe disability. And yet a recent Chinese series (Li 2000) reported 20 cases of typical CP after severe head injury observed over 8 years. At CT, 16 had brain hematomas at cortical and subcortical levels (14 were evacuated) and 4 brain infarctions in deep nuclei and corona radiata. It is quite possible that the true incidence is actually underestimated.

In the United States, 2 million cases severe enough to cause brain damage occur yearly (20% of all head injuries), but penetrating trauma has become rare after the enforcement of helmets and the introduction of airbags. Even in a war setting, helmets reduce the extent of damage and the limited extent of SI (the portion of the parietal cortex that has to be involved) ensures that CP would be rare.

Cancer most certainly represents an important cause of CP and, although data are very limited and in the absence of prospective studies, we may expect that roughly 2% of cancer patients suffer CP. Parietal tumors not infrequently trigger CP (especially meningiomas, but also gliomas, rather than metastases) (e.g., Bender and Jaffe 1958), but this goes often unrecognized. Thalamic tumors only rarely cause CP (Tovie *et al.* 1961), but this is not surprising: striatal tumors also only rarely cause extrapyramidal symptoms (see also Lozano *et al.* 1992). Worldwide 10 million cases of new cancers occur every year.

An underrecognized cause of CP is surgery (and particularly neurosurgery; Table 2.13), either via direct brain damage or strokes.

No quantitative data exist regarding differential incidences of CP between rapidly and slowly developing lesions.

In sum, in the United States alone, there should be more than a half million people suffering BCP.

3. Age of onset of CPSP (Table 2.3)
Although one prospective study on CPSP found no significant difference between the general stroke population and CPSP, the general impression from all other studies, both prospective and retrospective, is that CPSP affects younger patients (sixth decade versus seventh decade). However, this awaits confirmation.

4. Sex distribution of CPSP (Table 2.4)
Stroke is more common in men than in women (but deadlier in the latter) worldwide. We should thus expect more men than women complaining of CPSP. A prospective study showed that, although men were more affected than women by stroke, women were more affected than men by CPSP; however, the difference was not statistically significant. Other studies are at odds between them, but Nasreddine and Saver's systematic review on thalamic CPSP found a larger percentage of men suffering CPSP. Wallenberg's strokes are also more frequent in men, and CPSP also appear to predominate in them.

5. Time to pain onset (Table 2.5)
CPSP and CP in general can develop immediately or up to 10 years after the inciting event. In several cases, CPSP is a presenting symptom (roughly one fourth): we had a

TABLE 2.3. Age of onset (CPSP only)

Author	Number of pts	Age of pts (years, mean)	
		Stroke group	CPSP group
Graff-Radford et al. (1985)	25	63.2 (19−81, median 66)	55.7 (19−78, median 63)
Bogousslavsky et al. (1988)	40	56.8 (20−86, median 63)	62.6 (52−73, median 63)
Michel et al. (1990)	12 (parietal CP)		59.2 (39−75, median 51)
Tasker et al. (1991)	73		>50 (67.2% of pts)
Schmahmann and Leifer (1992)	6 (parietal CP)		46.3 (28−58, median 48)
Wessel et al. (1994)	18	66 (50−86, median 64.5)	69 (56−85, median 67)
Samuelsson et al. (1994)	39	67	69 (46−86) PSS
Andersen et al (1995)	87	69 (median) (40−79)	71.5 (median) (41−78)
Lampl et al. (1995)	139	68.7 (putaminothalamic hemorrhages)	
Mori et al. (1995)	104 (thalamic hematoma)	63.8 ± 10.7	nr
Chung et al. (1996)	175	61.2 (11−93)	
Bowsher (1996)	CVA 111		CVA 59.2 (40−78, median 59)
	SAH 19		SAH 46.1 (29−62, median 45)
Kim and Choi-Kwon (1996)	67	60 (27−83)	67 and 54 (2 pts)
Kim and Bae (1997)	17 (brainstem stroke)	61 (range 52−71)	
Nasreddine and Saver (1997)	180		60 (median) (18−85)
McGowan et al. (1997)	63	58 (24−84)	60 (40−78)
Paciaroni and Bogousslavsky (1998)	25	61.4 (39−89, median 63)	61.2 (39−80, median 63)
Kim and Choi-Kwon (1999)	41 LMI	57.8 (35−86, median 56)	(57.5 (47−76, median 55.5))
	14 MMI	60.4 (42−75, median 59.5)	(58.8 (48−70, median 56))

(continued)

TABLE 2.3 (continued)

Author	Number of pts	Age of pts (years, mean)	
		Stroke group	CPSP group
Kumral et al. (2001)	16	59.7 (35–85, median 58)	54
Bowsher (2001)	8	73.5 (40–96, median 74)	77 (69–91, median 77.5)
Lampl et al. (2002)	39		60.5
Weimar et al. (2002)	119	64.5 yrs (median, overall 63, range: 14–91)	62 (median)
Garcia-Larrea et al. (2002)	12 spinal 10 brainstem 18 thalamocortical		44.2 (25–61, median 47.5) 49.5 (36–67, median 42.5) 54.7 (26–72, median 55); nr in 2 pts Spinal vs. thalamocortical difference statistically significant (ANOVA, $p = 0.019$)
Widar et al. (2002, 2004)	43	66 (33–82)	60.9 (43–78, median 64)
Greenspan et al. (2004)	13		nr
Kemeda et al. (2004)	157	Medullary infarct, overall: 61.3 ± 12.4 yrs LMI 60.7 ± 12.4 yrs MMI 65.0 ± 12.3 (difference statistically significant, $p < 0.034$; no significant difference in the age of onset between men and women)	
Kong et al. (2004)	107	60.9 yrs	62.5
Widar et al. (2004)	43		67.6 (range 33–82) 30 men: 64 yrs (range 33–79) 13 women: 76 (range 54–82)

TABLE 2.4. Sex distribution (CPSP only)

Author	Pathology	Men		Women		Men/women ratio	
		Stroke	CPSP	Stroke	CPSP	Stroke	CPSP
Head and Holmes (1911)	Thalamic syndrome/LMI		7 (64%)		4 (36%)		1.75
Kameyama (1976)	Thalamic vascular lesions	26 (30%)		61 (70%)			0.42
Graff-Radford et al. (1985)	Non-hemorrhagic thalamic infarctions	14 (56%)	3 (75%)	11 (44%)	1 (25%)	1.27	3
Kawahara et al. (1986)	Small (<2 cm) thalamic hemorrhages	16 (43.2%)		21 (56.8%)		0.76	
Bogousslavsky et al. (1988)	Thalamic infarcts	19 (47.5%)	1 (33%)	21 (52.5%)	2 (67%)	0.9	0.5
Mauguière and Desmet (1988)	Thalamic vascular lesion		15 (63%)		9 (37%)		1.66
Leijon et al. (1989) and Boivie et al. (1989)	Stroke (same goup of CPSP pts for 2 different studies. Authors' statement: male dominance could not be explained by a difference in the incidence of stroke between men and women because stroke affected more women than men in Sweden. However, strong bias likely, given the selection criteria		20 (74%)		7 (26%)		2.8
Michel et al. (1990)	Cortical pain (MRI or CT confirmed lesion). 12 pts		8 (66.7%)		4 (33.3%)		2
Tasker et al. (1991)	CPSP: 73 personal consecutive cases		40 (55%)		33 (45%)		1.21

(continued)

TABLE 2.4 (continued)

Author	Pathology	Men		Women		Men/women ratio	
		Stroke	CPSP	Stroke	CPSP	Stroke	CPSP
Schmahmann and Leifer (1992)	Parietal lesion		3 (50%)		3 (50%)		1
Steinke et al. (1992)	Thalamic stroke	33 (53%)		29 (47%)		1.13	
	Infarct	6 (33%)		12 (67%)		0.5	
	Hemorrhage	27 (61%)		17 (39%)		1.58	
Wessel et al. (1994)	Thalamic stroke (CP in 10/18 pts, sex distribution not reported)	6 (33%)	nr	12 (66%)	nr	0.5	
Samuelsson et al. (1994)	Lacunar infarct syndrome. Pure sensory stroke (thalamic) in 10 cases. CSPS in 3 pts	20	5 (PSS)	19	5 (PSS)	1.05	1 (PSS)
Kumral et al. (1995)	Thalamic hemorrhages	34 (34%)		66 (66%)		0.51	
Andersen et al. (1995)	Acute stroke (prospective study)	110 (53%)	7 (44%)	97 (47%)	9 (56%)	1.13	0.77
	Pts with somatosensory deficits (SSD)	44 (50.5%)		43 (49.5%)		1.02	
Lampl et al. (1995)	139 putaminothalamic hemorrhages (among 279 consecutive pts with supratentorial hemorrhages)	88 (63.3%)		51 (36.7%)		1.7	
Mori et al. (1995)	104 thalamic hemorrhages	63 (60.5%)		41 (39.5%)		1.5	

Bowsher (1996)	Personal series of 138/156 CP pts						
	CVA		75 (54%)		63 (45%)		1.19
	SAH/post-neurosurgery		63 (57%)		48 (43%)		1.33
	Brain trauma		12 (52%)		11 (48%)		0.53
Chung et al. (1996)	Thalamic hemorrhages	75 (43%)	3 (100%)	100 (57%)	—	0.75	—
Kim and Bae (1997)	Pure or predominant sensory stroke due to brainstem lesion. 17 pts	13 (76.4%)	2 (100%)	4 (23.6%)	0	3.25	1.28
McGowan et al. (1997)	LMI (retrospective analysis)	45 (71%)	9 (56%)	18 (29%)	7 (44%)	2.5	1.23
Nasreddine and Saver (1997)	Meta-analysis		63 (55%)		51 (45%)		1.78
Yamamoto et al. (1997)	Brain CP (MCS pts series)		25 (64%)		14 (36%)		3
Paciaroni and Bogousslasky (1998)	Pure sensory thalamic stroke	17 (68%)	3 (75%)	8 (32%)	1 (25%)	2.12	1.21
Bowsher et al. (1998)	Subgroup of Bowsher (1996) pts		40 (55%)		33 (45%)		
Kim and Choi-Kwon (1999)	"Severe post-stroke paresthesias" in lateral and medial medullary infarction	43 (78.2%)	LMI 10 (71.4%) MMI 3 (60%)	12 (21.8%)	LMI 4 (28.6%) MMI 2 (40%)	3.58	2.5 / 1.5
Kumral et al. (2001)	Bilateral thalamic infarction	10 (62.5%)	1 (6.2%)	6 (36.5%)	0	1.66	—
Bowsher (2001)	Stroke	64 (67.3%)	5 (62.5%)	31 (32.6%)	3 (37.5%)	2.06	1.6

(continued)

TABLE 2.4 (continued)

Author	Pathology	Men		Women		Men/women ratio	
		Stroke	CPSP	Stroke	CPSP	Stroke	CPSP
Lampl et al. (2002)	Thalamic ventroposterior stroke		16 (41%)		23 (59%)		0.69
Weimar et al. (2002)	Stroke	77 (65%)	8 (73%)	42 (35%)	3 (27%)	1.83	2.66
Widar et al. (2002, 2004)	Stroke	30 (69.7%)		13 (30.2%)			
Greenspan et al. (2004)	CPSP		10 (77%)		3 (23%)		3.3
Kameda et al. (2004)	Lateral and medial medullary infarct	LMI: 122 (73%) MMI: 32 (78%) LMI + MMI: 5 (83%) Overall: 159 (74%)	nr	LMI: 45 (27%) MMI: 9 (22%) LMI + MMI: 1 (17%) Overall: 55 (26%)	nr	LMI: 2.7 MMI: 3.5 LMI+MMI: 5 Overall: 2.89	nr
Kong et al. (2004)	Stroke	68 (64%)	nr	39 (36%)	nr	1.74	nr
Widar et al. (2004)	Stroke	30 (70%)	nr	13 (30%)	nr	2.3	nr

TABLE 2.5. Timespan between stroke injury and CP onset

Author	Cumulative % of pts with CP within				Notes
	1 day	2 days–1 mo	1 mo–3 mos	> 3 mos	
Edinger (1891)					2 wks
Dejerine and Roussy (1906)		1 pt			Pain can arise during the acute period of the stroke, at the same time of the development of the hemiplegia, or can be delayed, arising some months after the stroke
Head and Holmes (1911)	50%	87%	(100%?)		Pain was the first symptom of stroke and preceded motor deficits in cases 5, 7 and 8; it developed early (hours) after the thalamic stroke in case 9, but it was delayed (days, weeks or months) in cases 10, 11, 12 and 13
Alajuanine et al. (1935)					CP in pontobulbar lesions is generally delayed (months) after the stroke (cases 2 and 3)
Garcin (1937) (review)					Wallenberg's syndrome (LMI): pain can be an initial feature, but in many cases develops days or months after the stroke, arising at the same time in face and contralateral limbs; often limb pain shows a delayed (weeks) onset compared to face pain
					Thalamic pain: it can be immediate or delayed more than one year after stroke
Riddoch (1938) (review)			1 pt		This author rejected, on the basis of published reports, the Lhermitte (1925) hypothesis that pain is apt to appear earlier with hemorrhages than with ischemic lesions
					In pontobulbar strokes pain usually coincides with stroke, but in some cases it may appear several days or more after stroke
Biemond (1956)					Cortical lesion
Silver (1957)					Cerebral AVM. CP appearance after 8 yrs
Hamby (1961)				1 pt	Reversible central pain (cortical origin)
Cassinari and Pagni (1969)					One pt developed central pain immediately after stereotactic coagulation at thalamic level
Fields and Adams (1974)	17%	50%		100%	Case report and review. Cortical pain, 8 pts, 2 missed data. Time span from immediate to 6–7 mos

(continued)

35

TABLE 2.5 *(continued)*

Author	Cumulative % of pts with CP within				Notes
	1 day	2 days–1 mo	1 mo–3 mos	>3 mos	
Schott et al. (1986)	75%				Thalamic stroke. Immediate pain development in 15/20 pts. Pain onset **delayed until 10 yrs after the stroke in one case**. Data in text and in tables not in agreement
Shieff and Nashold (1987)	63%				Series of 27 pts with the thalamic syndrome. 17/27 pts had their pain from the time of their initial stroke, while in 10 it developed after an interval of as long as 2 yrs, in 3 after a further stroke
Mauguière and Desmet (1988)	50%	75%	96%	100%	Thalamic syndrome, 30 pts. CP in 24/30 pts. Max. delay: 6 mos
Bogousslavsky et al. (1988)	0%	33%	100%	100%	Delayed onset (1 wk, 2 mos and 3 mos) of CP in 3/40 pts
Leijon et al. (1989)	15%	52%	78%	100%	Series of 27 pts. Pain onset: 4/27 on 1st day; 14/27 within 1 mo; 21/27 within 3 mos; 24/27 within 1 yr; 27/27 within 34 mos
Michel et al. (1990)	50%	58.3%	91.6%	100%	Retrospective study. 12 pts. Cortical CP. Lesion sparing the thalamus confirmed by means of MRI or CT scans with reconstruction. Very delayed onset (2 yrs) in 1 pt
Tasker et al. (1991)	29%	46%		100%	Series of 73 pts with CP of brain origin. Pain onset was delayed after an identifiable ictus in about two thirds of the cases, being less than 1 yr in 51% of the pts. The onset was immediate in 29% but >2 yrs in 4.2% of their cases
Schmahmann and Leifer (1992)	(17%)	33.3%		100%	Parietal pseudothalamic syndrome. 6 pts. Pain occurrence: 1 wk after a traumatic injury, 4 mos after resection of meningioma, and 3 wks, 6 mos, 1 and 4 (or 5) yrs after vascular accidents. Immediate hemiparesthesia in 1 case
Bowsher (1993)			75%		CPSP pts. Median time span: 3 mos. In some cases pain developed 24 mos after the stroke
Wessel et al. (1994)	0%	50%	70%	100%	10/18 pts with single thalamic infarct and CP. Pain onset within 1 mo in 5 pts; within 6 mos in all pts
Samuelsson et al. (1994)		100%			3 CPSP pts among 39 pts with lacunar infarct syndromes (pure sensory stroke). "Painful dysesthesia" developed gradually during the 1st mo after stroke
Kumral et al. (1995)	0%	100%			Prospective study. 100 pts with thalamic hemorrhage. Delayed (1 mo) thalamic pain: 3 pts Delayed (1 mo) thalamic pain plus chorea plus ataxia (thalamic syndrome): 6 pts

Study					Notes
Andersen et al. (1995)	?	63%	?	100%	Prospective study. The number of pts suffering from CP increased in time from 10 at 1 mo to 13 at 6 mos and to 16 at 1 yr after the stroke (end of follow-up)
Kumral and Celebisoy (1996)					1 thalamic stroke. CPSP **8 yrs after stroke**
Bowsher (1996)	?	40% (<1 wk)	?	100%	Personal series of 138/156 CP pts. Pain onset immediate (arguably less than a week from the inciting event) in 47 (+8 N/K, abbreviation not explained in the paper) pts (39.8% of cases). Delayed pain onset (from 1–2 wks **up to 6 yrs**) in 83 pts (60.1%) Average interval between stroke and delayed pain onset: CVA pts (63): 6.2 mos (range 0.08–72, median 3) SAH pts (16 pts): 4.4 mos (range 0.25–12, median 4)
Chung et al. (1996)	?	(see notes)	?		Thalamic hemorrhage. Paresthesia at onset: posterolateral lesion: 31/77 pts (40%). (Disagreement between data in text and in Fig. 8 [Fig. 8: 21% of paresthesia at onset]) dorsal lesion: 34% of pts "Thalamic syndrome" present at discharge from hospital (14 days after the admission), on average: posteromedial thalamic lesion: 25% of pts posterolateral thalamic lesion: 32% of pts dorsal thalamic lesion: 25% of pts
Nasreddine and Saver (1997)	18%	56%	71%	100%	Systematic review on thalamic syndrome. 180 pts with the site of the lesion documented by postmortem examination. Exclusion criteria: pts with tumoral/nonvascular etiology, and symptoms consisting solely of evoked dysesthesia without spontaneous pain. Information regarding the time from stroke to the development of pain available in 66 cases. Pain onset (% of pts, noncumulative): immediate: 18% within the first post-stroke wk: 18% 1 wk to 1 mo: 20% 1–3 mos: 15% 3–6 mos: 12% 6–12 mos: 6% >1 yr: 11%

(continued)

TABLE 2.5 (continued)

Author	Cumulative % of pts with CP within				Notes
	1 day	2 days–1 mo	1 mo–3 mos	> 3 mos	
McGowan et al. (1997)	?	75%	?	100%	Lateral medullary infarction (LMI). CPSP in 16/63 pts. Average time span between LMI and pain onset: 4 weeks (range 1–24). Pain onset was within 2 weeks in 3 pts, 1 mo in 9 pts and 6 mos in the remaining 4 pts
Yamamoto et al. (1997)				100%	39 CPSP pts. Interval between the onset of the inciting lesion and the occurrence of pain: 1–6 mos
Paciaroni and Bogousslasky (1998)		100%			25 pts with pure sensory syndrome in thalamic stroke CPSP in 4/25 pts after a mean of 10.5 days (range 2–15 days). Delayed pain in 2 pts, delayed pain and dysesthesias in 1 pt and delayed dysesthesia in 1 pt
Peyron et al. (1998)			33%	100%	9 LMI CPSP. Median stroke-pain delay 4 mos (range: 3–41)
Kim (1998)	40%		80%	100%	6 stroke pts. Early-onset CPSP contralateral to the ischemic lesion + delayed ipsilateral sensory symptoms mirroring the site of the most severe CPSP (without new ischemic lesions). In 1 pt unclear time span
Kim and Choi-Kwon (1999)	14.3% LMI 100% MMI	42.9% LMI	85.8% LMI	100%	Medullary infarction. LMI pts: onset of sensory symptoms immediate to 6 mos after the stroke. Among 14 pts reporting severe paresthesia/pain the onset of symptoms was immediate in 2 cases (14.3%), within 1 mo in 4 cases (28.6%) and between 1 and 3 mos in 6 cases (42.9%). In one pt (7.1%) symptoms developed after 6 mos and in one case the time span between stroke and the onset of symptoms was unknown. MMI pts: immediate development of sensory symptoms, if present, in all but 1 pt in whom they developed within 1 mo
Li (2000)					3–120 days after severe head injury (mean: 30.5 days)
Kumral et al. (2001)	0%	0%	100%		16 pts with bilateral thalamic infarction. CPSP in 1 pt 3 mos after the stroke
Bowsher (2001)		75%	100%		1 pt with possible CPSP was eliminated from study because pain appeared 108 mos (9 yrs, 4 yrs in the text) after stroke
Oliveira et al. (2002)			75%		Gradual onset in 77.5% of pts

Reference					Notes
Lampl et al. (2002)	0	14%	43%	100%	Prospective study. Primary end point of the study: evaluation of CPSP incidence and time span between stroke and pain. CPSP in 7/39 pts
Kim (2003)					Day CPSP occurred: 12, 36, 67, 70, 209, 246, 267. Median: 70 20 pts with CPSP or paresthesia after lenticulocapsular hemorrhage. Pain or paresthesia occurred 0–24 mos after the onset, more prominently in the leg than other body parts
Rossetti et al. (2003)					1 pt. Ipsilateral acute limb pain at stroke onset. MRI: infarction in the territory of the right anterior parietal artery. Basal ganglia, thalamus, and subthalamic region intact. Incidence of acute ipsilateral pain at the onset of stroke: 1/29 pts with hemiballismus-hemichorea (retrospective analysis of more than 4000 pts). Occurrence of hemiballismus with ipsilateral pain is specific for an anterior parietal artery stroke
Greenspan et al. (2004)		8%	46%	100%	13 consecutive CPSP pts. Mean latency from stroke to CPSP: 5.6 mos (1–12, median 4)
Hansson (2004)		53%		100%	Stroke pts. Data from Widar et al. (2002), Andersen et al. (1995) and Leijon et al. (1989)
Nakazato et al. (2004)		8 pts		8 pts	14 pts. Wallenberg syndrome, *unreliable* data (8 + 8 pts instead of 14)

patient who immediately suffered CP upon awakening from parietal glioma surgery; in one patient described in Garcin (1968), the onset was so sudden that the patient *"thought he had been hit on the face"* and Cassinari and Pagni (1969) reported one patient who developed CP immediately after stereotactic coagulation at thalamic level. However, a majority (half to three quarters) develops it within 3−6 months after the causative lesion. Pain onset delayed over 1 year is rare, but not exceptional: in such cases, the pain may sometimes commence after an infection, trivial accident or surgery (Tasker and Dostrovsky 1989). In some patients, the onset coincides with improvement of the sensory loss. The time of onset does not appear to depend on lesion level and early-onset (including immediate) and late-onset pains appear to be clinically identical. CP may also precede other neurological signs.

6. Side of the lesions (Table 2.6)

Right-sided lesions predominate among CPSP patients at both thalamic and cortical levels. This difference is most likely not due to a difficulty of communication after left lesions (moreover, right lesions may cause hemineglect and anosognosia more frequently). It should not depend on simple prevalence of right strokes either, since men, but much less women, show CPSP laterality.

7. Size of the lesion and CPSP (Table 2.7)

Data are available only for thalamic vascular strokes. The hypothesis that CP correlates with the size, rather than the site, of the lesion is a time-honored one, but available data are conflicting. There are several old reports in which the size of the thalamic lesion originating CP was noted at autopsy. Lhermitte (1936) suggested that CPSP is rare in patients in whom the thalamus is completely or almost completely destroyed by a large hemorrhagic lesion. However, Garcin (1937), quoting Lhermitte and Schuster, stated that the volume of the lesion did not seem to correlate with the presence or the absence of CP in thalamic syndrome. Nevertheless, he noted that CP develops more frequently when the thalamic nuclei are affected by larger or multiple hemorrhages, especially with involvement of the lateral nucleus. More recently, after the introduction of new imaging technologies (CT, MRI), the site and the volume of the lesions have been reported in papers dealing with thalamic stroke. In some papers the authors also reported the occurrence of CPSP, allowing the evaluation of the lesion volume in CPSP cases. Apparently, the volume of the lesion in patients with thalamic CPSP does not seem to differ from the expected volume in thalamic hemorrhage, nor between patients with somatosensory deficits with and without CPSP. In conclusion, it would seem that CPSP can follow both small and large lesions and the site of the lesion is more important than its size. However, other data strongly suggest that total destruction of the thalamus is incompatible with a CP generator on that side (Chapter 7).

8. Pain distribution

Contrary to the notion that CP is diffuse and difficult to localize, patients can usually describe the location of their pain. Its distribution corresponds somatotopically to the site of the lesion: e.g. after lower medullary infarction (Wallenberg's syndrome), CP, when present, is projected to the ipsilateral hemiface, tongue, gums and inner

TABLE 2.6. Side of lesion

Author	R/L ratio	Men/women ratio	Notes
Fields and Adams (1974)			All reported, well-examined cases of cortical CP are on the right side of the brain (including their case)
Kameyama (1976)	1.07 (whole group) 3 (CPSP)	0.42	Thalamic stroke. 87 pts. Right-sided lesions: 45/87 (51.7%). Left-sided lesions: 42/87 (48.3%). CPSP: spontaneous pain in 9/45 right-sided lesions (20%) and 3/42 left-sided lesions (7%). Dysesthesia in 13/45 right-sided lesions (27%) and 12/42 left-sided lesions (29%)
Walshe et al. (1977)	0.8		18 cases of thalamic hemorrhage among 146 pts with CT-confirmed intraparenchymal brain hemorrhage. Right-sided lesions in 8 cases and left-sided in 10. Men/women ratio not reported
Graff-Radford et al. (1985)	1.09 (whole group) 3.5 (posterolateral lesions)	1.27	25 pts with nonhemorrhagic thalamic infarctions. Dysesthesia only in 4/9 posterolateral thalamic infarction
Schott et al. (1986)	2.2 (whole group) 1.8 (CPSP) 8 (no CPSP)		Laterality reported in 29/35 pts with thalamic stroke. Right-sided lesion: 20 pts. Spontaneous or provoked CPSP in 20 pts. Right side affected in 13 cases. Right-sided lesion in 8/9 pts without CPSP
Kawahara et al. (1986)	1.3 (whole group)	0.76	Small (<2 cm) CT-confirmed thalamic hemorrhages. Right-sided lesion: 21/37 pts (56.7%). Left-sided lesions: 16/37 pts (43.2%). Type of hemorrhage: anterolateral: 3R/1L; posterolateral: 15R/13L; medial: 2R/1L; dorsal: 1R/1L. Dysethesia/paresthesia in 6 posterolateral stroke pts
Bogousslasky et al. (1988)	2.18 (general population)	0.9	Prospective study. 40 pts with a CT-proven "pure" thalamic infarct. Right-sided infarct: 24 pts (60%); left-sided infarct: 11 pts (27.5%); bilateral infarct: 5 pts (12.5%)
	3.5 (inferolateral lesions)		Inferolateral infarct: right-sided: 14/18 pts (78%); left-sided: 4/18 pts (22%)
	0.5 (pts with CPSP)		CPSP pts: Right-sided infarct: 1/3 pts (33%); left-sided infarct: 2/3 pts (66%)
Michel et al. (1990)	11	2	Retrospective study. 12 pts with cortical CP (MRI or CT confirmed lesion). Right-sided lesions: 11/12 pts; left-sided lesions: 1/12 pts
Tasker et al. (1991)	4.5		Series of 73 personal consecutive CPSP pts. Side of the body affected by pain: right 43.9% of cases; left 53.4%. Bilateral pain was present in 2.7% of cases. In 11 pts with thalamic pain the thalamic lesion was right-sided in 9 cases and left-sided in 2. There was a thalamic + suprathalamic lesion in 5/9 cases There were 1 small and 1 large left-sided lesions and 1 small and 3 large right-sided lesions
Schmahmann and Leifer (1992)	0.2	1	Parietal pseudothalamic pain syndrome: 6 pts 5 left-hemisphere lesions; 1 right-hemisphere lesion

(continued)

TABLE 2.6 *(continued)*

Author	R/L ratio	Men/ women ratio	Notes
			Authors' note: left-hemispheric predominance in this series may be simply coincidental
Hirato *et al.* (1993)	0.8	0.8	9 CPSP pts (4 men, 5 women). 3 thalamic lesions (2R, 1L); 3 putaminal lesions (1R, 2L); 1 combined thal/putam (L); 2 cortical lesions (1R, 1L). R/L (overall): 4R, 5L
Wessel *et al.* (1994)	1.25 (whole group) 1.5 (CPSP)	0.5	Thalamic infarct. 18 pts. Right-sided lesion in 10 cases (R/L ratio 1.25). CPSP in 10 pts: right thalamus affected in 6 cases
Samuelsson *et al.* (1994)	1.16 (whole group) 0.43 (PSS)		Lacunar infarct syndromes. Pts collected from a series of 100 consecutive pts. Pure sensory stroke (thalamic) in 10 cases. CPSP in 3 cases of PSS Whole group: right-sided lesions: 21; left-sided lesions: 18 PSS: right-sided lesions: 3; left-sided lesions: 7
Andersen *et al.* (1995)	2.2 (general population) 2.5 (112 pts without SSD) 1.75 (55 pts with SSD) 2.2 (16 pts with CPSP) 1.6 (pts with CPSP without crossed symptoms)	1.13	Prospective study on CPSP incidence after any stroke

Characteristic of CT-scan according to abnormalities in sensibility

		Somatosensory deficits (SSD)		
	Overall population: 183 pts	Absent (112 pts, + 8 CT scan missing/ normal)	Present, CPSP absent (55 pts, + 16 CT scan missing/ normal)	CPSP (16 pts)
Right-sided lesions	126 (69%)	80 (71%)	35 (64%)	11 (69%)
Left-sided lesions	57 (31%)	32 (29%)	20 (36%)	5 (31%)

Comparison of pts with a single acute lesion on CT scan

	Overall population: 31 pts	Somatosensory deficits without pain (20 pts)	CPSP (11 pts)*
Right-sided lesions	20 (64.5%)	11 (55%)	9 (82%)
Left-sided lesions	11 (35.5%)	9 (45%)	2 (18%)

* 10 pts in the original Table V.
Pts with a single acute CT-confirmed lesion: pts with CPSP: R/L ratio: 4.5; pts with sensory deficits but without CPSP: R/L ratio: 1.22. Crossed neurological signs attributable to brain-stem lesions in 3 pts with CPSP.
Authors' conclusion: No statistically significant difference. Lesions giving rise to CPSP can be both right- and left-sided.

Author	R/L ratio	Men/ women ratio	Notes
Kumral *et al.* (1995)	1.04 (general population)	0.5	Thalamic hemorrhage. Right lesions in 51%; left lesions in 49% of pts (anterolateral: 9R/12L; posterolateral: 28R/27L; medial: 8R/7L; dorsal: 6R/3L). CPSP in 9 pts

Author	R/L ratio	Men/women ratio	Notes
Mori et al. (1995)	1.6		Thalamic hematoma. 104 pts. 86 survivors at 6 mos. CPSP in 6 pts (R/L ratio not reported). Right-sided lesions: 65, left-sided lesions: 39. 9/65 (13.8%) pts with right-sided and 9/39 (23.1%) pts with left-sided lesions died
Chung et al. (1996)	0.83 (whole group)		Posterolateral thalamic hematoma. 77 pts. Dejerine–Roussy syndrome in 32% of pts. Right-sided lesion in 35/77, left-sided lesion in 42/77 pts. Hemineglect observed in 20 pts with right-sided hematoma and language abnormalities in 18 pts with left-sided lesion
Kim and Choi-Kwon (1999)	1.23 (general population) 1.14 (thalamic stroke)	1.3	Unilateral stroke. 67 pts
Bowsher (1996, 1998)	See notes	1.32	Retrospective study on pts with CP Dominant side lesions: 57/111 pts (51%, not 54% as calculated by the author) with CPSP after CVA (Dom/Non-dom ratio: 1.05) 9/19 pts (47%) with CPSP after SAH (Dom/Non-dom ratio: 0.9). Dominant side affected in 66/130 CPSP pts (51%) (Dom/Non-dom ratio: 1.03). Right-sided MRI-confirmed thalamic involvement in 14/34 CVA pts (41%) (R/L ratio: 0.41)
Nasreddine and Saver (1997, 1998)	1.72 2.15 (men); 1.2 (women)	1.23	Systematic review on thalamic pain 180 pts. 114 right-sided (63%), 66 left-sided lesions (37%) (statistically significant difference, $p < 0.001$) Updated data (1998): 216 pts, 129 right-sided (60%), 87 left-sided lesions (40%) (statistically significant difference, $p < 0.006$) *Authors' conclusion:* Right-sided lesions predominate among reported cases of thalamic pain syndrome. Subgroup analysis suggests men contributed more than women to this asymmetry (43 right-sided and 20 left-sided men vs. 28 right-sided and 23 left-sided women)
McGowan et al. (1997)	1.03 (general population)	2.5	MRI-confirmed LMI. Mainly retrospective analysis. Right-sided infarcts in 32 pts; left-sided in 31
Kim and Bae (1997)	1.12		Pure or predominant sensory stroke due to MRI or CT confirmed brainstem lesion. 17 pts. 9 right-sided lesions, 8 left-sided lesions
Kim (1998)	5	2	6 CPSP pts (4 men, 2 women). 2 thalamic infarcts (right-sided), 1 lenticulocapsular hemorrhage (left-sided), 2 medial medullary infarcts (right-sided), 1 pontine infarct (right-sided). Early-onset contralateral CPSP followed by delayed ipsilateral to the lesion painful sensory symptoms
Paciaroni and Bogousslasky (1998)	0.92 (general population)	2.12	Pure sensory syndrome in thalamic stroke. 1 pt with CPSP
Peyron et al. (1998)		2	9 pts with LMI

(continued)

TABLE 2.6 *(continued)*

Author	R/L ratio	Men/ women ratio	Notes
Kim and Choi-Kwon (1999)	1.23 (LMI) 1.33 (MMI)	3.6 (overall popula- tion)	55 consecutive pts with lateral or medial medullary infarction Right-sided LMI: 23 pts (56%). Left-sided LMI: 18 pts (44%) Right-sided MMI: 8 pts (57%). Left-sided MMI: 6 pts (43%)
Li (2000)	3.6		8 pts with SHI CP had left limb pain, 3 right limb pain, 2 left hemiface/tongue/limbs pain, 1 left hemiface/tongue
Kumral et al. (2001)	Bilateral	Bilateral	16 consecutive pts with simultaneous bilateral infarction. CPSP in 1 pt
Garcia-Larrea et al. (2002)	1 (brainstem) 1.22 (thalamo- cortical)	nr	42 (consecutive) selected pts. CP from spinal (12 pts), brainstem (10 pts) and thalamocortical lesion (20 pts) Right-sided brainstem lesions: 5/10 (50%) Right-sided thalamocortical lesions: 11/20 (55%)
Weimar et al. (2002)	1	2.66	119 consecutive pts (from a stroke unit); survival > 1 yr. Clinical reexamination of pts with probable CPSP, + sensory testing for all somatic modalities Comparison of 11 pts (3 women, 8 men) with and 108 pts without CPSP 1 yr after stroke: Left hemispheric stroke: 27% vs. 23% Right hemispheric stroke: 27% vs. 24% **Infratentorial stroke: 27% vs. 12%** No visible stroke: 18% vs. 41%
Greenspan et al. (2004)	0.85 (overall) 1 (thalamic) 2 (cortical subcortical)		13 consecutive CPSP pts. Right-sided lesions: 6 pts (46%); left-sided lesions: 7 pts (54%) Right-sided thalamic lesions: 2/4 pts (50%) Right-sided cortical-subcortical lesions: 4/6 pts
Kong et al. (2004)	1.38	1.74	107 post-stroke pts (39 women, 68 men) out of 475 pts attending the outpatient clinic of a rehabilitation center Side of hemiplegia: left 58 (54%), right 42 (38%), bilateral 7 (8%). 13 CPSP pts (side of lesion not reported)
Willoch et al. (2004)	1.5	1.5	5 CPSP pts (2 women, 3 men). 3 R strokes (2 ischemic [VP thalamus + mediobasal part of occipital lobe; posterior thalamus + mesial temporal lobe], 1 hemorrhagic [midbrain, affecting medial lemniscus, spino-trigemino-thalamic tract and reticular formation]), 2 L strokes (1 ischemic [posterior thalamus + border zones of PCA bilaterally], 1 postoperative hemorrhage [hemangioma in the L inferior parietal lobe, bordering occipital and temporal lobes]) Pain side/distribution 3 pts L hemibody (in 1: face spared) 2 pts R hemibody

TABLE 2.7. Size of the lesion

Author	Mean volume of the lesion	Notes
Kameyama (1976)	nr	In his series of 11 pts with VPL lesions extending to nucleus centrum medianum thalamic pain never developed *Author's conclusion:* CP is rare in cases with large thalamic lesions.
Kawahara (1986)	4 mL or less	6 cases of "paresthesia and/or dysesthesia" among 37 pts with small (less than 2 cm in mean diameter) thalamic hemorrhages. Assuming approximately spherical lesions, their (calculated) volume was about 4 mL or less
Leijon *et al.* (1989)	32.7 mL (range 0.5–144.4) **BS:** 2.6 mL (range 2–4.3) **TH:** 18.1 mL (range 0.6–144.4) **ET:** 73.2 mL (range 47.2–99.2) **UN:** 0.8 mL (range 0.5–3.	Group of 27 CPSP pts. BS: brainstem lesions (8 pts). TH: thalamic lesions (9 pts). ET: supratentorial extrathalamic lesions (6 pts). UN: unidentified supratentorial lesions (4 pts) Thalamic lesions extended beyond the thalamus in 7/9 cases
Kumral *et al.* (1995)	33% <4 mL 67% >4 mL	Thalamic hemorrhage. 100 pts. Small hemorrhages in 33 pts; large hemorrhages (>2 cm in diameter and/or 4 mL in volume) in 67 CPSP in 9 pts (8 with large hemorrhages and 1 with small hemorrhage) 6 posterolateral hemorrhages (1 small, 5 large) in 6 pts, anterolateral, medial (small) and dorsal (large) in 3 pts
Samuelsson *et al.* (1994)	Lacunar infarcts	39 pts. 3 CPSP in 10 pts with pure sensory stroke (posterolateral thalamus). Mean diameter of the lesions: Pure sensory stroke (9 lesions): 9 mm Sensorimotor stroke (9 lesions): 15 mm Pure motor stroke (14 lesions): 16 mm
Andersen *et al.* (1995)	Median volume of the lesions: **pts without SSD:** 2 mL (range 0–96) **Pts with SSD without pain:** 1 mL (range 0–200) **CPSP pts:** 16 mL (range 0–210)	Prospective study Volume of the lesion evaluated on CT scan. Larger lesions in CPSP pts (difference statistically significant), but no demonstrable difference in single acute lesion size between CPSP pts and pts with sensory deficits (SSD) but without pain *Author's conclusion:* Pts with CPSP have larger lesions since larger lesions affect by chance the spino-thalamo-cortical pathway more often.

(continued)

TABLE 2.7 (continued)

Author	Mean volume of the lesion	Notes
Mori *et al.* (1995)	Volume of hematoma (mm³) among survivors: Within thalamus: 3 ± 3 Extending to IC: 9 ± 6 Extending to midbrain or putamen: 18 ± 12	Thalamic ematoma. 104 pts. 86 survivors at 6 mos. CPSP in 6 pts (within thalamus hematoma: 2, extending to the IC: 3, extending to midbrain and putamen: 1) Statistically significant difference among all hematoma size
Chung *et al.* (1996)	Mean length of the hematoma's largest diameter and corresponding volume: **anterior type:** 17 mm (95%CI 10.6–22.5): 2.5 mL **posteromedial type:** 25 mm (95%CI 21.4–28.1): 8.2 mL **posterolateral type:** 31 mm (95%CI 28.4–32.9): 15.5 mL **dorsal type:** 24 mm (95%CI 21–25.9): 7.2 mL **global type:** 37 mm (95%CI 24.2–40.9): 26.4 mL	Thalamic hemorrhage. 175 consecutive pts. Mean volume calculated assuming a spherical shape **anterior type:** 11 pts; posteromedial type: 24 pts; posterolateral type: 77 pts; dorsal type: (32 pts; global type: 31 pts. The global type was large enough to occupy nearly the entire area of the thalamus **Paresthesia at onset:** posterolateral type: 21% (as reported in fig. 8b, in text it is stated 31/77 pts, i.e. 40%) dorsal type: 34% **Delayed thalamic syndrome:** posteromedial type (volume 8.2 mL): 25% of pts posterolateral type (volume 15.5 mL): 32% of pts dorsal type (volume 7.2 mL): 25% of pts
McGowan *et al.* (1997)	nr	LMI 52 pts. Extent of the infarction (MRI scans) evaluated in a blind fashion. Size of the infarction graded 0–4 according to a predetermined scoring scale (0 = normal, 4 = LMI plus ventrobasal cerebellar infarction plus brainstem infarction beyond the lateral medulla). Statistical analysis performed *Author's conclusion:* The different MRI infarct size scores had no relationship with CPSP.
Paciaroni and Bogousslasky (1998)	nr	Pure sensory thalamic stroke. 25 pts CPSP in 4/25 pts Thalamic infarcts were very small. Pts without CPSP had a median involvement of 2 nuclei (range 1–5)

aspect of cheek and often, but not always, contralaterally below the collarbone, diffusely or sectorially (arm and rarely the trunk and leg), simultaneously or at different intervals, in keeping with damage to the spinal nucleus and tract of the trigeminal nerve and the crossed STT. Exceptional simultaneous involvement of both sides of the face is explained by involvement of the descending root of the trigeminal nerve of one side and the crossed quintothalamic pain fibers coming from the other side (Riddoch 1938).

CP is always segmentally distributed, supporting a role of somatotopically organized structures. Roughly 40% of all BCP patients complain of hemibody pain (hemipain), with or without the hemiface. In all other cases, CP is restricted to one or more body parts, e.g., the hemiface, one hand, one foot, a quadrant of the body, or the mouth and hand (the cheiro-oral syndrome), without a transition zone; the face and arm are most affected, and the leg least, reflecting greater cortical representation, but a hemiface singly is affected in roughly 10% of the cases. The pain may vary in site ("wander"), disappearing from one limb only to arise in another, and intense pains in the limbs may be found simultaneously with only paresthesias in the face, or vice versa (Garcin 1937; Riddoch 1938).

The area of pain (spontaneous and evoked and rarely only evoked) may match the sensory and/or motor deficit, but may also be patchy, i.e., confined to a fraction of the disabled region, even after lesions causing extensive loss of somatic sensibility (e.g., Michel *et al.* 1990; Tasker *et al.* 1991); in contrast, CP is never localized to an unaffected area. CP is experienced as superficial (projected to the skin), deep (originating in muscle and bone) or both in varying proportions.

9. Quality of pain (Table 2.8)

Most patients experience one or more pain qualities simultaneously (two to four), in the same or different body regions (e.g., burning in leg and aching in face or, for example, in Wallenberg's syndrome dysesthesias to the hemiface and shooting pains to the limbs and trunk or vice versa) and seemingly identical lesions may cause different combinations of pain qualities in different patients. CP can have any quality, although some qualities are commoner; bizarre qualities are the exception rather than the rule. Variation in pain qualities is highest in CPSP and SCI CP. Attempts to correlate various pain descriptors with some pathophysiology have failed. The most common pain qualities appear to be burning, aching, lancinating, pricking, lacerating and pressing (but also shooting, stabbing, squeezing, cramping, throbbing, tearing, smarting, cutting, pulling, crushing, sore, splitting, icy feeling, stinging, "like a tight armor," "sitting heavily on a ball," "like a flash of lightning"). Dysesthetic pain is common in MS and incomplete SCI (including post-cordotomy), but, upon close questioning, may turn out to consist of a number of specific pain qualities. A burning quality is not a hallmark of CP, and in the landmark Danish paper (Andersen *et al.* 1995), lacerating was the commonest descriptor of pain. The more introspective point out that their symptoms bear no relation to anything they have experienced in the past. Whereas the majority have pain that can be described, several have no pain at all, but an unpleasant and difficult-to-describe sensation that drastically reduces their quality of life; moreover, there may be no sharp transition from non-painful to painful dysesthesias. Some patients complain of pruritus, singly or in combination of

TABLE 2.8. Pain quality

Muscle spindle pain	A cramp or contraction, with burning. There are sometimes areas of constant cramping sensation, usually in a single muscle belly, as well as diffuse burning when the muscle takes on a load. Weight-bearing while sleeping or resting on a surface also causes great soreness, so that pts feels like they have been sleeping on rocks. (This, plus the burning dysesthesia from touching bedclothes, can make sleeping a torment.) Pts may describe muscle spindle pain as "drawing" or "pulling" or "crushing"
Burning	A chemical, not a purely physical burn
	Terms used: mentholated burning like the skin of my legs has been destroyed and the charred flesh turned up at the edges like in a dry lake bed a sick burn, like that inflicted by a toxic chemical a scalding, scathing torment, like in hell
Cold	like touching dry ice so that it burns my hand tells me the skin of my legs is cold but it feels like burning like I am touching an incredibly cold pipe in a freezing night, so that it drains the flesh and burns me like a dentist is touching the nerve in my tooth, only very cold
Metallic	like tinfoil under my skin creepy, like chewing tinfoil
Wetness	When I am wet and sweaty, my skin is really sensitized and the burning lights up and I feel wet and uncomfortable underneath the burning
Dysesthesia in the aggregate	"I feel like I am being put on ice and then put into a fire with a million ice picks plunged into my body" (Bette Hamilton, one of Dr. Kevorkian's clients): this includes the burn, the cold, the metallic, and adds the lancinating component of CP
	"often intolerable . . . crushed feeling, scalding sensation, as if boiling water was being poured down the arm, cramping, aching, soreness, as if the leg was bursting, something crawling under the skin, pain pumping up and down the side, as if the painful region was covered with ulcers, as if pulling a dressing from a wound, as if a log of wood was hanging down from the shoulder, as if little pins were sticking into the fingers, like a wheel running over the arm, cold stinging feeling" (Head and Holmes 1911)
	"boiling hot, deep as though in the bones, showers of pain like electric shocks or red-hot needles evoked by touch, as though the arm and leg were being twisted, continuous sensation of pins and needles, a strange sensation of the limbs being abnormally full" (Loh *et al.* 1981)
	"as if knives heated in Hell's hottest corner were tearing me to pieces" (Holmes 1919)
Circulatory	Pins-and-needles
Visceral (peristaltic)	Burning in the bladder, fullness or nausea in the gut ("like my bowels will explode"), heightened sense of distension and urgency with flatus or stool
Pruritus	This may occur singly or combined with other qualities

other above-cited qualities (Table 2.9; Canavero *et al.* 1997). Paresthesias can also be the main complaint. Numbness is experienced by many; it can occur with both total loss of tactile sensibility, but also normal thresholds to touch, and sometimes describes patients' paresthesias or dysesthesias.

According to Dr. McHenry (www.painonline.org), himself a CP patient, patients when asked to describe their pain quality sound like pain imbeciles and will only tell of the components if they "listen" very carefully, and then only with cues from the examiner. The result is that clinicians receive the false impression that CP is singular when it is plural, especially in symptoms other than dysesthetic burning. The patient of necessity borrows verbal descriptors from nociceptive pain, but these may mislead the examiner, leading to conflicts that the patient cannot explain and decreased credibility. Burning dysesthesia is an amalgam of pain sensations, but most closely corresponds to the second pain that follows, for example, touching a hot stove. There is nearly always a cold component, and frequently there is a metallic quality, as well as a sensation of wetness.

10. Intensity of pain

Intensity varies widely between individuals, and severe pain is commoner among paretics rather than plegics; the suicidal people are usually paretic. After lenticulocapsular stroke, intensity tends to be maximal in the leg rather than in the arm or face (Kim 2003). Generally speaking, CP tends to be worst in areas of most severe initial sensory loss, while its evoked components are usually worst in areas of retained or only mildly impaired sensibility. Globally, most patients consider the pain to be severe or even excruciating, although some of them rate the pain intensity rather low on rating scales. However, even when low or moderate, CP can be assessed as severe because it causes much suffering and burden due to its irritating character and constant presence. Pain can be assessed as a worse handicap than, for example, severe motor impairment. It is difficult to say if intensity of pain is worse with lesions at some levels rather than others, since published studies lack adequate power. In our experience, there appears to be no meaningful difference among suprathalamic, thalamic, brainstem or cord lesions. Intensity can be constant or more often may fluctuate spontaneously, even paroxysmally, or following aggravating or mitigating stimuli. Interestingly, variation in intensity may differ between pain qualities in the same patient. In its more extreme, intractable form, the patient is motivated to commit suicide. For most patients, the intensity of CP is sufficient to interfere with daily activities and is a potential or active factor in the development of depression, along with neurologic disabilities, themselves a risk factor; depression may, in turn, increase the perceived intensity and affective quality of the pain.

11. Components

Patients with CP demonstrate three types of pain: (1) a constant spontaneous component (almost all); (2) an intermittent (every day, with pain-free intervals lasting a few hours at most), brief (seconds to minutes), intense, spontaneous component (about 15%), generally shooting, shock-like or lancinating and with a similar distribution to that of steady pain; when present, it can be the major complaint; and (3) evoked pain (65%), that is, hyperesthesia, hyperpathia,

TABLE 2.9. Central neurogenic pruritus due to brain lesions (excluding MS)

Authors	Sex/age	Trigger	Onset	Sensory findings	Site	CT/MR	Drugs	Effect	Notes
King et al. (1982)	F 58	SAH (basilar tip aneurysm) wrapping. Also: stenosis 90% right ICA	Post-operative, over several weeks	Pain temperature hypesthesia	left limbs, left trunk (both pruritus and hypesthesia)	Hypodensity of posterior limb internal capsule/ lateral aspect of frontal and temporal lobes (right)	Carbamazepine	Reduction in intensity, frequency and duration	Also occasional paroxysmal sensations of warmth in the same distribution of pruritus. EEG: focus of intermittent slow activity + sharp waves + spikes in frontotemporal region. Episodes of pruritus *uncorrelated* with slow + sharp activity
Sullivan and Drake (1984)	M 43	Nocardia abscesses (2) F (right) no mass effect	Not specified	Pin sensibility decreased Occasional touch allodynia (perceived as pruritus)	Left limbs, left trunk (both pruritus and hypesthesia)	No lesion on sensory axis	Phenytoin + cyproheptadine. Carbamazepine	Lessen paroxysms but pruritus more persistent improvement	EEG: mild diffuse slowing + irregular polymorphic right frontotemporal delta rhythm. Itching *uncorrelated* to EEG changes. Further complaints: painful fits
Massey (1984)	M 36	Infarct	Not specified	Hemianesthesia	Left (hemisoma)	Hypodensity in middle cerebral artery territory	5 of these pts treated with carbamazepine or amitriptyline. However, all 9 relieved at 3 mo follow-up (in F 67, amitriptyline 50 mg + benadryl)		EEG: no focus associated to pruritus
	M 54	Hemorrhage	Not specified	?	Left (hemisoma ?)	Hypodensity in internal capsule			
	F64	Infarct	Not specified	Hemianesthesia	Right (hemisoma)	Hypodensity in middle cerebral			

Reference	Sex/Age	Type	Onset	Sensory signs	Pain location	Imaging	Treatment	Outcome
						artery territory (parietal)		
	M 72	Infarct	NS	Hemianesthesia	Left (hemisoma ?)	Hypodensity in internal capsule		
	M 68	Infarct	Not specified	Hemianesthesia	Right (hemisoma ?)	Hypodensity in internal capsule		
	M 61	Infarct	Not specified		Left (hemisoma ?)	Hypodensity in middle cerebral artery territory		
	F 62	Hemorrhage	Not specified	?	Right (hemisoma ?)	Hypodensity in internal capsule		
	M 76	Infarct	Not specified	Pinprick sensibility decreased (left hemisoma)	Left forearm and leg (pruritus)	Hypodensity in internal capsule + middle cerebral artery territory — focal		
	F 67	Infarct	Post-operative, over c.1 mo (carotid surgery)	Hemianesthesia (pruritus bilateral worse on left)	Left hemisoma	Hypodensity in middle cerebral artery territory + internal capsule		
Shapiro and Braun (1987)	F 74	Infarct	Days	Normal, except poor 2-point discrimination (on left)	left ear, cheek, ala nasi, upper lip, neck, upper back, knee	Hypodensity (superficial) in parietal lobe	Amitriptyline (20 mg/day)	Significant but incomplete — spontaneous disappearance

(continued)

TABLE 2.9 (continued)

Authors	Sex/age	Trigger	Onset	Sensory findings	Site	CT/MR	Drugs	Effect	Notes
Procacci and Maresca (1991)	F 82	?	Not specified	Hyperpathia	Bilateral (starting on the left)	Negative (also at MRI)	Antihistaminics + psychotropics	Ineffective	Intense pruritus, 2 yr long, worse in the morning
Canavero et al. (1997)	M 37	SAH	2 weeks	Not available	Left nose and throat	Not available	54 drugs incl. amitriptyline at full dosage. Propofol test. IT baclofen	Ineffective. Diazepam 10–25 mg transitorily effective	
Kimyai-Asadi et al. (1999)	F 74	Right thalamic stroke	Several weeks	Normal (?)	Various localized areas of the left trunk and extremities	Right thalamic stroke	Topical therapies (moisturizers, emollients)	Alleviation of each episode of pruritus	Episodic pruritus. Right side spared. Oral medications refused
	M 69	Right MCA stroke	Several days	Left-sided hemiplegia	Left thigh	Infarction of the territory of the middle cerebral artery	Amitriptyline (50 mg/day)	Effective (or spontaneous resolution?)	Localized, unremitting pruritus, interfering with sleep. Pruritus resolved in a week

Central neurogenic pruritus due to spinal cord (excluding MS) lesions

Authors	Sex/age	Trigger	Onset	Sensory findings	Site	CT/MR	Drugs	Effect	Notes
Vuadens et al. (1994)	F 69	Cavernoma at T1 (MRI)	Not specified	Dysesthetic area inner aspect right arm	6 yr long pruritus + also aching pain Itch appeared late and preceded CP by at least 4 yrs		Not specified	Not specified	

Reference	Sex/Age	Lesion	Onset	Itch/pain description	Clinical course	Imaging	Treatment	Response	Comments
Sandroni (2002)	F 55	Cavernoma at T9–10	Sudden	Pain plus intense itch; then pain abated, and itch spread. Itch appeared on the 9th year of symptoms (pain)	Mid-back (itch); Groin (pain); spread to whole lower abdomen below T9		Lidocaine patch 5%	Marked relief. No response to H1 blockers and steroids. Topiramate ineffective on both itch and CP. Other AD/AED ineffective	Previous episodes of typical CP in affected hypesthesic areas, each spontaneously regressed
Dey et al. (2005)	M 54	Cavernoma at C3–4	Gradual	Unilateral, focal itch (after pain)	Excision at first completely relieved both CP and itch. 3 mos postop, neck and shoulder pain recurred, radiating down left arm to base of left thumb, spreading over 2 yrs to whole hand. Pain changed from intermittent and stabbing to constant and burning. Itch recurred 2 yrs postop	Normal postop MRI	Lidocaine patch 5%, EMLA cream and gabapentin; Opioids; TCAs, SSRIs, AEDs (OXCBZ, CBZ, zonisamide, tiagabine, levetiracetam), IV lidocaine, stellate ganglion block with lidocaine; TENS and acupuncture	Moderately relieved itch; Improved pain but not itch; Itch unrelieved; Worsened the itch	Both itch and pain improved by distraction. Scratching temporarily relieved itch although worsening the pain. Some itch was felt deep within the biceps area of upper arm; temporary relief without pain exacerbation by squeezing biceps

In all pts other causes of pruritus were excluded by thorough investigation. The only dermatological findings were due to scratching. Pruritus in all came in paroxysms or bouts, intermittent or continuous

The undetailed report by Andreev and Petkov describes pruritus of the nostrils (6 pts) as almost pathognomonic of a brain tumor infiltrating the base of the fourth ventricle (see in Canavero et al. 1997)

Another report of localized pruritus appears in Johnson et al. (2000) (reference not available).

MS: Multiple sclerosis

hyperalgesia and/or allodynia (Tasker 2001). Any single patient may, however, complain of only one of these three components. Only a minority of CPSP patients has their spontaneous CP absent for up to a few hours each day.

Shooting (lancinating) pain is the most distinct, most severe and most startling, but it does not cause the most suffering, because the pain is limited to the surface area affected and can often be eliminated by shifting position or rubbing the area; this pain shoots from distal to proximal sites. The phenomenon is most dramatic early in the disease and tends to diminish with time, leading to false notions of drug benefit. It is indistinguishable clinically from the "lightning pains" of tabes dorsalis. Lancinating pain is said to originate where mini-fasciculations occur (Dr McHenry, painonline.org).

Paretics display the greatest number of CP components, unlike plegics and MS patients (although the ones they have can be severe). Gradients can be observed, namely spontaneous pain tends to be distal (i.e., where sensory loss becomes greatest) and evoked pains proximal (i.e., where sensory loss is present but least marked).

12. Evoked pains

The spontaneous discomfort of CP is often (roughly 60%) accompanied by certain unpleasant effects induced by somatosensory stimuli, and which, by definition, cannot occur in an area of complete somatosensory interruption; it is unusual in the complete absence of clinically detectable sensory loss (about 7% in Tasker *et al.* 1991). Infrequently, these can be the only symptoms, i.e., in the absence of constant pain (3/27 in the series of Shieff (1991) and 7% in the series of Tasker [2001]), and may first be noticed after several years with the disease. These abnormally unpleasant sensations (pain, dysesthesias, paresthesias) are usually unbearable and evoke violent emotional and defensive reactions, generally being referred to as the worst component of CP; often poorly localized, they may be elicited either by normally non-painful stimuli, namely touch (including caresses and others; see below) – but not, at least initially, deep pressure – vibration, moderate cold and heat (*allodynia*) or by mildly to moderately painful stimuli, particularly sharp objects plus noxious cold and heat (*hyperesthesia: hyperalgesia and hyperpathia*) delivered to an area of nearly (but not) always elevated threshold to stimuli of one or more somatosensory modalities (thermal, mechanical static and dynamic). Hyperalgesia may be less frequent in brainstem CP. These evoked pains are elicited most prominently by a single sensory modality, a little more often than by several (Tasker 2001). Riddoch (1938) and others noted how pain can be evoked by simple pressure in areas of analgesia to pinprick. Also, even in the presence of nearly abolished pinprick sensibility, firm pinching or repeated pinpricks may be felt as painful. Head and Holmes (1911) also noted how pressure (deep tissue pain) with an algometer could evoke discomfort in cases with complete analgesia to pinprick (as reemphasized by Mailis and Bennett 2002). In patients with complete thermanesthesia, extremes of heat and cold may evoke disagreeable nonthermal sensations (Riddoch 1938). Allachesthesia is allodynic pain in an area other than that stimulated. According to the IASP nomenclature (1994), hyperpathia (a term first introduced by Foerster) is "a painful syndrome, characterized by an abnormally painful reaction to a stimulus, especially a repetitive stimulus, as well as an increased threshold." Riddoch (1938) (wrongly), but also Head and Holmes (1911), considered these to be the cardinal feature of CP: "The sensation evoked is abnormal. The painful sensation develops explosively. There is usually little relation between the strength of the stimulus and the amount of sensation excited: it is 'nearly all or nothing.' Moreover, there is no refractory period for hyperpathic responses." The effective stimulus may include all somatosensory stimuli or only a specific type of input (such as cold or draft, the light touch of clothing or pinprick, even smoke). These grossly unpleasant sensations may demonstrate temporal or spatial spread.

Simple neurologic sensory tests characterize *radiation of pain or dysesthesia* (to body areas not directly in contact with the pain-evoking stimulus: "in a hot room... if one rubs the whiskers of the face with the palm of the hand, burning is felt in the ulnar forearm. Sitting on a chair until the burning is prominent on points of contact, burning is also felt in the lateral thigh which is not in contact with the fabric of the chair"), present in half the cases, *after-sensations* (the persistence of pain long after the stimulus and the arrival of primary afferent impulses that evoke pain), seen in about 40% of cases, and prolonged *temporal summation* (the gradual build-up of pain with repeated stimulation) (Garcin 1937; Riddoch 1938). Radiation of sensations from the stimulus site and spatial and temporal summation appear to be more common in CP than in PNP. Although response latencies can be normal, anomalous summations may be seen: *slow temporal* (pain or dysesthesias start after a delay which, during the daytime, the patient can anticipate and avoid: "if occlusive touch is applied to the skin, within minutes, evocation of the spontaneous dysesthetic burning occurs. The stimulus may be roughness, but the patient perceives it as heat. The search for ever 'cooler' shoes may be launched when what is needed is smooth leather, not the sueded tongue which is common"), *very slow temporal* (starting after hours: "as to confinement or weight-bearing it renders a night's recumbency as feeling like the bed was hard as rocks. As to exercise, it means the muscle soreness the day after exertion is overwhelming"), *delayed with overshoot* (this is not a temporal delay: rather it is a heightened threshold for pain, which, when reached, overshoots wildly, most easily seen in the response to sharp objects. A normal will note graded sharpness as painful before a CP patient will, but because the pin in pinprick testing is so sharp, this delay is often missed at examination), *spatial* (an unexpected increase in pain as the area of stimulus is increased: it appears never to have been tested in CP). *Wind-up pain* (increasing pain with increasing numbers of pinpricks, i.e., temporal summation) has been reported in CP (see also Bowsher 2005).

In other words, provoked pain is characterized by late onset and poor localization, generally radiates from the stimulated point to the entire half of the body (one third of cases) or lesser body areas and persists for an unusually long time after stimulation has ceased. Evoked pains have a distribution which is less widespread than that of steady or intermittent pain. As a rule, somatic stimuli can cause or aggravate pain only when applied to the affected side, but sometimes even the stimulation of the normal side gives rise to exacerbation of pain (synesthesalgia).

Patients may wear as little clothing as possible over affected areas and seek a narrow window of room temperature, or alternatively wear gloves to avoid contact with the painful hand.

Paradoxical burning on cold stimulation is reported by some patients with CP (e.g., Berglund *et al.* 2001; Bowsher 2005). According to the review of Greenspan and colleagues (2004, and references therein), all studies report a large proportion of CP patients with cool (about 50%) or warm hypesthesia, with *no more than 23%* (but 50% in the series of Attal *et al.* 2000 and 56% in that of Andersen *et al.* 1995) showing cold allodynia (see also Morin *et al.* 2002) and very few or no cases of heat allodynia (e.g., 3/16 in Attal *et al.* 2000). In their personal series, two patients with bilateral warm hypesthesia also had bilateral cold hypesthesia, with same-side prevalence; cold allodynia occurred uncommonly among patients with cold hypesthesia (2/11), both unilateral CPSP, who also had bilateral cold hypesthesia. Interestingly, the patient with normal cold detection threshold had the most extreme cold allodynia (in this case, cold allodynia was evoked at temperatures cold enough to activate receptors in the cool pathway, but not those of the supposed heat-pinch-cold pathway). Tactile allodynia is reported by about 40% of patients. Hair sensation is usually unaffected and has never been reported to cause burning.

A review of all published cases and case series of CP over a century shows CP exacerbation by environmental changes (wind, weather changes, low atmospheric pressure, altitude, cold or warm temperatures), emotional stress (sudden fear, joy, anxiety, depression, others), tiredness, smell, loud noises, sad or distasteful music, (sudden) bright light, movements (including vibrations and changing position) and physical activity (e.g., walking, non-strenuous activity, isotonic—isometric muscle contraction of one or more muscles together, with ensuing activation of muscle stretch receptor afferents: this so-called movement/kinesthetic/proprioceptive allodynia, seen in about 10—20% of patients, can hinder rehabilitation and virtually paralyze some patients), visceral stimuli (e.g., a full urinary bladder or rectum, drinking cold and warm water, passing urine, cough, Valsalva maneuver), the thermal grill, smoking (and even the curling of cigar smoke along the fingers), intellectual concentration, inactivity (such as attempts to sleep), merely blowing on the skin and combing the hair. Less commonly, similar stimuli may reduce the pain. Dyskinesias and other anomalous motor reactions can also worsen CP. Rarely, an overresponse to pleasant stimuli or relief by pleasant stimuli (e.g., warmth or orgasm) may also be found (Riddoch 1938); for instance, Biemond (1956) described a patient who drew a passing sensation of pleasure with cold drinks and ice creams.

Table 2.10 gives a summary of studies focusing on all discussed clinical features.

13. Somatosensory findings (Tables 2.10—2.12)

Dejerine and Roussy (1906) concluded that persistent loss of superficial sensation ("*hémianesthésie superficielle persistante*") to touch, pain and temperature, associated with a more pronounced and persistent loss of "deep" sensibility, was typical of "thalamic pain." Sometimes, superficial hemianesthesia was replaced by hyperesthesia. They also noted a predominantly distal hemianesthesia (or hypesthesia), less pronounced proximally on the limbs, slightly exceeding the midline. Pain and thermal sensibility were reduced, but not totally abolished. Patients could not recognize the nature of the stimulus and the site of the stimulation and complained of dysesthesia, topoanesthesia and topoanalgesia, with a delayed perception of the stimuli. In many cases these troubles of superficial sensibility were subtle,

TABLE 2.10. Clinical features (selected studies)

Three-quarters of pts reported pain in one half of the body, except the face in a large majority. The largest variability in pain location was found in pts with low brainstem lesions: two of these had alternate laterality, with pain in the face on one side and in the contralateral arm and/or leg. A few pts have pain only in one leg or arm. Contrary to the notion that CP is diffuse and difficult to localize, all the pts could describe well the location of the pain. CPSP is experienced as superficial or deep or both in almost equal proportions

Quality of pain:

Burning: 59% (brainstem lesions: 75%, thalamic lesions: 22%), aching: 30%, pricking: 30% (unidentified lesions: 50%) Lacerating: 26% (brainstem lesions: 0%, thalamic lesions: 44%), other: 41% (thalamic lesions: 67%)

Tasker *et al.* (1991)

73 personal consecutive CPSP cases. Pain distribution showed no predilection for any particular part of the body.

CP may involve one side of the body maybe with a side preference or, in a small minority of cases, both sides (2.7%)

Pain location	% of cases			
	Unilateral			Bilateral
	Right	Left	Total	
Face	5.5	4.1	9.6	1.4
Face, patchy body	15.1	9.6	24.7	
Hemibody (+head)	15.1	16.4	31.5	
Body only	1.4	0	1.4	
Patchy body only	9.6	20.6	30.2	1.4
Overall			97.3	2.7

The hand alone was affected in one pt.

Pts demonstrated 3 types of pain:
steady spontaneous: 98.6% of cases
burning: 64.4%
aching: 38.6% (aching, bruising, sore, throbbing, pulling, pressing, swelling, cramping, rushing, tight, grabbing, pinching, tearing)
dysesthesic: 31.6% (numb, tingling, fuzzy, stinging, itchy)
cold: 10.6%
intermittent lancinating spontaneous: 16.4% of cases (more prevalent with brainstem lesions)
evoked (hyperesthesia, hyperpathia and/or allodynia): 64.9% of cases (unusual in the absence of clinically detectable sensor loss) hyperpathia–allodynia affected hemibody in 89% of pts in which it was present and was patchy in 11%. It was evoked by single-modality in 35.4% of cases and by multiple modalities in 54.2%

Correlation of pain type with lesion site (40 cases)

	Lesion site	BS	TH	TS	SU	D	UI
	No. of pts	14	6	6	11	1	2
Pain type (%)	Constant	100	83.3	100	100	100	100
	Intermittent	21.4	0	0	9.1	0	0
	Evoked	71.4	83.3	50	90.9	0	100

BS: infratentorial, brainstem; TH: thalamus only; TS: thalamus + supratentorial; SU: supratentorial sparing thalamus; D: diffuse; UI: none seen with imaging, presumably supratentorial.
No preferential factors associated with intermittent and evoked pain.

Michel *et al.* (1990)

Retrospective study. Cortical CP. 12 pts. Cortical lesion sparing the thalamus confirmed by means of MRI or CT scans with reconstruction

Spontaneous pain in 10/12 pts; evoked pain in 5/12 pts. 2 pts without spontaneous pain had evoked pain. Hemibody pain in 5/12 pts (+ head in 2 pts; patchy spontaneous pain in 2 pts). Limb pain: 7 pts (forearm/hand: 5 pts, calf/foot: 2 pts). Patchy pain only: 2 pts

(continued)

TABLE 2.10 *(continued)*

Shieff (1991)

Group of 27 pts with the thalamic syndrome. Pain was seldom reported in a dermatomal pattern, more commonly (and less distinctly) in terms of body parts, either singly or in combination; face and arm most affected, and the leg least, reflecting greater thalamic representation of the upper limb and face. Pts usually complained of pain in anesthetic or hypoesthetic areas, but not invariably: 4 had spontaneously arising pain without any sensory change, and 3 had hyperpathia alone

---

Schmahmann and Leifer (1992)

Parietal pseudothalamic pain syndrome. 6 pts

Quality of pain:
Burning: 4/6 pts
Aching: 2/6 pts
Freezing, ice-like, cold: 3/6 pts
Dull: 2/6 pts

Pain location:
Right hemibody: 3/6 pts (2 right, 1 left)
Right arm and hand (+ face to a lesser extent in 1 pt): 2/6 pts
Right arm and leg: 1/6 pts
Allodynia: 2/6 pts
Pain exacerbated by cold and damp weather: 1/6 pts
Touch-provoked dysesthesias: 1/6 pts
Arm and hand principally affected

Andersen et al. (1995)

Prospective study on CPSP incidence in an unselected stroke population. 267 pts. Survivors able to communicate at 1 yr: 191 pts. CPSP in 16 pts

Distribution of pain:
Hemibody: 6/16 (37.5%)
Upper extremity: 5/16 (31.2%)
Upper + lower extremities: 5/16 (31.2%)

Pain severity:
Mild: 6/16 (37.5%)
Moderate: 7/16 (43.7%)
Severe: 3/16 (18.8%)

Pain type:
Burning: 3/16 (18.8%)
Freezing: 3/16 (18.8%)
Aching: 4/16 (25%)
Lacerating: 8/16 (50%)
Squeezing: 3/16 (18.8%)

Other: 2/16 (12.5%)

Constant pain in 14 pts. Exacerbating or provoking external or emotional factors in 7 pts. 15/16 pts had dysesthesia or allodynia on sensory testing. Other symptoms in additional pts: spontaneous paresthesia and evoked dysesthesia to touch and cold: 1 pt; evoked dysesthesia and shoulder pain with spontaneous resolution: 1 pt; severe pain in the right eye + Horner syndrome with spontaneous resolution: 1 pt (brainstem infarction)

Bowsher (1996, 1998, 2001) Studies with serious interpretive problems

156 CP pts from a personal series. 112 CVA pts, 19 SAH pts, 4 postoperative infarct pts, 3 brain trauma, 4 MS pts, 1 AVM pt, 3 syringo-bulbomyelia pts, 3 spinal ischemic pts, 7 postcordotomy pts. Demographic data reported for 148 pts

Distribution of pain (131 pts: 112 CVA and 19 SAH):
limbs: 30 pts (22.9%)
upper limb: 14 pts (10.7%)

lower limb: 10 pts (7.6%)

face+hemibody: 27 pts (20.6%)

hemibody below face: 21 pts (16%)

face+limbs: 9 pts (6.9%)

face+upper limb: 5 pts (3.8%)

face+lower limb: 2 pts (1.5%)

face both legs: 1 pt (0.8%)

face only: 8 pts (6.1%)

other: 4 pts (3%)

Types of pain *(121 pts: 102 CVA and 19 SAH):*
burning or scalding: 59 pts (48.7%)

aching or throbbing: 44 pts (36.3%)

shooting or stabbing: 10 pts (8.3%)

painful pins and needles: 8 pts (6.6%)

Allodynia in 66/92 (71.7%) CVA pts and 11/14 (78.6%) SAH pts (unknown allodynic status in 10 CVA pts and 4 SAH pts due to dysphasia or unreliable responses)

Types of allodynia *(106 pts: 92 CVA and 14 SAH):*
tactile: 57 pts (53.7%)

movement: 22 pts (20.7%)

thermal: 20 pts (18.8%)

tactile+movement: 12 pts (11.3%)

tactile+thermal: 9 pts (8.5%)

thermal+movement: 1 pt (0.9%)

no allodynia: 29 pts (27.3%)

More than 1 type in some pts

Exacerbating factors *(115 pts: 100 CVA and 15 SAH pts):*
cold: 58 pts (50.4%)

stress: 54 pts (46.9%)

stress+cold: 32 pts (27.8%)

orgasm: 10 pts (8.7%)

others (stress ± cold ± warm ± orgasm; exercise/fatigue): 10 pts (8.7%)

Clinical sensory impairment *(105 pts: 92 CVA and 13 SAH pts):*
pinprick: 85 pts (80.9%)

tactile: 56 pts (53.3%)

thermal: 83 pts (79%)

all three: 37 pts (35.2%)

Area of sensory impairment > painful area; max impairment in the region of max pain; thermal and pinprick impairment ≫ tactile impairment; lesser thermal and pinprick impairment in minimal pain areas

73 CPSP pts (included above). 6 pure sensory strokes. Correlation of MRI findings with pain characteristic

Type of pain *(70 pts):*
burning: 32 pts (45.7%)

non-burning (aching, throbbing, cramp-like etc.): 30 pts (42.8%)

burning AND non-burning: 8 pts (11.4%)

No correlation between type of pain and site of the lesion. Burning pain more common in pts with lesions apparently confined to white matter; non-burning pain more common in pts with lesions apparently confined to gray matter (uncertain conclusion). Pts ≥ 70 yrs: burning pain in 3% of cases; non-burning pain in 25% of cases ($p = 0.03$, t-test)

(continued)

TABLE 2.10 *(continued)*

Allodynia *in 41/70 pts (58.5%):*
pure mechanical: 25/70 pts (35.7%)

pure thermal: 9/70 pts (12.8%) (usually cold; warm and cold in 2 pts)

mixed: 7/70 pts (10%)

movement allodynia: 9/41 pts (21.9%) (7 VPL lesions, 1 parietal lesion)

Pain intensity:
Median pain intensity: 45 VAS units (range 0–80)

Pts with principally **aching pain** (27 cases): median pain intensity: 38 VAS units (range 0–80, pain absent in 2 pts with fluctuating pain)

Pts with principally **burning pain** (18 cases): median pain intensity: 50.5 VAS units (range 13–84)

Difference between the 2 means statistically significant ($p = 0.03$)

No difference in pain intensity according to pain extent or location

Site of pain and most painful region

Site of pain	Lesions site (most painful region)			
	Purely supratentorial	VPL	Other, including brainstem	Infratentorial
Hemibody + face	22 (?)		15	
Hemibody	34		19	
Restricted to the face or one limb or less	(proximal limb)	12 (face)	6	(proximal limb)
Cheiro-oral		2		
Crossed			7	

CPSP in old people (median age: 77.5 yrs). 8 pts (!). Burning pain in 25% of pts. CPSP pts in the present survey appear to have a statistically significant tendency to have non-burning pain than younger hospital-referred subjects (data from the analysis of 35 pts with CPSP, reference study not indicated, but see Bowsher *et al.* (1998) reporting burning pain in only 3% of pts 70 yrs old or more)

NB: z-test for proportion of pts with burning pain: Bowsher (1996) (51%) vs. this survey, $z = 1.053$, $p = 0.292$ (NS); Bowsher *et al.* (1998) (45.7%) vs. this survey, $z = 0.742$, $p = 0.458$ (NS)

Kim and Bae (1997)

17 pts with pure or predominant sensory stroke due to MRI or CT confirmed brainstem lesion. Paramedian dorsal pontine: 15 pts, dorsolateral pons: 1 pt, lateral midbrain: 1 pt. Follow-up: 1 mo–3 yrs

Paresthesia (numbness or tingling sensation) starting in a part of the body (hand or foot) and then spreading to other parts (hemibody) was the initial and main complaint in all pts

Sensory symptoms (almost) completely resolved in 5 pts. Paresthesia usually persisted in the others. In 2 pts (12%) paresthesia worsened, became painful and was often exacerbated by cold weather or fatigue, mimicking the so-called "thalamic pain syndrome" (follow-up: 18 mos, 3 yrs)

Normal spinothalamic sensation in both pts. Impaired lemniscal sensation in 1 pt.

6 pts complained of bilateral perioral or facial symptoms, in 2 cases extending to hemibody. Hemibody involvement in 4 (+2) pts

Nasreddine and Saver (1997)

Systematic review. 180 pts. Pain after thalamic stroke. Pain features available in many instances

Pain type:
painful paresthesias: 100% of pts (as required by inclusion criteria)
non-painful spontaneous paresthesias: 90% of pts (18/20)
allodynia (evoked dysesthesias): 86% of pts (51/59)
hyperalgesia: 84% of pts (41/49)

Distribution of pain (50 pts):
arm: 93%
leg: 74%
face: 66%
trunk: 28%

Simultaneous involvement pattern (% of cases):
face, arm, trunk, leg: 24%
arm, leg: 22%
face, arm, leg: 16%
arm alone: 12%

Other features (% of pts):
weakness ipsilateral to pain: 58% (70/120)
hemiataxia: 34% (24/70)
choreoathetosis: 26% (18/70)
visual field deficit: 21% (16/77)

Right/left frequency difference not significant

MacGowan et al. (1997)

CPSP and Wallenberg's LMI. LMI in 63 pts; CPSP in 16 pts (25.4%); 11 additional pts complained of rare (less than twice monthly) non-painful dysesthesias in a limb or cheek. Two pts with crossed sensory deficits without pain suffered from a compulsive urge to scratch and pick their painless cheek and developed escoriated ulcers; one pt with CPSP did the same

Characteristics of CPSP (% in 16/16 pts):

Pain type:
Spontaneous pain: 100% (16/16) (as required by inclusion criteria)

Spontaneous pain + allodynia: 75% (12/16)

Allodynia:
cold induced: 75% (12/16)
additional mechanical: 37.5% (6/12)

Pain description:
burning: 87.5% (14/16)

electrical: 50% (8/16)

constant: 100% (16/16)

intermittent allodynic exacerbation: 100% (16/16)

Impairment of sensory modalities (QST on *contralateral* cheek) (% of CPSP pts and control)

Thresholds	CPSP (9 pts)	No CPSP (10 pts)
Innocuous thermal		
Normal	88.8%	30%
Absent/elevated	11.1%	70%
Noxious thermal		
Normal	88.8%	20%
Absent/elevated	11.1%	80%
Pressure pain		
Normal	100%	40%
Absent/elevated	0%	60%
Combined		
Normal	88.8%	0%
Absent/elevated	11.1%	100%

(continued)

TABLE 2.10 *(continued)*

The presence of a pain state could be predicted (100% specificity, 89% sensitivity) by the presence of normal threshold to thermal and pressure pain stimuli contralateral to the side of the infarct (crossed quintothalamic tract spared)

Distribution of pain:
ipsilateral cheek + contralateral arm and leg: 37.5% (6/16)

ipsilateral cheek only: 31.2% (5/16)

contralateral arm and leg: 18.7% (3/16)

contralateral arm only: 12.5% (2/16)

In Nakazato *et al.* (2004), pain location after brainstem stroke: hypalgesic side of the face (early onset, ipsilateral to the lesion in 9 pts, typical lesion) and extremities (delayed onset, contralateral to the lesion in 5 pts, ventral type)

Paciaroni and Bogousslavsky (1998)

Thalamic stroke. Pure sensory syndromes in pts among 3628 included in the Lausanne Stroke Registry

Symptoms during the stroke:
pain and/or dysesthesias in 7/25 pts

contralateral paresthesia in 18/25

Delayed pain and/or dysesthesias: 4/25 pts (16%)

Site of symptoms:
Hemibody (including face): 13 pts

Perioral+hand: 4 pts

Face+upper limb: 3 pts

Perioral+hand+foot: 1 pt

Other: 4 pts

Oliveira *et al.* (2002)

40 pts. CPSP.

Continuous pain in 85% of cases. Burning pain in 71.7% of cases

Pain type:
hyperalgesia: in 22.5% of pts

hyperpathia: in 75% of pts

thermal-tactile-kinesthetic allodynia: in 75% of pts

Myofascial syndrome in 67.5%, having segmental distribution in 57.5% and predominating in supratentorial extrathalamic lesion group (highly significant)

Somatosensory deficits:
Thermosensory deficits in all pts

Kim (2003)

20 pts with CPSP or paresthesia after lenticulocapsular hemorrhage (LCH)

Symptoms description *(in various combinations):*
numb, cold, burning, aching, swollen, squeezing

Pain severity:
Mean VAS score: 5.6

CPSP was distinctly more severe in the leg than in the arm or face in the majority of the pts. It was limited to the lower leg or even to the foot area in half of them. Among the admitted pts, the initial sensory deficit was also relatively severe in the lower extremities (results consistent with the previous observation that the severity of CPSP was closely related to the degree of initial sensory deficit in pts with LMI). **A leg-dominant sensory deficits or CPSP was noted**

The leg-dominant pattern of CPSP, rarely associated with lesions occurring at other locations, appears to be one of the characteristics of CPSP after LCH

CPSP usually developed some time after the onset, tended to persist, and partially responded to medications.

These characteristics are consistent with CPSP that developed in pts with stroke occurring in other regions

Greenspan *et al.* (2004)

13 CPSP pts. Ongoing pain was commonly characterized by more than one descriptor in each pt:

thermal quality (burning, cold): 53% overall

burning and cold: 38%

hot and cold: 15%

mechanical quality (sharp/stabbing, pressure/heavy, tightness, squeezing): 77% overall

sharp/stabbing: 33%

pressure/heavy: 33%

tight/squeezing: 7% each

Svendsen *et al.* (2005)

Study on sensory function and quality of life in MS pts with pain, MS pts without pain (+ healthy control subjects). 50 MS pts with pain (MSPp) randomly recruited from a previous epidemiological MS study. Mean MS duration: 12 yrs. CP in 29 MSPp (58%). Mean CP duration: 7 yrs

CP findings (% of pts):
Site

Face: 0%, back: 17%, chest: 7%, upper limbs: 10%, lower limbs: 65%

Temporal pattern:
Constant: 76%, Intermittent: 24%

Pain intensity (VAS 0–100 mm, mean values):

Least: 17, Worst: 86

CP descriptors:

Tingling, tiring, taut, burning (in 12/29 CP pts vs. 1/15 with musculoskeletal pain, p = 0.034), dull, grueling

Aggravating factors (in descending % incidence):

Cold, same body position for a long time, touch (e.g., clothes), physical strain, body movements (incl. walking), warmth, tiredness, stress, loud noise

Alleviating factors (in descending % incidence):

Physiotherapy (incl. massage and extension), analgesic, rest, cold, warmth, change of position, body movements

Results of examination:

MSPp had more commonly decreased sensation to touch, warmth, vibration and/or position sense and increased sensation to touch or pinprick than pts without pain, but no difference in decreased cold or pinprick sensation. All CP pts had signs of spinothalamic dysfunction (increase/decrease in pinprick and/or temperature sense)

CP pts vs. musculoskeletal pain pts:

No difference in detection or pain threshold for temperature, tactile stimulation, vibration, pressure. Cold and/or mechanical allodynia in 11/29 CP pts vs 1/15 pts with musculoskeletal pain ($p = 0.035$). No other differences in QST

Authors' conclusion: More than half of MS pts suffer from CP, which is associated with mechanical or thermal hyperalgesia. Allodynia is more common in MS pts with CP.

TABLE 2.10a. Somatosensory troubles in Head and Holmes' cases of thalamic pain

	5	6	7	8	9	10	11	12	13
Case no.	5	6	7	8	9	10	11	12	13
Sex	F	M	F	M	M	F	F	M	M
Age	51	49	60	64	59	65	52	65	43
Side of pain	L	R	L	L	L	L	R	L	R
Tactile sensibility (Von Frey)	−	0	=	=	−	−−	−−	0 −−(head)	−−
2-point discrimination	0	nt	=	=	−−	nt	−−	nt	nt
Localization of stimuli	−−	nt	=	=	=	nt	=/−	0	nt
Threshold for prick	=	++	=	=	=	+	+	++	++
Unpleasant response to prick	+	++	+	+	+	++	+	++	++
Threshold for painful pressure	=/+	++	− (sole)	−−	=	− (palm, sole) = (hand) + (shin)	+	++ = (sole)	++ −− (sole)
Unpleasant response to pressure	+	++	++	++	+	++	++	++	++
Sensibility to heat	−	0	=	= (shifting)	.	0	=	0	0
Sensibility to cold	−	0	=	= (shifting)	.	0	=	0	0
Unpleasant response to extreme heat	+	++	+	++	+	+	=	nr	++
Unpleasant response to extreme cold	+	++	+	++	++	++	nr	++	++
Pleasant response to mild warmth	nr	nr	nr	nr	++	nr	nr	nr	nr
Unpleasant response to visceral stimulation	+	nr	nr	nr	nr	nr	nr	+	++
Unpleasant response to tickling/scraping	nr	nr	0	=/+	+	++	++	+	++
Appreciation of vibration	nr	nr	−		−	−−/0	−	0	−−/0

0, lost; =, unchanged (no difference between affected and unaffected side); −, diminished; −−, strongly diminished; +, increased; ++, strongly increased; nt, not tested; nr, not reported. Head and Holmes objectively analyzed sensory loss and dissociation of sensibility in pts with lesions of the CNS at spinal, mid-brain, thalamic and cortical level by means of an instrumentation that in some cases was designed expressly for this purpose. Results on the affected part were always compared with results obtained in the unaffected similar part of the body. Data were recorded as accurately and objectively as possible. Light touch was examined first by applying a wisp of fine cotton wool avoiding any deformation of structure. For determining the threshold for light touch the authors employed

Von Frey's graduated hairs ranging from 8 to 110 g/mm². They always performed 16 contacts in 1 minute, avoiding rhythmicity. The series of tests were performed without word exchange; hallucinatory responses were also recorded. Pressure-touch was tested by *contact with the observer's finger* provided that its surface temperature was similar to that of the part to be examined. The threshold for pressure-touch was determined by a *pressure-aesthesiometer*. Specific and as accurate as possible methods were used to test the faculty of localization, the threshold for the appreciation of roughness, the ability to discriminate two simultaneous contacts, the power of recognizing the posture of any part of the body, the power of appreciating passive movements and the power of appreciating weight, size, bi-dimensional shape, three-dimensional form, texture and consistence of objects. The power of recognizing vibration was tested by means of a *tuning-fork, beating 128 Hz*, also noting the duration of the sensation. Tickling and scraping were employed to evaluate the affective component of sensation.

Superficial sensibility to pain was tested first by pricking with a *sharp steel pin or needle* and a comparison between normal and affected parts was always performed. Being well aware that this test was subject to a source of error due to the reduction of the power of recognizing the size (sharpness) of the stimulating object, in cases with slight disturbances of pain sensation, they determined the threshold for pain by means of an aesthesiometer (algesimeter). They also noted that if a pain-spot was not directly stimulated, the same pressure was reported as touch. Finally, pressure-pain was tested by means of a *Cattell algometer*, measuring the amount of pressure (kg) on a standard area necessary to evoke pain. Results of the test on the affected part were always compared with results in the similar unaffected part of the body.

The **thermal sensibility** was examined by means of *silver tubes filled with hot or cold water*. The temperature of the water at the moment of testing was read on a *thermometer*. The authors determined the threshold for heat and cold on similar parts of the body, as well as the power to distinguish the relative warmth or coldness of two tubes. Moreover, the sensation evoked by neutral temperature was compared with that of a distinctly cold or warm tube. They also observed the effect of extreme heat (50°C or more) and cold (15°C or less) and compared the sensation evoked on normal and abnormal parts of the body. To study the affective component of thermal stimuli, they employed large glass tubes (4 cm in diameter) filled with water at various temperature. They also noted that the temperature tests were liable to lead to erroneous conclusions due to the tendency to call all sensations evoked during the testing either hot or cold. Pts with thalamic lesions and capable of no thermal appreciation were more liable to call "hot" every thermal stimulus and even repeated pricking. This confusion was more likely to occur in pts with over-response to affective stimuli. In many pts it was also difficult to determine the extent of the neutral zone between heat and cold threshold, as pts possessed no word which expressed this neutral sensation ("nothing but a touch").

They reported data on one pt with SCI (Brown—Séquard paralysis) without CP, 3 cases of brainstem lesion (1 of them with CP following a Wallenberg's syndrome), 9 cases of thalamic lesion (thalamic syndrome) and 5 pts with cortical lesions (1 of them reporting pain during sensory epileptic attacks). Their conclusions on neurological features in thalamic syndrome were however based on data on 24 pts. In their opinion, the essential feature of thalamic syndrome is the tendency to react excessively to unpleasant stimuli (over-reaction).

In the pt with CP following *Wallenberg's syndrome* the sensibility to light touch (cotton-wool, Von Frey's hairs), the appreciation of roughness (Graham—Brown aesthesiometer) or of two simultaneous contacts and the power of recognizing vibration were not different between the two sides of the face, even if the pt complained that all forms of touch were less vivid over the affected (right) side. The affected side of the face was insensitive to superficial pain (prick), but pressure-pain was not lost (the Cattell algometer gave approximately equal readings on the two sides). Both heat and cold were appreciated on the two halves of the face and the thresholds were the same, but heat seemed hotter over the affected side while cold seemed less cold. On the body there was no difference in appreciation of touch, roughness and vibration but sensations were more vivid on the normal (right) half of the body. Heat and cold could be appreciated, but heat seemed hotter on the affected (left) half of the body and cold seemed less cold. The left half of the body, except an area in the left perineum, penis and scrotum, was insensitive to prick. The pressure of the algometer necessary to evoke pain was considerably higher on the affected hemibody than in the normal half. The left testicle was insensitive to the pressure.

Somatosensory troubles in their pts suffering from *thalamic syndrome* are summarized in the table above.

As of loss of superficial and *"deep" sensibility*, "in some pts with thalamic syndrome this loss is so insignificant that it can be discovered by measurement only, so we can imagine the existence of the over-reaction without it." Even if all pts with over-reaction had a more or less recognizable sensory loss, the excessive response bears no relation to the extent of the accompanying loss of sensation. They noted that the *appreciation of posture and recognition of passive movements* is impaired more frequently than any other sensory quality. The amount of this loss varies from a scarcely measurable defect to a complete loss of these sensibilities.

Tactile sensibility was frequently diminished and in some cases totally lost, but generally a threshold could be obtained, especially increasing the strength of the stimulus. Tactile threshold, measured with Von Frey's hairs, was unchanged between the two halves of the body in 5 cases, but in the majority of the cases it was raised on the affected side. In few cases only the affected parts were totally insensitive to the tactile hairs and also to pressure-aesthesiometer. In some pts, the consecutive contacts (especially with increasing strength) caused widespread tingling that made conclusive demonstration of the threshold impossible. Determination of tactile threshold was also prevented by the occurrence of involuntary (induced) movements, with accessory sensations misinterpreted as stimulation.

(continued)

TABLE 2.10a (continued)

Many pts (50% of cases) could not recognize the *position* of a stimulated spot. In many cases where tactile sensibility was diminished, the inability was maintained even with pricks or painful pressure, to which the pt was sensitive. Pts could be at a loss where they were touched, or could refer touch to wrong areas. When the posture was not recognized and the power of localization was lost, pts recognized the stimulus as a change within the part of themselves and did not refer the discomfort to the action of an external agent. Moreover, when localization was affected, unpleasant sensations could spread widely over the affected part: for instance, they noted that a prick on the hand could cause a painful sensation in the cheek or side.

In no instance among 22 pts the threshold for pinprick pain was lower on the affected body side; it was identical on both sides in 13 cases and raised in 9 cases, in whom a stronger stimulus was needed to produce a sensation of prick. Yet most pts (20/22) showed an over-response to prick.

They also attempted to measure the amount of pressure evoking pain, comparing the 2 sides of the body. They noted that the same pressure produced more disagreeable discomfort and increased reaction on the affected side in every one of 24 pts tested. Moreover the pain developed explosively, as the pressure increased over a certain point. They noted that the threshold for pressure pain was frequently lower on the affected side of the body (15 cases), but it was higher in 3 cases and unchanged in 6 cases. No pts showing a lowered threshold for painful pressure did show a lower threshold for pinprick pain. Yet, the response on the affected half of the body was excessive in all 24 pts. They also stated that excessive pressure (especially on a bone) normally caused discomfort rather than pain, and that distressing sensation differs profoundly from the pain produced by a prick, even if both stimuli were perceived as painful. They concluded that pressure pain contain some sensory factors to which the affected half of the body is peculiarly susceptible and the over-reaction was due to this increased susceptibility, rather than increased sensibility to pain (as demonstrated by the fact that threshold to pinprick may be raised in pts with lowered threshold to pressure). A reduced sensibility to pain delays the appearance of the over-reaction, but, as the stimulus is strong enough to cause pain, the discomfort greatly exceeds that produced over the unaffected part.

Sensibility to heat and cold could show all degrees of change from total loss to a slight increase of the neutral zone. Thermal appreciation could be unaltered, even if, in the majority of cases, it was diminished or lost and threshold for the appreciation of heat and cold were never lowered and could be the same on both sides of the body or be raised. The threshold for thermal stimuli and the range of discrimination was normal and was the same on the 2 sides of the body in 37.5% of cases (9/24 pts). In these pts could appear an over-response to pleasurable heat. However, in many cases, the appreciation of heat and cold was abolished and ice and water over 50°C evoked only discomfort on the affected side. The threshold for heat-induced over-reaction was about 40—45°C in most pts, but in some cases temperatures of 55—60°C were needed. The threshold for cold-induced over-reaction was generally below 15°C. The evoked sensation was the same whichever of the two extremes was used and the pt cannot recognize the cause of the unpleasant sensation. This over-reaction could occur both in pts in whom the threshold for the appreciation of heat and cold was identical on the two halves of the body and in cases where the sensibility to heat and cold was completely lost: 22 out of 24 pts with thalamic syndrome showed an excessive response to extreme heat and cold. Even though, in many cases, only heat above 50°C and cold below 15°C (or melting ice) evoked the over-reaction, in some cases with lesser thermal serangement, temperatures below 26°C and above 40°C evoked this indiscriminate response from the affected half of the body.

Some pts, with less severe impairment of thermal sensibility, could recognize temperature above 38—40°C as warm and those below 26—28°C as cold. However, any temperature that could be appreciated was "hotter" or "colder" on the affected side than on the unaffected one, perhaps due to the increased affective reaction.

They also stated that it was unlikely that pts had an actual increase in sensibility to temperature, but they simply translated the increased discomfort into terms of greater cold or heat; moreover, in pts suffering from thalamic lesions, the power of appreciating either heat or cold cannot be lost singly.

In other words, heat and cold are not dissociated; if one form of sensation is lost, the other will be gravely disturbed.

The loss of thermal sensibility generally affected intermediate temperatures, yielding a sensation of pleasant warmth. However in several pts able to appreciate mild heat (34°C), the application of water at 38°C on the affected part evoked a higher degree of pleasure than the same application over the unaffected part. In one case, excessive pleasure could be converted into excessive discomfort as soon as water temperature exceeded 46°C. In a few pts when thermal sensibility was abolished, warmth applied over a sufficiently large surface evoked a feeling of pleasure, even if the pt did not recognize it was warm and extreme hot or cold evoked great discomfort.

Head and Holmes analyzed the effects of visceral stimulation in pts suffering from thalamic syndrome by comparing the effect elicited by squeezing testicles (without pinching the scrotum). They noted that in many pts the discomfort was more intense and the cremasteric movements were more brisk after squeezing the testicle of the affected side. They also noted that even when pinprick pain threshold on the glans penis were the same on both sides, the discomfort described by the pts was greater after pricking of the affected half.

66

Pts complaining of thalamic pain could complain of unpleasant sensations after scraping the palm or the sole of the foot, or moving a rough object over the skin or even rubbing the hairs over the affected part of the body. Sometimes, these sensations were not painful, but very unpleasant and frequently they spread from the stimulated area to the entire limb or half of the body. Examination with a *Graham–Brown aesthesiometer* (to estimate the appreciation of roughness) frequently induced this anomalous response. Nevertheless, the threshold of appreciation of roughness was never lowered. It was always unchanged or increased, but in the large majority of the pts the aesthesiometer induced greater discomfort on the affected side. Occasionally even the vibration of the tuning fork was able to give rise to similar spreading sensations. In pts characterized by an over-response to painful stimuli tickling was also unpleasant and induced greater reaction.

The vibrations of a tuning fork were generally appreciated on both halves of the body, but in almost every case for a shorter time on the affected side. In many cases, the pt complained that vibrations were "not so plain" or tuning fork vibrated less rapidly on the affected side. Only in few cases (in whom most other sensations were gravely affected), the affected half of the body was insensitive to this stimulus. They noted that a shortened appreciation of the vibration of a tuning fork is associated with the over-response to painful stimuli, independently of the unpleasant feeling-tone evoked by vibration.

Response to pleasurable stimuli (p. 133):

"We were anxious to discover if sensations, normally accompanied by a pleasurable feeling-tone, also produced a similar over-reaction. Unfortunately, the greater number of methods … either produce discomfort or … an entirely indifferent sensation. But in the milder degrees of heat we possess a **measurable stimulus** (!!) endowed with a pleasant feeling-tone … In a few cases when thermal sensibility was abolished, warmth applied over a sufficient large surface evoked a feeling of pleasure … One of our patients found a hot-water bottle pleasant and soothing to the affected foot, but did not recognize that it was warm until he touched it with some normal part … Many patients found the warm hand of the observer unusually pleasant on the abnormal side, although no such manifestations of pleasure were produced when it was applied to the normal part of the body. In one case … the patient could not recognize any thermal stimulus as such, and yet over the affected half of the body … water at from 38°C to 48°C evoked intense pleasure. Temperature of 50°C and above, or of 18°C and below, caused great discomfort [three cases are described and "several patients" referred to]. So far we have been unable to find any temperature which produces a sensation of pleasurable cold."

Behavior of the affected half of the body in states of emotion (p. 135):

"A highly educated patient confessed that he had become more amorous since the attack, which had rendered the right half of his body more responsive to pleasant and unpleasant stimuli. 'I crave to place my right hand on the soft skin of a woman. It's my right hand that wants the consolation. I seem to crave for sympathy on my right side.' Finally he added, 'My right hand seems to be more artistic.'"

TABLE 2.10b. Review of somatosensory abnormalities in Head and Holmes' published cases, Head and Holmes (1911)

24 CP pts.

As far as the loss of superficial and "deep" sensibility is concerned, "in some patients with thalamic syndrome this loss is so insignificant that it can be discovered by measurement only, so we can imagine the existence of the over-reaction without it." Even if all pts with over-reaction had a more or less recognizable sensory loss, the excessive response bears no relation to the extent of the accompanying loss of sensation

Tactile threshold (von Frey's hairs):
identical on both sides: 5/24 pts (20.8%)
raised or lost or undetermined on the affected side: 19/24 pts (79.2%) *

Tactile sensibility was frequently diminished and in some cases totally lost, but generally a threshold could be obtained, especially increasing the strength of the stimulus. In few cases only the affected parts were totally insensitive to the tactile hairs and also to pressure-aesthesiometer

Threshold for pinprick pain:
identical on both sides: 13/22 pts (59.1%)
raised on the affected side (a stronger stimulus was needed to produce a sensation of prick): 9/22 pts (40.9%)
lower on the affected side: 0/22 pts (0%)
Over-response to prick: 20/22 pts (90.9%)

Threshold for thermal stimuli and range of discrimination:
raised on the affected side: 15/24 pts (62.5%)
normal and identical on both sides: 9/24 pts (37.5%)
lower on the affected side: 0/24 pts (0%)

Sensibility to heat and cold could show all degrees of change from total loss to a slight increase of the neutral zone. Thermal appreciation could be unaltered, even if, in the majority of cases, it was diminished or lost. The loss of thermal sensibility generally affected intermediate temperatures.
In pts with normal threshold could appear an over-response to pleasurable heat. In pts with abolished appreciation of heat and cold, ice and water over 50°C evoked only discomfort on the affected side. In pts suffering from thalamic lesions, the power of appreciating either heat or cold could not be lost singly. In other words, heat and cold are not dissociated; if one form of sensation is lost, the other will be gravely disturbed.

Threshold for heat-induced over-reaction:
about 40—45°C in most pts (55—60°C in some cases)

Threshold for cold-induced over-reaction:
generally below 15°C
The evoked sensation was the same whichever of the two extremes was used and the pt could not recognize the cause of the unpleasant sensation

Threshold for pressure pain:
lower on the affected side: 15/24 pts (62.5%)
identical on both sides: 6/24 pts (25%)
raised on the affected side: 3/24 pts (12.5%)

Visceral stimulation (comparison of the effects elicited by squeezing testicles without pinching the scrotum):

In many pts the discomfort was more intense and the cremasteric movements were more brisk after squeezing the testicle of the affected side. Even when pinprick pain threshold on the glans penis were the same on both sides, the discomfort described by the pts was greater after pricking of the affected half

Vibrations of a tuning fork (128 Hz):
Generally appreciated on both halves of the body, but in almost every case for a shorter time on the affected side; vibrations "not so plain" or tuning fork vibrating less rapidly on the affected side. Only in few cases (in whom most other sensations were gravely affected) the affected half of the body was insensitive to this stimulus. A shortened appreciation of the vibration of a tuning fork was associated with the over-response to painful stimuli, independently of the unpleasant feeling-tone evoked by vibration

---

* In some pts the consecutive contacts (especially with increasing strength) caused widespread tingling that made conclusive demonstration of the threshold impossible. Determination of tactile threshold was also prevented by the occurrence of involuntary (induced) movements, with accessory sensations misinterpreted as stimulation.

TABLE 2.11. Somatosensory troubles in the review of De Ajuriaguerra (1937)

	Lehmitte/Claude	De Ajuriaguerra/Lehmitte	Roussy/Foix	Davidson/Schick	Foix
Pt's sex	F	F	M	M	M
Age	49	nr	nr	53	nr
Side of the cortical lesion	L	R	R	R	L
Somatosensory troubles contralateral to the lesion					
Tactile sensibility	− (hand, radial)	− − (hand, ulnar)	− − (hemibody)	− (hemibody)	− (=foot)
Pinprick sensibility	− (cheiro-oral)	nr	− − (hemibody)	− (hemibody)	− (=foot)
Thermal sensibility	+ (cheiro-oral)	− (hand, ulnar)	0 (hemibody)	− (hemibody)	nt
Hyperesthesia (over-reaction)	Y	Y	Y (hemibody)	Y	nr
Allodynia	Y	nr	nr	Y	nr
Localization	nr	−	− − (hemibody)	−	nr
Sense of position	nr	0	− − (hemibody)	nr	nt
Vibration	nr	nr	nr	−	=
Site of the lesion (autopsy)	nr	nr	Cortical/subcortical fronto-parieto-temporo-occipital	Parieto-temporo-insular	Fronto-parieto-temporo-occipital + insula
Thalamic lesion(s)	nr	nr	N	N	N

0, lost; =, unchanged (no difference between affected and unaffected side); −, diminished; − −, strongly diminished; +, increased; nt, not tested; nr, not reported.

TABLE 2.12. Somatosensory findings in selected series

Kameyama et al. (1976): Thalamus

87 pts with Vc thalamic vascular lesions randomly selected from a routine autopsy series

Sensory findings (even if this was not clearly stated, it seems that "hypesthesia" meant a reduction of superficial and deep sensibility for all modalities).

Sensory deficit: No. of pts (%)	Pts with right-sided lesions and deficit	Pts with left-sided lesions and deficit
Hypesthesia: 76/87 (87%)	39/45 (87%)	37/42 (88%)
Deep sensibility: 11/87 (13%)	7/45 (16%)	4/42 (10%)
Dysesthesia: 25/87 (29%)	13/45 (27%)	12/42 (29%)
CP: 12/87 (14%)	9/45 (20%)	3/42 (7%)

Lesion confined to	Sensory disturbances–no. of pts (%)			
	Hypesthesia	Deep sensibility	Dysesthesia	CP
Vc	33/38 (87%)	2/38 (5%)	14/38 (37%)	6/38 (16%)
Vc + internal capsule	26/31 (84%)	5/31 (16%)	9/31 (29%)	4/31 (13%)
Vc + pulvinar	18/19 (95%)	3/19 (16%)	2/19 (11%)	2/19 (11%)
Vc + centrum medianum	10/11 (91%)	3/11 (27%)	1/11 (9%)	0/11 (0%)

Even if CP seems more common in pts with right-sided thalamic lesion, hypesthesia, abnormalities of deep sensibility and dysesthesia seems equally frequent in pts with left-sided or right-sided thalamic lesion

Graff-Radford et al. (1985): Thalamus

25 pts with CT-confirmed non-hemorrhagic thalamic infarction

Site of the lesion	No. of pts		Sensory deficits			
	25 non-hemorrhagic thalamic infarction		Decreased sensibility to pinprick and to light touch	Decreased proprioceptive sensibility	Reduction in vibratory perception	Dysesthesia
Posterolateral thalamic infarction	9 (+ posterior cerebral artery infarct in 4 pts)		8/9 pts*	5/9 pts[†]	4/9 pts	4/9 pts
	Probable complete geniculothalamic infarction	4/9 pts (PCA infarct in 4/4 pts)		4/4 pts		1/4 pts
	Partial geniculothalamic infarction	5/9 pts	3/5 pts	1/5 pts 0/5 pts[‡]	0/5 pts	3/5 pts[§]
Anterolateral thalamic infarction	5			0/5 pts[¶]		
Medial thalamic infarction	3			0/3		
Lateral thalamic/ posterior limb of the internal capsule lesion	8		4/8 (pinprick)	1/8 (light touch)		0/8 pts

* On the foot only in 1 case and on the lower face only in 1 case.

[†] On the foot only in the same case with decreased pain and tactile sensibility.

[‡] The 3 pts with reduction in pinprick and light touch sensation had normal proprioception. No abnormality in pinprick, light touch and proprioceptive sensibility in 1 pt.

[§] One of them with normal vibration sense and 2 of them with normal vibratory and proprioceptive sensibility.

[¶] Transient proprioceptive loss in one case.

	No. of pts		Somatosensory evoked responses	
Site of the lesion	25 non-hemorrhagic thalamic infarction		Unilateral median nerve stimulation of the affected arm	Median nerve stimulation of the non-affected arm or bilateral median nerve stimulation
Posterolateral thalamic infarction	9 pts			
	Probable complete geniculothalamic infarction	4 pts (PCA infarct in 4/4 pts)	No response after P14 (brainstem) in both hemispheres	Normal response in the unaffected hemisphere and a N17 wave over the affected hemisphere*
	Partial geniculothalamic infarction	5 pts; SER in 2 pts	Normal N17, N19 and N20. Delayed N29, N32, N34 and N60†	
Anterolateral thalamic infarction	5 pts; SER in 4 pts		Delayed N17, N19 and N20 over the frontal, central and parietal areas, respectively. In 2 cases N29, N32 and N34 were delayed. N60 was delayed in all cases in the central region, but the response varied over the parietal area. In one case there was only a delay of N60	
Medial thalamic infarction	3 pts		The most consistent delay noted was in the N60	
Lateral thalamic/ posterior limb of the internal capsule lesion	8 pts; SER in 7 pts		All had normal N17 and delayed N60. However, wave N19, N20, N29, N32 and N34 were very variable, in an heterogeneous manner	

* In one pt (left deficit) bilateral stimulation produced some ipsilateral responses over the right hemisphere (side of the infarct) due to ipsilateral response.

† In 2 pts the SER could not be interpreted. In one case arm had normal sensation (only leg had decreased sensation) and SER were normal.

The **clinical hallmark** of a lesion involving the whole **geniculothalamic** distribution is loss of sensation in all primary modalities: pts may have associated dysesthesia, hemiparesis, hemianopia and choreiform movements. A geniculothalamic lacune in Vc caused "pure hemisensory loss" (contralateral sensory loss involving part of the body for the modality of pain and light touch, but not proprioception or vibration). Occasionally there may be dysesthesia, but no motor signs. There are little or no accompanying neuropsychological deficits. Electrophysiological findings in complete geniculothalamic infarction with loss of both proprioception and pain sensation correspond to an absence of SERs of all waves after P14 (i.e., N17, N19, N20, N29, N32, N34 and N60) in the hemisphere ipsilateral to the lesion. In contrast, a lacune in the same territory corresponds to an intact N17, N19 and N20 response, but a delayed or absent N32, N34 and N60 waves. Sensory loss is rare in tuberothalamic infarction. In anterior choroidal infarction sometimes there is sensory loss for pinprick and light touch, but not proprioception or vibration. Neuropsychological evaluation: few abnormalities unless there was concomitant PCA infarction

Schott et al. (1986): Thalamus

43 pts with CP from thalamic or thalamocapsular lesions

Study on somatosensory deficits and SSEP

(continued)

TABLE 2.12 *(continued)*

	Thermal and pain sensibilities	Tactile sensibility	Vibration sense	Stereognosis	Kinesyesic sensibility	SSEP
Normal	5 pts	5/15 pts	8/15 pts	6/15 pts	4/15 pts	5 pts
Impaired	7 pts	6/15 pts	5/15 pts	4/15 pts	6/15 pts	12 pts (abnormal)
Abolished	16 pts	3/15 pts	1/15 pts	4/15 pts	4/15 pts	12 pts

One pt had a reduced sensibility to all modalities over the arm and absence of sensibility to all modalities over the leg

Hyperpathia in 18/20 pts (9 pts not tested). **Tactile allodynia** in 13/20 pts

Mauguière and Desmedt (1988): Thalamus

Results of somatosensory examination in 30 pts with thalamic syndrome (some possibly already included in Shott *et al.* 1986). Pain affecting 24 pts (entire hemibody: 14 pts; extremities only: 10 pts)

Somatosensory findings in 24 CPSP and 6 pain-free stroke pts

	Touch and joint position sense	Vibration sense	Pain sensibility	Temperature sensibility
Unaffected	8/24 (0/6)	9/24 (0/6)	15/24 (1/6)	14/24 (1/6)
Reduced	8/24 (0/6)	13/24 (0/6)	9/24 (3/6)	9/24 (2/6)
Lost	8/24 (6/6)	2/24 (6/6)	0/24 (2/6)	1/24 (3/6)

Somatosensory findings and SEP in 24 CPSP*[†‡] pts and 6 pain-free stroke[§] pts

		SEP		
Somatosensory findings (N: normal; I: impaired; L: lost		Normal	Abnormal	Abolished
Touch and joint position sense	N	8/8[‡]		
	I		6/6[†]	2/10*
	L			8/10*
				6/6[§]
Vibration sense	N	4/8[‡]	2/6[†]	3/10*
	I	4/8[‡]	4/6[†]	5/10*
				0/6[§]
	L			2/10*
				6/6
Pain sensibility	N	5/8[‡]	6/6[†]	4/10*
				1/6[§]
	I	3/8[‡]		6/10*
				3/6[§]
	L			2/6
Temperature sensibility	N	6/8[‡]	4/6[†]	4/10*
				1/6[§]
	I	2/8[‡]	2/6[†]	5/10*
				2/6[§]
	L			1/10*
				3/6[§]

* 10 pts showed a complete loss of contralateral cortical SEPs components, but preservation of P9 (brachial plexus), P14 (medial lemniscus) and N18 (brainstem nuclei) far-fields. All these pts complained of **spontaneous burning/crushing pain.** Hyperpathic overreaction in 7 of them. Thalamic infarction involved the geniculothalamic territory in 6 cases. Three pts had a posterior thalamic hemorrhage and 1 pt a capsulothalamic hematoma.

† 6 pts had abnormal contralateral cortical SEPs, with prolonged latency and/or decreased voltage. These pts complained of **painful paresthesia** and showed hyperpathic overreaction to repeated touch. Four pts had a geniculothalamic artery territory infarct and 2 pts a capsulothalamic hemorrhage.

‡ In 8 pts contralateral cortical SEPs showed no difference between affected and unaffected side. These pts complained of painful paresthesia and allodynia/hyperpathia. **None of them had spontaneous pain.** The thalamic lesion involved the anterolateral thalamus in 2 cases, the caudal pole of posterior thalamus in 1 case and the posterolateral thalamus in 5 cases.

§ In **6 pain-free pts** contralateral parietal and frontal SEPs components were absent after median nerve stimulation on the affected side, but P9, P14 and N18 components were unaffected. On CT all pts showed a focal posterolateral thalamic infarction (geniculothalamic territory). Concomitant occipital infarct in 5/6 pts.

Bogousslavsky et al. (1988): Thalamus

Clinical findings and long-term follow-up of 40 pts with a CT-proven "pure" thalamic infarct

Sensory disturbances	Type of thalamic infarct				
	Inferolateral (thalamogeniculate artery, Vc n.) (18 pt)	Tuberothalamic (VA+VL nn.) (5 pts)[†]	Posterior choroidal (3pts)[‡]	Paramedian (unilateral: 9, bilateral: 5 pts)[§]	Total (40 pts)
(Hemi)sensory symptoms or signs at the time of infarction (impaired sensibility)	17 (94.4%)*	4 (80%)	1 (33.3%)	5 (35.7%)	27 (67.5%)
	alone	alone	alone	alone	alone
Tactile					
Temperature	5	3	1	4	13
Pain	11[¶] (61.1%)　(27.8%) [1 (3.6%)]	1 (20%)　(60%)	0　(33.3%)	1 (7.1%)　(28.6%)	13 (32.5%)　(32.5%)
Position					
Vibratory					

* No impaired consciousness; neuropsychologic dysfunction in 1 pt; CPSP in 3 pts. In 1 pt only pain sensibility impaired.

[†] Neuropsychologic dysfunction as main disturbance: dysphasia (left-sided infarct, 4 pts), hemineglect (right-sided infarct).

[‡] Motor, sensory or neuropsychologic dysfunction mild or absent. In 1 pt hemibody numbness.

[§] Consciousness impairment followed by neuropsychological disturbances. Sensory loss less common than motor. Painful intolerance to light in 1 pt.

[¶] CPSP developed in 3/27 pts with sensory dysfunctions. All cases had a nondissociated hemisensory loss involving the elementary modalities.

CPSP seen only in pts with inferolateral thalamic (thalamogeniculate) infarction lesioning Vc. No dissociated sensory loss. Best predictor of CPSP: severe hemianesthesia involving all elementary sensory modalities

Boivie et al. (1989): Thalamus (Study with serious limitations)

27 CPSP pts. Referral to pain clinic

Exclusion criteria: severe dysphasia, dementia or confusion, presence of nociceptive, PNP or psychogenic pains

4 pts groups, according to the localization of the lesion based on clinical and CT evaluation:
brainstem CPSP (8 cases)
thalamic CPSP (9 pts, but only 2/9 pts had lesion restricted to the thalamus; the other had lesions extending into the lateral capsule and basal ganglia)
supratentorial extrathalamic CPSP (6 pts)
CPSP from unidentified lesion (4 pts).

Hemibody pain in 20/27 pts; dominant pain quality: burning, aching, pricking, lacerating (with differences between the 4 groups).

Mean VAS score: 2.5–7.9 (depending on stroke location)

Somatosensory deficits were studied by means of clinical sensory tests and quantitative methods. The examination was carried out 3 yrs (mean) after the stroke. The tests were performed during 2 or 3 sessions in standardized regions of the body (hands and feet included for all tests). In all tests, the contralateral unaffected side of the body was used as control. No pt had higher threshold for vibration and warmth–cold on the control side. No pt had hyperesthesia on the control side

(continued)

TABLE 2.12 *(continued)*

Methods of examination

Sensibility	Clinical sensory tests By means of	Site	Quantitative methods By means of	Site
Tactile	Strokes of cotton wool	Cheek, dorsum of the hand and dorsum of the foot	15 nylon filaments (Von Frey hairs)*	Cheek, pulp of index finger, dorsum of the foot
Thermal (warmth)			Thermotest apparatus[†]	Cheek, tenar eminence and dorsum of the foot
Thermal (cold/warmth)	Round surface (3.9 cm^2) of a tuning fork of room temperature	Cheek, dorsum of the hand and dorsum of the foot	Thermotest apparatus	Cheek, tenar eminence and dorsum of the foot
Pain (pinprick)	Light prick with a pin	Cheek, dorsum of the hand and dorsum of the foot		
Pain (heat)			Thermotest apparatus	Cheek, tenar eminence and dorsum of the foot
Pain (cold)			Thermotest apparatus	Cheek, tenar eminence and dorsum of the foot
2-point discrimination	Compass	Pulp of index finger and dorsum of the foot		
Vibration thresholds			Vibrameter[‡]	Second metacarpal and first metatarsal
Dermolexia	Drawing digits by a blunt probe	Tenar eminence and dorsum of the foot		
Kinesthesia	Asking the pts to identify passive joint movements performed manually	Index finger and big toe		

* Filaments ranging from 10 mg to 300 g. The weakest stimulus that the pt identified >50% of the times was taken as the perception threshold.

[†] The stimuli were given by a 2.5 × 5 cm plate fixed to the skin. This plate could be heated or cooled in a controlled manner. The difference between the thresholds for perception of warmth and cold was used as the threshold for innocuous temperature.

[‡] Vibrating at 100 Hz with constant probe pressure. The mean detection threshold of 3 consecutive tests was taken as the measured variable.

The presence of numbness, paresthesias, spontaneous or evoked dysesthesias, hyperesthesia, allodynia, radiation of perceived sensation, delay in the perception of a stimulus, prolonged after-sensation and summation of repeated stimulation for 15 s was also recorded.

In the clinical examination of touch, cold and pinprick the results were classified as normal, hypo- or hyperesthetic. In the quantitative examination the affected side had to have at least twice as high a threshold as the control side to be considered pathologically raised. The abnormality was classified as slight to moderate if the threshold was 2–5 times higher than on the control side and severe if it was more than 5 times higher

	Normal Clinical	Normal Quantitative	Hypoesthetic or 2–5 times higher Clinical	Hypoesthetic or 2–5 times higher Quantitative	Hyperesthetic or >5 times higher Clinical	Hyperesthetic or >5 times higher Quantitative
Tactile[‡]	15	48	48	23	37	29
Thermal*						
warmth		0		19		81
cold	7		41		52	
Pain						
pinprick[†]	4		37		59	
heat[§]		7		15		78
cold						
2-point discrimination[¶]	65		13		22	
Vibration thresholds[‖]		59		7		33
Dermolexia	56		17		28	
Kinesthesia[•]	63		37		na	

(% of pts with normal and raised thresholds on the side of pain)

* Reduced or lost sensibility for innocuous temperature: 27/27 pts (severe defect in 80% of cases); decreased sensibility for noxious temperature: 25/27. Raised threshold differences: warmth = cold: 17 pts (63%); warmth > cold: 8 pts (30%); warmth < cold: 2 pts (7%); no temperature appreciation (0–50°C) in 70% of pts. Cold sensibility clinically abnormal in 93% of pts. In pts unable to perceive warmth at all, but still able to perceive heat, a sudden burning sensation was perceived as the temperature reached the threshold. In some pts thermal stimuli evoked paresthesia or dysesthesia,

but not cold or warmth and sometimes warmth evoked a cold sensation or vice versa. Cold hyperesthesia: contradictory results between clinical test and Thermotest. With quantitative Thermotest no pt revealed a reduced threshold for cold or heat pain, but 5/22 (23%) pts had cold allodynia when tested with a metal object of room temperature. All but 2 pts were hypoalgesic to temperature pain. The authors were unable to demonstrate major differences between the four groups in the frequency, severity and patterns of the abnormalities in thermal sensibility, but thalamic pts had a slight tendency to be more affected than the others.

† Pinprick threshold could not be determined. Impaired sensibility to pinprick in 26/27 pts. Hyperalgesia in almost 60%. Hyperalgesia was more common in pts with thalamic lesion and least common in pts with brain-stem lesion. Hypoalgesia in 37%. All but 1 pt abnormal sensibility to pinprick (96%).

‡ Normal threshold in only 1/9 thalamic pts, but in 6/8 brainstem pts. Examination with cotton wool: abnormal touch sensibility in 85% of cases. Quantitatively raised threshold in 52% of cases.

§ Noxious heat and cold perception was decreased in 25 of 27 pts.

¶ Sensibility to touch was more severely affected in thalamic pts, as was 2-point discrimination and kinesthesia.

‖ 41% of pts had a raised vibratory threshold (more impaired in thalamic pts than other groups).

Qualitative sensory abnormalities

		% of pts
Numbness		67%
Paresthesia		41%
Dysesthesia		
	Spontaneous	85%
	Evoked	41%
Hyperesthesia		88%
	Pinprick	64%
	Cold	56%
	Touch	48%
Allodynia		23%
Radiation of pain		50%
After-sensation		45%

All data in this study referred to the region where the sensory abnormality was most pronounced, which appeared to be identical to the region of maximal pain in most pts, but this fact was not systematically investigated. However, tests were performed in standardized regions of the body, so most pts should have had maximal sensory abnormalities and/or pain just on cheek, pulp of index finger, thenar eminence and dorsum of the hand and foot, **an unlikely event. In conclusion, it is difficult to understand from what body area results were elaborated: the standardized one, that with maximal sensory abnormalities or, unlikely, that with maximal pain.**

Authors' conclusion: Some kind of sensory abnormality on the affected side was present in 27/27 CPSP pts. All pts had abnormal temperature and pain sensibility, with a severe deficit in most cases, without differences between groups. The only specific sensory sign common to all pts was decreased or lost sensibility to innocuous warmth and cold. Sensibility to low threshold mechanical stimuli (vibration, tactile sensibility and joint movements) may be normal. Neither the level of the lesion along the neuraxis nor concomitant injury to the medial lemniscal pathway is crucial for the development of CPSP.

Michel *et al.* (1990): Cortex

Retrospective study. 12 pts. Cortical lesion sparing the thalamus confirmed by means of MRI or CT scans with reconstruction. Electrophysiological study: SEPs (median and posterior tibial nerves stimulation), flexion reflex RIII

Sensory abnormalities

Sensibility	% of pts		
	Normal	Impaired	Lost
Tactile	25	58.3	16.7
Thermal	8.3	75	16.7
Pinprick	16.7	75	8.3
Pallesthesia	41.6	50	8.3
Kinesthesia	58.3	25	16.7
Stereognosis	66.7	8.3	25
SEPs (median nerve stimulation on the affected side, N20). (Not done in 1 pt)	25	25 (reduced amplitude)	41.7 (absent)
SEPs (tibial posterior nerve stimulation on the affected side, 3 pts)			100
RIII (5 pts)	60	40 (increased threshold)	

(continued)

TABLE 2.12 *(continued)*

Sensory abnormalities matching pain distribution. In 7/12 pts all the modalities were impaired (hemianesthesia in 1 case, thermal and pinprick hypoesthesia in 6 cases). In 5 pts the lemniscal sensibility was normal or near normal, but thermal and pinprick (3 cases) or thermal sensibility alone (2 cases) were impaired

Tasker *et al.* (1991): Brain sites

64 out of 73 (87.6%) personal consecutive pts had clinically detectable sensory defect

Somatosensory function affected		% of pts		
Hemihypoesthesia	All modalities	46.5% (usually involving half of the body: isolated spinothalamic loss: 26%)		
	Dissociated sensory loss	20.5%		
		Pain and temperature sensibility mainly loss	8.2%	
		Pain and temperature sensibility spared:	5.5%*	
			Isolated tactile hypoesthesia	1.4%
			Reduced touch, position, vibration and hyperesthesia, allodynia	2.7%
			Tactile hypoesthesia (face), hyperesthesia, allodynia (hemibody)	1.4%
		Isolated hyperpathia ± allodynia	6.8%	
Facial hypoesthesia		6.9%†	All modalities	1.4%
			Dissociated sensory loss	5.5%
No clinically detectable somatosensory abnormality		5.5%		
Evoked pain in the absence of sensory loss		6.8%		

* No deficits of thermoalgesia.

† Three cases with infratentorial brainstem lesions with dissociated sensory loss in the face and contralateral body (hypoesthesia in the face and hypoalgesia in the body) complained only of facial pain.

Pain distribution correlated with sensory abnormalities. Dissociated sensory loss was more frequent with lesions too small to visualize, thalamic lesions and infratentorial brainstem lesions

Correlation of sensory loss with lesion site (40 cases)								Correlation of evoked pain with sensory loss (48 cases)*	
	Lesion site	BS	TH	TS	SU	D	UI	Evoked pain (% of pts)	
	No. of pts	14	6	6	11	1	2		
								% present	% absent
Sensory loss (%)	None	14.3	16.7	16.7	0	0	0	8.3	20.0
	Spinothalamic	35.7	16.7	0	9.1	100	50	33.3	36.0
	Multimodal	50.0	66.7	83.3	90.9	0	50	58.3	44.0
Evoked pain (%)		71.4	83.3	50	90.9	0	100	Unusual in the absence of clinically detectable sensory loss	

BS: infratentorial, brainstem; TH: thalamus only; TS: thalamus + supratentorial; SU: supratentorial sparing thalamus; D: diffuse; UI: none seen with imaging, presumably supratentorial.

* In the previous original table, 47 cases (64.9% of 73 pts). 48 cases = 65.7% of 73 pts.

Schmahmann and Leifer (1992): Cortex

Parietal pseudothalamic pain syndrome. 6 pts. CT confirmed lesions. Thalamus always spared

	Handedness	Pain site	Sensibility		
			Pinprick	Thermal	Tactile
1	R	R Arm and leg	I	I	N, Al
2	R	R Arm and hand (face)	Lo	Lo	N
3	R	R Hemibody	I	I	N
4	L	L Hemibody	I	I	I
5	L	R Hemibody	I	I	I
6	R	R Arm and hand	I	I	N, Al

I: impaired; Lo: lost; N: normal; Al: allodynia present.

Sensory abnormalities	No. of pts (%)	
	Normal	Decreased
Pinprick		6/6 (100)
Temperature		6/6 (100)
Touch threshold*	4/6 (66.7) 2[†]	2/6 (33.3)
Vibration*	4/6 (66.7)	2/6 (33.3)
Proprioception*	4/6 (66.7)	2/6 (33.3)
Graphesthesia	1/6 (16.7)	5/6 (83.3)
	Present	Absent
Temporal summation	4/6 (66.7)	2/6 (33.3)
Spatial summation	4/6 (66.7)	2/6 (33.3)

* Touch, vibration and proprioception always associated.

[†] No. of pts with hyperpathia.

Authors' conclusion: Arm and hand principally affected. Alteration of pinprick and temperature sensation in the affected areas in all pts. Impaired touch, vibration and proprioception only in 2. Temporal or spatial summation of touch and pinprick (producing uncomfortable dysesthesia or increase in burning/ice sensations) in 3.

Wessel *et al.* (1994): Thalamus

18 pts with a single ischemic thalamic lesion and sensory disturbances and/or CP in the opposite hemibody

3 pts groups:

pts with somatosensory deficits, CP and abnormal SEPs (classic thalamic syndrome: 6 pts)

pts with somatosensory deficits, no CP (1 yr follow-up) and abnormal SEPs (analgetic thalamic syndrome: 8 pts)

pts without somatosensory deficits, CP and normal SEPs (pure algetic thalamic syndrome: 4 pts)

Sensory clinical examination for: touch, heat and cold temperature, pinprick, joint position, vibration. Non-affected mirror side acted as control. SEPs recorded after median and tibial nerve stimulation. Abnormalities defined with respect to normal laboratory values. Thalamic infarction classification on CT scans: anterolateral (tuberothalamic artery), posterolateral (geniculothalamic artery), paramedian (interpeduncular profunda artery). Pts with other stroke types excluded from study

(continued)

TABLE 2.12 *(continued)*

Sensory disturbances

		Posterolateral (10 pts)		Anterolateral (2 pts)		Paramedian (2 pts)		Capsulothalamic (4 pts)		Total (18 pts)	
		No CP	CP	No CP	CP	No CP	CP	No CP	CP	No CP	CP
Sensibility		6 (60%)	4 (40%)	0	2 (100%)	0	2 (100%)	2 (50%)	2 (50%)	8 (45.5%)	10 (55.5%)
Tactile											
	Normal		2 (50%)		2 (100%)						4 (40%)
	Reduced	3 (50%)					2 (100%)	1 (25%)	1 (25%)	4 (50%)	3 (30%)
	Lost	3 (50%)	2 (50%)					1 (25%)	1 (25%)	4 (50%)	3 (30%)
Temperature											
	Normal		3 (75%)		2 (100%)	1 (50%)			1 (25%)		7 (70%)
	Reduced	5 (83.3%)	1 (25%)			1 (50%)		2 (50%)	1 (25%)	7 (87.5%)	3 (30%)
	Lost	1 (16.7%)								1 (12.5%)	
Pinprick											
	Normal		2 (50%)		2 (100%)			1 (25%)		1 (12.5%)	4 (40%)
	Reduced	4 (66.7%)	2 (50%)				2 (100%)	1 (25%)	1 (25%)	5 (62.5%)	5 (50%)
	Lost	2 (33.3%)							1 (25%)	2 (25%)	1 (10%)
Position											
	Normal		2 (50%)		2 (100%)		2 (100%)		1 (25%)		7 (70%)
	Reduced	5 (83.3%)	2 (50%)					2 (50%)	1 (25%)	7 (87.5%)	3 (30%)
	Lost	1 (16.7%)								1 (12.5%)	
Vibratory											
	Normal		2 (50%)		1 (50%)		2 (100%)				5 (50%)
	Reduced	3 (50%)	1 (25%)		1 (50%)			1 (25%)	2 (50%)	4 (50%)	4 (40%)
	Lost	3 (50%)	1 (25%)					1 (25%)		4 (50%)	1 (10%)
Hyperpathia (tactile allodynia?)			2 (50%)		1 (50%)				2 (50%)		5 (50%)
Median SEP											
	Normal	1 (16.7%)	2 (50%)		2 (100%)		2 (100%)		1 (25%)	1 (12.5%)	7 (70%)
	Abnormal	5 (83.3%)	2 (50%)					2 (50%)	1 (25%)	7 (87.5%)	3 (30%)
Tibial SEP											
	Normal		2 (50%)		2 (100%)		2 (100%)				6 (60%)
	Abnormal	6 (100%)	2 (50%)					2 (50%)	2 (50%)	8 (100%)	4 (40%)

Severe damage of the major somatosensory relay region (Vc or intralaminar thalamic nuclei) as shown by the clinical, SEPs and CT findings in the group 2 pts **may be incompatible with the occurrence of CP.** A less extensive damage with preserved but abnormal SEPs could release the mechanism for CP. In pts with pure algetic syndrome the lemniscal system and the Vc relay seem intact. CT evidence of paramedian or anterolateral thalamic infarct (occurring in this series only in pts with CP) may predict the development of CP. Pts with a loss of cortical SEPs and a posterolateral thalamic infarct probably will not develop CP

Samuelsson *et al.* (1994): Brain lacunae

39 stroke pts with MRI confirmed lacunar syndromes (from occlusion of a single small perforating artery) from 100 consecutive pts. Pure sensory stroke (PSS): 10 pts; sensorimotor stroke (SMS): 12 pts; pure motor stroke (PMS): 17 pts.

MRI findings: SMS and PMS were predominantly lenticulocapsular. PSS were predominantly thalamic. Symptoms over face + hand + leg in 23 pts, over face + hand in 4 pts, over hand + leg in 12 pts. The prognosis of sensory impairment was favorable except for **3 CPSP pts**

Clinical examination: touch, pinprick, vibration, kinesthesia, graphesthesia. Quantitative thermal testing (QTT) aimed at evaluating perception thresholds for cold, warmth and heat pain. QTT performed with a Thermotest. Thresholds obtained bilaterally from the cheek, hand (thenar/hypothenar eminence) and leg (L5 dermatome). Temperature limits: 10-50°C. Unaffected side used as control. Follow-up and repeated test up to 1 yr after stroke onset (17 pts)

Sensory examination (affected vs. unaffected side)

Sensibility		Lacunar syndrome		
		PSS (10 pts)	SMS (12 pts)	PMS (17 pts)
Pinprick	Decreased	10	12	
	Normal			
Touch	Decreased	10	8	
	Normal		4	
Vibration	Decreased	4		
	Normal	6	12	
Kinesthesia	Decreased	1		
	Normal	9	12	
Graphesthesia	Decreased			
	Normal	10	12	
Quantitative assessment of thermal thresholds (QTT)				
Cold	Decreased*		C, H, L	H, L
	No difference			C
Warmth	Decreased*		C, H, L	
	No difference			C, H, L
Heat pain	Decreased*		C, H, L	H
	No difference			C, L
Residual sensory symptoms (3 mos)		10[†]	6[‡]	
CPSP		3 (severe: 2)[§]	0	

* Statistically significant difference between symptomatic and asymptomatic side. C: cheek; H: hand; L: leg.

[†] At 1 yr complete recovery in 1 pt; minor residual symptoms in 6 pts. Decreased sensibility to pinprick and touch in all 6 pts. No pain reduction at 1 yr follow-up.

[‡] Generally sensory symptoms more pronounced in the hand. Sensory symptoms resolution within 3 mos in all but 6 pts (still present at 1 yr). Decreased sensibility to pinprick in all 6 pts; decreased sensibility to touch in 4/6.

[§] Decreased sensibility to pinprick and touch in all pts. Dyskinesthesia and reduced vibration perception resolved within 6 mos after stroke.

Thalamic infarcts predominated among the pts with the most pronounced sensory (QTT) abnormalities

Pts with PSS and SMS ($n = 22$) had significant thermal hypoesthesia on the affected side (all tested modalities). Thermal anesthesia in 5 pts. Thermal thresholds outside the range tested (10-50°C) in all 3 pts who later developed CPSP. Pts with PMS (by definition without signs of sensory dysfunction on clinical examination) had thermal hypoesthesia for cold and heat pain in the hand and for cold perception in the leg

Thermal perception (including thermal anesthesia) generally improved over time, but 1 yr after the stroke there was still a statistically significant reduction for warmth and heat pain perception in the hand and leg

Authors' conclusion: Data confirm an involvement of spinothalamic-mediated sensory modalities in PSS and SMS. QTT may be a more sensitive test than SEPs for detection of sensory impairment in lacunar infarcts. Spinothalamic-mediated sensory modalities are also impaired in pts with PMS. The study suggests a gradual transition from intact sensibility to subclinical and clinical apparent sensory dysfunction.

(continued)

TABLE 2.12 *(continued)*

Triggs and Beric (1994): Brain strokes

6 of 48 stroke pts with functionally limiting dysesthesias induced by repetitive light touch, joint movement or neuromuscular electrical stimulation

Lesion location: cortical (parietal) stroke: 2 pts; MCA infarction: 1 pt; thalamic infarction: 1 pt; brainstem infarction: 2 pts. Sensory loss in all pts

Clinical and quantitative sensory testing:
light touch perception: Von Frey hairs (threshold = lowest stimulus intensity detected >50% of trials)
vibration threshold (clavicle, 2nd metacarpal, 1st metatarsal, anterior tibia): vibrameter
thermal sensibility (cervical, thoracic, lumbar and sacral dermatomes): thermotest stimulator

Sensibility	Threshold on symptomatic side in 6 pts		
	Normal	2–5 times higher	>5 times higher or perception absent
Tactile (light touch)	4	1	1
Thermal Temperature discrimination		2	4
Pain*			
Thermal pain perception		4	2
Pinprick sensibility		4	2
Vibration	3	2	1
Graphesthesia	3	1	1 (1 pt not tested)
Position sense	3	3	0

* Non-consensual impairment in thermal pain perception and pinprick sensibility in 2 pts.

QST found substantial impairment of pinprick and temperature sensibilities in all pts. Sensibilities attributable to dorsal column function were relatively preserved

Naver *et al.* (1995): Brain strokes

Study aimed at evaluating incidence and mechanisms of symptoms interpreted as unilateral disturbances of autonomic function (coldness, dryness, sweating and trophic changes). 37 consecutive pts (19 men, 18 women, mean age 58 ± 13 yrs) with acute monofocal stroke. Control group of 15 pts aged 64 ± 15 yrs with a single TIA. Site of the lesion: hemispheric in 26 pts, brain stem in 11 pts

Examination of:
temperature perception thresholds (by means of Thermotest)
skin temperature (by means of an electronic thermometer)
evaporation rates (by means of an evaporimeter)
skin blood flow responses (by means of laser Doppler flowmeters)

Vasomotor reflexes evoked by means of a single deep breath, arousal and mental stress.

Results over the affected side of the body (contralesional side) in stroke pts:

Pain: 16.2% (6 pts)
Unpleasant sensation of coldness in 43% of cases (7 brain stem infarcts, 9 hemispheric infarcts). Pinprick sensation reduced in all these pts
Unpleasant sensation of warmth in 8% of cases (3 hemispheric infarcts; 1 pt with brain stem infarct complained of contralateral coldness and ipsilateral warmth)
Subjective symptoms of temperature asymmetry and hypalgesia (to pinprick) in 51% of cases (19 pts). Quantitative temperature test made only in 11 pts (8 cases unreliable responses due to neglect or aphasia). 11/11 impaired temperature perception over the hand; 10/11 impaired temperature perception over the foot. Significant higher thermoneutral zone (over the ipsilateral **asymptomatic** side too). **CPSP** pts: **hypalgesia** in 6/6; impaired temperature perception in the affected side (thermotest): 3 /3 (cooperating pts):
Skin temperature: lower (statistically significant difference between affected and non-affected side only in pts with hemispheric lesions)
Relatively lower basal skin blood flow and asymmetrical vasomotor responses

Excess of evaporation (pts with brain stem lesions; ipsilesional in hemispheric stroke)

Vasomotor reflex asymmetries (weak vasodilator or vasoconstrictor reflexes) in 34% of cases

The detected abnormalities correlated significantly with:

sensations of unilateral (contralesional) coldness

hypalgesia (contralesional)

thermohypesthesia (contralesional)

anatomical lesions in spino-thalamo-cortical pathways

Vasomotor asymmetries are probably due to lesions of descending uncrossed vasomotor pathways. Subjective coldness may be due to disturbed central processing. **Impaired pinprick sensation and temperature perception** may occur in pts with or without CPSP

Vestergaard *et al.* (1995): Brain strokes

Unselected consecutive group of 11 CPSP pts (5 women, 6 men) surviving more than 1 yr after stroke. MRI verified ischemic infarctions in all pts (suprathalamic: 11/11 pts (bilateral: 2 pts), solely extrathalamic: 6 pts, thalamic: 5 pts (bilateral: 1 pt); brainstem/cerebellum: 7 pts [bilateral: 1pt]). Right-sided pain in 4 pts, left-sided in 5 pts, crossed symptoms in 2. Constant pain in 7 pts, intermittent pain in 4

Pain rating: VAS scale and Danish version of the McGill Pain Questionnaire (MPQ). Median VAS: 3.3 (range 0–7). Median pain severity (0–5 scale): when worst: 4 (range 2–5), when least: 1 (range: 0–3)

Sensory examination was carried out in the painful area, using the contralateral mirror area as reference. Results statistically evaluated

Sensibility			Sensory tests performed by means of
Tactile		Von Frey hairs (0.2–10 mg)	Mechanical sensory detection threshold ≥ 50% of stimuli perceived. Temporal summation to brush (allodynia): Von Frey hairs mounted on a rotating axis (0.16 and 1.5 Hz)
Thermal	Warmth Cold }	Thermotest (computerized version)*[†]	Cut-off limit: 52–10°C. Determination of warmth and cold detection thresholds from a baseline temperature of 30°C and 1°C/s rate of change
Pain	Heat Cold }	Thermotest (computerized version)	Determination of heat and cold pain detection thresholds from a baseline temperature of 30°C and 2°C/s rate of change
	"Pinprick"	Argon laser*	Brief argon laser stimuli over an area of 7 mm^2; 200 ms duration. Pain threshold defined as distinct pinprick sensation

* Sensory tests were carried out at the maximum pain site which in all pts involved the thenar eminence. Sensation was graded as: normal, increased or decreased with respect to the non-affected contralateral thenar eminence. Argon laser stimuli were also delivered at the thenar eminence.

[†] Warmth and cold detection thresholds examined in both hands before determination of heat and cold pain detection thresholds. Random examination sequence. Thresholds calculated as the mean of 8 determinations. Subjects with severe sensory loss: cut-off limits values included in calculation if <50% of stimulations reached the cut-off limits; otherwise cut-off limit used as threshold. Determination of pain-free sensitivity range: by means of calculated warm and cold sensibility indexes. Qualitative sensation (from "cold pain" to "heat pain") and presence of cold allodynia also evaluated.

Clinical sensibility examination			Normal	Hypesthesia	Hyperesthesia
			% of pts		
Touch			0	100	0
	Allodynia				
	Not present	Present			
	45.4	54.6			
Temperature	20°C		0	54.5	45.5
	40°C		0	80	20
	Cold allodynia				
	Not present	Present			
	45.5	54.5			
Pinprick			0	80	20

(continued)

TABLE 2.12 *(continued)*

In one pt touch, 40°C temperature and pinprick not ratable (aphasia). If evoked dysesthesia is included, 88% of CPSP pts with somatosensory deficits had allodynia/dysesthesia to cold (but only 3% of non-CPSP pts with somatosensory deficits; see Andersen *et al.* [1995]).

Quantitative sensibility examination		Detection thresholds		
		% of pts		
		Affected > not affected	Not affected > affected	No difference
Touch[†]		45.4 (markedly only in 27.2)	27.2 (markedly only in 9.1)	27.2 (equal or almost equal in 54.5)
Temperature[‡]	Warm	100 (median values: 43.5 vs. 33.4°C)*	0	0
	Cold	90.9 (median values: 20.6 vs. 28.3°C)*	9.9	0
	Heat pain	90.9 (median values: 48.9 vs. 44.4°C)*	9.9	(almost equal in 36.3)
	Cold pain	45.4	18.2	36.3% (no threshold on either side above 10°C in 4 pts)
Pinprick[§]		54.5 (markedly only in 27.2)	(9.1)	36.3 (equal or almost equal in 72.3)

* Statistically significant difference.

† No tactile sensation in 2 pts. Pain aggravation from rotating Von Frey hairs (allodynia) only in 1 pt.

‡ Warm detection threshold was higher in the pain area in 100% of cases, and all pts except 1 had increased cold detection threshold. Warm sensibility index was lower on the affected side in all pts. Cold sensibility index was lower on the affected side in 73% of cases, higher in 9% and identical in 18%. The qualitative experience of temperature stimuli (10–45°C) showed marked individual differences.

§ No correlation between pain detection threshold and VAS.

Sensibility change affected the hemibody in 8/11 pts; in 3 was smaller. In 8 pts the pain area was smaller than the area of changed sensibility, whereas in 3 the areas of changed sensibility and pain were identical. Thus 100% of pts had pain in the body part with sensory abnormalities. 78% of pts showed abnormal evoked sensations with temperature stimuli in the 10–45°C range (from altered to paradoxical sensations: cold stimuli evoked painful heat sensations but never vice versa, see original Fig. 4)

An increased threshold to warm and cold detection is a consistent feature in this study. An abnormal mechanical detection threshold is a less consistent feature. There is a discordance between clinical examination results for touch and pain (100% of pts with changed sensibility) and qualitative examination (altered thresholds in 36 and 27% respectively). Sharp needle and laser stimuli could engage different central neurons. Damage to the spino-thalamo-cortical pathway is a necessary condition in CPSP

Andersen *et al.* (1995): Brain strokes

Examination of sensibility in 207 stroke pts surviving 6 mos or longer and able to communicate

Sensory examination:
touch: cotton wool
temperature: metal roller, 20 or 40°C
pinprick

Sensibility to touch, temperature and pinprick evaluated in the face, forearm, hand, lower leg and foot. Contralateral side as control. Sensation graded as normal increased or decreased with respect to the non-affected side. Somatosensory deficits found in 87 pts (42%)

Sensory examination in 71 pts with somatosensory deficits without pain and 16 pts with CPSP

Sensibility	Normal	Decreased	Increased	Allodynia	Dysesthesia	Allodynia and/or dysesthesia	Not ratable
Touch							
No CPSP	5	65	1	0	0	0	0
CPSP	2	12	1	9 (56%)*	8 (50%)*	12 (75%)*	1*
Temperature							
20°C							
No CPSP	28 (39%)	37	6 (8%)	0	2 (3%)	2 (3%)	0
CPSP	1 (6%)*	8	7 (44%)*	9 (56%)*	12 (75%)*	14 (88%)*	0
40°C							
No CPSP	30 (42%)	38 (54%)	3	0	0	0	0
CPSP	1 (6%)*	13 (81%)*	1	0	0	0	1*
Pinprick							
No CPSP	2	67 (94%)	2 (5%)	0	0	0	0
CPSP	1	11 (69%)*	3 (19%)*	-	-	-	1*

* Statistically significant difference between no CPSP pts and CPSP pts.

No differences with pts without sensory deficits for age, sex, disposing disease or history of previous stroke, bar more acute onset extremity paresis and more disability.

Bowsher (1996), Bowsher et al. (1998): Brain strokes (These papers suffer from severe limitations in clarity of data reporting)

105 CPSP pts (92 post CVA; 13 post SAH). No clinically evident sensory deficit in 1 pt. Area of sensory impairment > painful area. Greatest impairment in the region of greatest pain. Thermal and pinprick impairment > tactile impairment. The change in large fiber sensations was the same in areas of maximal and minimal pain. Changes in pinprick and thermal sensations were less in areas of minimal pain

Sensory deficits on clinical examination

	% of 105 pts				
	Global	Alone	+ Tactile	+ Pinprick	+ Thermal
Tactile	53.3	1.9	-	8.6	7.6
Pinprick	80.9	6.7	8.6	-	30.4
Thermal	79	8.6	7.6	30.4	-
Tactile + pinprick + thermal		35.2			
Thermal + pinprick	67.6	30.4			
Thermal and/or pinprick	97.1				

Quantitative sensory tests in CVA-SAH pts (mirror two sides)

	Perception thresholds		
	Affected = non-affected	Affected < non-affected	Affected > non-affected
Tactile	10	4	
2-point discrimination	4		
Pinprick	2	5	
Pinch	4	8	
Warm	2	6	
Cold	2		4
Hot pain	2	6	
Skin temperature	4	9	

(continued)

TABLE 2.12 *(continued)*

Statistically significant difference between median values for areas of maximum and minimum pain in comparison with their mirror areas for all tested modalities except vibration. However only pinprick, warm and cold deficits reached a significant difference between areas of maximal and minimal pain.

Brainstem lesions vs. supratentorial lesions: significant differences only for warm and hot pain thresholds.

73 CPSP pts. 6 pure sensory strokes. Correlation of MRI findings with sensory abnormalities

Differences in sensory perception: Allodynic pts

	Perception threshold differences		
	Allodynic CPSP pts (mechanical allodynia)	Allodynic CPSP pts (thermal allodynia)	Non-allodynic CPSP pts
Allodynic CPSP pts (mechanical allodynia)	–	NS	NS
Allodynic CPSP pts (thermal allodynia)	NS	–	NS*
Non-allodynic CPSP pts	NS	NS*	–
Pain-free control stroke subjects	NS	Perception threshold significantly higher in allodynic CPSP pts (with the exception for hot pain)	Perception threshold significantly higher in non-allodynic CPSP pts for: sharpness, warmth and cold

* Only difference between allodynic CPSP pts and non-allodynic CPSP pts: greater deficit for warmth ($p = 0.05$). NS: not significant.

Sensory perception thresholds were measured in the maximally painful areas and their contralateral mirror areas in CPSP pts with supratentorial lesions (including the Vc) and infratentorial lesion and in stroke pts without CP (controls)

Statistical analysis of threshold difference between maximally affected region and its contralateral mirror area

Sensibility	Vc vs. controls	Brainstem vs. controls	VPL vs. brainstem
Tactile (Von Frey hairs)	NS	NS	NS
Pinprick (weighted needles)	Vc > controls	Brainstem > controls	NS
Warm (Thermotest)	NS	Brainstem > controls	Brainstem > Vc
Cold (Thermotest)	Vc > controls	Brainstem > controls	NS
Hot pain (Thermotest)	NS	Brainstem > controls	NS (brainstem > Vc, $p = 0.05$)

Statistical analysis of threshold differences between maximally affected region and its contralateral unaffected mirror area

Sensibility	Tactile (Von Frey hairs)	Pinprick (weighted needles)	Warm (Thermotest)	Cold (Thermotest)	Hot pain (Thermotest)
Vc vs. controls	NS	Vc > controls	NS	Vc > controls	NS
Brainstem vs. controls	NS	Brainstem > controls	Brainstem > controls	Brainstem > controls	Brainstem > controls
Vc vs. brainstem	NS	NS	Brainstem > Vc	NS	NS (brainstem > Vc, $p = 0.05$)
Burning pain vs. non-burning pain vs. controls	NS	Burning pain > controls	Burning pain > non-burning pain (=controls)	Burning pain > non-burning pain (=controls)	NS
Tactile allodynia vs. no allodynia	NS	NS	NS	NS	NS

Wallenberg's syndrome. Thresholds:

raised to a greater extent in the pts whose pain was principally burning than in those in whom it was principally non-burning

significant elevations of threshold for touch, sharpness, warm (but not for cold or for hot pain) between brainstem CP and painless stroke pts

The touch threshold was the only one that differed significantly between brainstem CP and Vc CP, being affected much more by Vc lesions

Kim and Choi-Kwon (1996): Brain strokes

67 consecutive pts with acute unilateral stroke. Routine neurologic examination included conventional sensory test

Sensory impairment (decreased sensibility)	Stroke location			
	Cortico-subcortical, 14 pts*	Lenticulocapsular, 24 pts	Thalamic or thalamocapsular, 15 pts[†]	Brainstem, 14 pts[‡]
Spinothalamic modalities (pinprick, temperature)	5 (50%)	7 (29%)	13 (87%)	9 (64%)
Vibration	3 (30%)	7 (29%)	11 (73%)	4 (29%)
Tactile sensibility	4 (40%)	7 (29%)	12 (80%)	3 (21%)

* 4 pts not evaluated; decreased spinothalamic modalities + vibration + tactile: 3 pts; decreased spinothalamic modalities + tactile: 1 pt.

[†] Decreased spinothalamic modalities + vibration + tactile: 10 pts; decreased spinothalamic modalities + tactile: 2 pt; decreased spinothalamic modalities + vibration: 1 pt.

[‡] Decreased spinothalamic modalities + vibration + tactile: 3 pts; decreased spinothalamic modalities + vibration: 1 pt.
LMI pts had selective sensory impairment of the spinothalamic modalities.

Chung et al. (1996): Thalamus

175 consecutive pts with thalamic hemorrhage. Analysis of neurological findings in pts with 5 different types of hematoma

Lesion site	No. of pts	Sensory features (% of pts)		
		Thalamic syndrome	Hypesthesia	Paresthesia at onset
Anterior	11	0	0	0
Posteromedial*	24	0	33	25
Posterolateral[†]	77	21	65	32
Dorsal[‡]	32	34	72	25
Global[§]	31	0	55	0

* Hematomas often ruptured into the 3rd ventricle and extended to mesencephalon (extension associated with worst prognosis). Sensory manifestation uncommon. High fatality (54%).

[†] Most frequent type (44% of cases). Large hematomas were often rupturing into the lateral ventricle and frequently extending into the posterior limb of the IC. Marked sensorimotor signs. Case fatality 35%, permanent neurologic sequelae frequently resulted.

[‡] Frequent posterolateral extension into the adjacent subcortical white matter. Sensorimotor symptoms were common.

[§] Clinically and radiologically similar to posterolateral type but very large size. Severe sensorimotor signs almost always present.

Casey et al. (1996): Brain sites

Study on laser-evoked cerebral potentials (LEPs) and sensory function in CP pts. 20 outpts selected. Lesion localization clinically and radiologically (MRI, CT) identified. Reproducible LEPs in 11 subjects (55% of the original population). 7 men, 4 women. Mean age 67 yrs (range 51–82)

Site of the lesion:
cortex: 3 pts (27%)
thalamus: 2 pts (18%)
brainstem: 6 pts (55%)

Mean duration of the lesion: 58 mos. CP referred to body parts neurologically affected by CNS infarction and rated on a VAS (0–10). Average VAS rating: 6.9. No analgesic allowed during the test period.

Neurologic examination:
Infrared CO_2 laser stimulation over the dorsum of the hand, in all pts. Beam diameter 9 mm (64 mm^2)
Side-to-side comparison. Laser pulse rating: 0: no sensation, 1: warm sensation, 2: pricking pain, 3: pricking pain followed by burning

(continued)

TABLE 2.12 *(continued)*

Median nerve routine SEPs (in 8 pts)

Thresholds for warmth and thermal pain, tested using a contact thermode. Stimuli delivered randomly to the volar surface of the forearm. Baseline 30°C. 8 different discrete intensities (from 33 to 52°C), of 5 s duration

Deep pain threshold, evaluated by means of a pressure algometer (0.5 cm in diameter) applied to the first metacarpal of each hand (volar aspect, 1st interosseous space)

Side-to-side differences considered abnormal if exceeding 3SD from the mean for normal subjects

Normative data: warmth threshold: 33.3 ± 3.3°C, heat pain threshold: 48.3 ± 1.6°C, deep pain: 2.8 ± 0.8 kg

Side-to-side differences in warm, heat pain and deep pain thresholds and perceived intensity of laser pulse perception

| | Greater thresholds for | | | Reduced laser pulse perception |
	Warmth	Heat pain	Deep pain	
Affected side	11/11 (100%)	5/11 (45%)	5/11 (45%)	7/11 (64%)
Unaffected side	0/11	6/11 (55%)	5/11 (45%)	4/11 (36%)
No difference			1/11 (9%)	

| | Side | | | | | | | |
	Affected	Unaffected	Affected	Unaffected	Affected	Unaffected	Affected	Unaffected
Symmetrical LEPs (5 pts)*	5/5 (100%)	0/5	1/5 (20%)	4/5 (80%)	2/5 (40%)	3/5 (60%)	2/5 (40%)	3/5 (60%)
Asymmetrical LEPs (6 pts)†	6/6 (100%)	0/6	4/6 (67%)	2/6 (33%)	3/6 (50%)	3/6 (50%)	5/6 (83%)	1/6 (17%)‡

| | Pts with 3 or more SD from the normal right–left differences | | | | | | | |
	Affected	Unaffected	Affected	Unaffected	Affected	Unaffected	Affected	Unaffected
Symmetrical LEPs	1/5 (20%)	0	1/5 (20%)	0	0	0	0	3/5 (60%)
Asymmetrical LEPs	3/6 (50%)	0	0 (2 pts = 3)	0	0	0	5/6 (83%)	1/6 (17%)

* LEPs amplitudes < 3 SD of that evoked from the unaffected side.

† LEPs amplitudes > 3 SD of that evoked from the unaffected side.

‡ Increased sensitivity to laser stimulation on the pathological side.

All pts had normal tactile and kinesthesic sensation bilaterally; one had slightly reduced vibratory sense bilaterally

Six pts (54%) had abnormal thermal and deep pain sensory function as determined by QST or LEPs. Including pinprick, 9/11 pts had somatosensory abnormalities. Five pts had LEPs amplitudes < 3 SD of that evoked from the unaffected side; all but 1 had symmetrical warm, heat and deep pain thresholds. The remaining pts had elevated warm and thermal pain thresholds and an increased laser sensory rating on the pathological side and slighty reduced LEPs on the abnormal side. Three pts had increased laser pulse sensitivity on the affected side, 2 hypoalgesia and 1 hyperalgesia to pinprick. Six pts had LEPs amplitudes > 3 SD and showed significant elevations of warmth, deep or thermal pain thresholds and/or reduced laser sensory ratings on the affected side. Laser stimulation on the affected side failed to evoke either N or P potential in these 6 pts. Seven pts had increased warm, heat and deep pain thresholds or reduced laser sensory ratings on the affected side and had more frequently asymmetrical LEPs. Pts with asymmetrical LEPs showed a higher proportion of pinprick hypoalgesia compared to those with symmetrical LEPs. (83% vs. 40%) LEPs sensory ratings were reduced on the affected side in 5 pts, but 4 pts reported greater sensory ratings on the affected side. No pt had significant higher LEP amplitude following stimulation of the affected side. One pt with increased sensibility to laser stimulation had decreased LEPs (see Wu *et al.* 1999)

Authors' conclusion: Pts with reduced LEPs had homolateral elevated heat pain and warmth thresholds and reduced laser sensory ratings when compared with the unaffected side. The observation that some pts reported greater laser sensory ratings on the affected side suggests that some of the CNS lesions associated with CP may produce heat hyperalgesia revealed exclusively by infrared laser stimulation. Reduced LEPs amplitude was related only to a loss of pain and temperature sensation.

Nasreddine and Saver (1997): Thalamus

Somatosensory deficits in 180 thalamic stroke pts from the literature:
in at least one modality: 85% of pts
no sensory deficit across all modalities in 15 pts

Clinical sensory impairment is not a necessary condition for the development of spontaneous pain

Impairment of sensory modalities (% of pts):
temperature: 59% (51/86)
light touch: 68% (81/120)
painful pinprick: 63% (47/75)
position: 58% (55/95)
vibration: 47% (45/95).

Different sensory modalities impaired with approximately equal frequency across the population; there was no right/left predominance of sensory impairments

Kim and Bae (1997): Brainstem

Pure or predominant sensory stroke due to MRI or CT confirmed brainstem lesion. 17 pts. Lesions: paramedian dorsal pontine: 15 pts, dorsolateral pons: 1 pt, lateral midbrain: 1 pt. Follow-up: 1 mo–3 yrs

Paresthesia (numbness or tingling sensation) starting at a part of the body (hand or foot) and then spreading to other parts (hemibody) initial and main complaint in all pts. Sensory symptoms (almost) completely resolved in 5 pts. Paresthesia usually persisted in the others. In 2 pts (12%) CPSP (follow-up: 18 mos, 3 yrs). 6 pts complained of bilateral perioral or facial symptoms, in 2 cases extending to hemibody. Hemibody involvement in 4 (+2) pts

Clinical features*	No. of pts (%)		
	Normal	Abnormal	Selective impairment
Paresthesia	0	17 (100%) (present)	
Spinothalamic sensation (pinprick, temperature)	13 (76%)	4 (24%)	1 (6%)[†]
Vibration sense	8 (47%)	9 (53%)	7 (41%) lemniscal sensation
Position sense	9 (53%)	8 (47%)	
Residual painful paresthesia	–	2[‡] (12%)	

* Equivocal absence of objective sensory deficits in 2 pts.

‡ Equivocal absence of objective sensory deficits in 1 pt. Normal spinothalamic sensation in both pts. Impaired lemniscal sensation in 1 pt.

† Pt with a somewhat laterally situated pontine lesion (without CP).

Authors' conclusion: Paresthesia is a sign suggestive of (medial) lemniscal sensory pathway, due to small lesions of the paramedian pontine area. Perioral bilateral symptoms suggest a trigeminal involvement.

MacGowan et al. (1997): Brainstem

Retrospective analysis of 63 pts with MRI-confirmed LMI (Wallenberg's syndrome). Clinical sensory deficit scored according to the degree of loss of sensation to pinprick and cold tuning fork (0 = no deficit, 1= reduced responses, 2 = no response). QST (thermal and pressure) in 19 pts (9 CPSP, 10 no CPSP), on standard areas (medial surface of the cheek, palmar surface of the first metacarpophalangeal joint, dorsal surface of the first metatarsophalangeal joint). Thermal stimuli sequence: 36, 40, 44, 48, 38, 42, 46, 50°C. Pressure stimuli: increments of 250 g/s of a plastic tip (1 cm in diameter), until pain was reported or limits were reached (2 kg on the face, 4 kg on the hand and foot)

Normative data:

Thermal thresholds (from 32 healthy controls): responses graded as: nothing, warm, hot (42 ± 4°C), very hot, faintly painful (46 ± 2.1°C), painful

Mean pressure pain thresholds (from 12 healthy controls): 1068 (±332) g on the cheek; 2045 (±590) g on the hand; 2100 (±693) on the feet

Data in agreement with previous reports

(continued)

TABLE 2.12 *(continued)*

Pts responses grading:

innocuous thermal threshold =

ELEVATED: thermal stimulus ≥ 46°C not reported as HOT

ABSENT: thermal stimulus ≥ 50°C not reported as HOT

noxious thermal threshold =

ELEVATED: thermal stimulus ≥ 48°C not reported as FAINTLY PAINFUL

ABSENT: thermal stimulus = 50°C not reported as PAINFUL

ALLODYNIA: thermal stimulus < 46°C reported as PAINFUL

pressure pain thresholds =

ELEVATED: pressure > 1500 g on the cheek and 3000 g on the hands and feet not reported as PAINFUL

ABSENT: pressure > 2000 g on the cheek and 4000 g on the hands and feet not reported as PAINFUL

All pts but 9 had sensory impairment. CPSP correlated significantly with the degree of clinical sensory loss (CPSP in 0/27 pts scored 0 or 1, 12/29 (41.4%) pts scored 2, 4/7 (57.1%) pts scored 3), but was not related with the infarct size

QST was performed in 19 pts (9 with CPSP, 10 without CPSP)

Quantitatively determined sensory threshold (LMI, 19 pts, contralateral cheek)

		Whole group	CPSP pts (n = 9)	No CPSP (n = 10)
Innocuous thermal threshold				
	Normal	11(57.8%)	8 (88.9%)	3 (30%)
	Impaired (elevated/ absent)	8 (42.1%)	1 (11.1%)	7 (70%)
Noxious thermal threshold				
	Normal	10 (52.6%)	8 (88.9%)	2 (20%)
	Impaired (elevated/ absent)	9 (47.3%)	1 (11.1%)	8 (80%)
Pressure pain thresholds				
	Normal	13 (68.4%)	9 (100%)	4 (40%)
	Impaired (elevated/ absent)	6 (31.6%)	0	6 (60%)
Innocuous thermal + noxious thermal + pressure pain thresholds all combined				
	Normal	8 (42.1%)	8 (88.9%)	0
	Impaired (elevated/ absent)	11 (57.9%)	1 (11.1%)	10 (100%)

The cheek contralateral to the infarct, a clinically silent area, had elevated or absent thresholds in all pts without CPSP, but had normal threshold in CPSP pts. The detection of normal contralateral cheek to both heat and pressure stimuli were 89% sensitive and 100% specific for the presence of CPSP. Abnormalities in the face contralateral to the infarct are referable to the crossed trigeminothalamic tract in the medullary reticular formation, medial to the infarcted lateral medulla. CP correlated with unilateral, but not bilateral thermosensory loss

Peyron *et al.* (1998): Brainstem

Lateral medullary infarct (Wallenberg's syndrome). 9 selected right-handed pts with unilateral CP. MRI detectable infarct in 8 pts, involving PICA in 2 cases

Isolated allodynia in 5/9 pts. Spontaneous pain and allodynia in 4 pts. Hyperpathia in 4 of the 5 allodynic pts. All pts were studied for pain and both lemniscal and extralemniscal sensory modalities. Reduced vibration sensation on the painful lower limb only in 1 pt. Normal SEPs in 5 out of 5 tested pts at the time of PET study (previous absent P14 in 1 pt, followed by complete recovery). Pain evaluated by means of a VAS (median: 4, range 2–5)

Distribution of hemisensory abnormalities	Number of pts				
	Patchy	UL	LL	H	HF
Thermal hypesthesia		1*	2[†]	4	2
Allodynia (cold, light touch)	1	2*	3[†]	2	1
Spontaneous pain			3		1

UL: upper limb; LL: lower limb; H: hemibody; HF: hemibody + face (crossed).

* Including trunk and part of the thigh.

[†] Including inferior abdomen in 1 case and face in another.

Clinical data

	Number of pts		
	Normal	Impaired	Not done
Lemniscal sensibility	8	1*	
SEPs	4	1[†]	4
	Absent	Present	Trigger*
Allodynia		9	C+T 5
			C+T+V 3
			C+T+H 2
Hyperpathia	5	4	Pr 4

* Hypopallesthesia (lower limb, site of pain).

[†] Initial P14 abolition (recovered).

C: cold, T: touch, V: vibration, H: hot; other allodynic stimuli: pressure, movement, pricking, electrical, radiation, burning (!), dorsal column stimulation burning, bruise (1 pt).

Pr: pricking; other hyperpathic stimuli: burning, electrical. Summation in 2/4 pts with pricking hyperpathia (!). In the same pt, allodynia severe or mild depending on area stimulated.

Kim (1998): Brain and brainstem

6 CPSP pts. Early-onset CPSP contralateral to the ischemic lesion (thalamus, lenticulocapsular area, brainstem) followed by delayed ipsilateral sensory symptoms with onset of mild ipsilateral pain mirroring the site of the most severe CPSP (without objective sensory deficits). No new ischemic lesions

Aggravating factors (both side):

movements, fatigue, cold water, cold or humid weather

Pain descriptors:

Burning: pts 1, 3, 4, 6

Aching: pt 1

Pressing: pts 2, 4

Squeezing: pts 2, 4, 5

Bursting: pt 5

Pricking: pt 6

Cold: pt 6

Paciaroni and Bogousslavsky (1998): Thalamus

Thalamic stroke. Pure sensory syndromes in 25 pts among 3628 included in the Lausanne Stroke Registry. Clinical symptoms strongly suggestive of pure thalamic sensory stroke with normal findings on CT or MRI scans in other 34 pts. Delayed pain and/or dysesthesias: 4/25 pts (16%)

Symptoms during the stroke:
pain and/or dysesthesias in 7/25 pts
contralateral paresthesia in 18/25

(continued)

TABLE 2.12 *(continued)*

Sensory dysfunction on clinical examination

	Clinical features		
Sensibility	Lost/impaired	Preserved	CPSP
Pinprick ⎫			
Thermal ⎬	24	1	4*
Tactile ⎭			
Vibratory	16	9	
Position	13	12	
Stereognosis/graphesthesia	12	13	

Numbness in 24 pts, complete anesthesia in 1 (without CP).

Pinprick, thermal and tactile loss consensual in 24 pts.

* Transient pain sensation in 4 other pts.

Kim and Choi-Kwon (1999): Brainstem

Medullary infarction. 55 consecutive pts (41 LMI, 14 MMI single first MRI confirmed infarctions). Comparison between long-term sensory sequelae of LMI and MMI. Mean follow-up 21 mos

Neurological examination: pinprick, temperature (cold tuning fork), vibration sense, position. Deficits categorized as mild (sensory perception >70%), moderate (sensory perception <70%, >30%), severe (sensory perception < 30%). Contralateral side as control. Trigeminal sensation compared with intact limb (possible bilateral impairment)

Nature and intensity of sensory symptoms assessed with a modified McGill–Melzak Pain Questionnaire and VAS

Sensory characteristics

		LMI		MMI
Sensory symptoms description		Face (%)	Body/limbs (%)	Body/limbs (%)
Burning		35	27	
Cold		22	38	10
Numbness		39	29	60
Squeezing				30
Sensory abnormalities				
	Acute stage§	61	79	83*
	Residual	56	83	71
Pattern of sensory abnormalities				
Crossed	Acute stage	39		
	Residual			
Contralateral trigeminal	Acute stage§	21		
	Residual	17		
Bilateral trigeminal	Acute stage§	12		
	Residual	2		
Ipsilateral trigeminal	Acute stage§			
	Residual	36		
Isolated hemibody/limb	Acute stage§	24		
	Residual	27†		
No abnormalities	Acute stage§	3		
	Residual			
Severity of sensory symptoms (burning, cold, squeezing, electrical)‡		VAS > 5	VAS > 5	VAS > 5
		35 (8/23)	29 (10/34)	40 (4/10)

* Decreased vibration or position sense in 80%, paresthesia 17%; mild spinothalamic impairment 17%.

† Symptoms restricted to regions below certain levels of trunk/leg in 9 pts (22%) or to arm/upper trunk in 2 pts (5%).

‡ Pts complaining only of "numbness/heaviness" excluded. Median VAS values: LMI: face: 3; body/limbs: 3. MMI: body/limbs: 5.

§ Acute stage: face: 23 LMI and 1 MMI pts, body/limbs: 34 LMI pts, 10 MMI pts.

Severity of residual sensory symptoms was significantly related to initial severity of objective sensory deficits. Most cited aggravating factors in LMI: cold environment > body movements > stress. Heat was reported as aggravating factor in 4 pts, rest in 2 pts

83% of LMI pts had body/limbs residual sensory symptoms (53% face): if "pain" defined as sensory symptoms more severe than grade 5 or 6, about one quarter would have qualified. Yet, majority of pts did not describe their symptoms (even if severe) as pain: thus, post-stroke paresthesia might be a more appropriate description for post-stroke sensory sequelae

Sensory symptoms most important residual sequelae in LMI pts and the second most important in MMI; the nature, the mode of onset and aggravating factors differ between the 2 groups, probably in relation to a selective involvement of the spinothalamic tract in the former and of the medial lemniscus in the latter

Kumral *et al.* (2001): Thalamus

16 consecutive pts with bilateral simultaneous MRI confirmed thalamic infarction. 1 CPSP pt with bilateral thalamo-geniculate infarction

Neurological examination

Impaired sensibility	No. of pts			
	Infarct territory			
	Thg (3 pts)	Pm (8 pts)	Pm + Thg (3 pts)	Po + Thg (2 pts)
Light touch	3Bi	3R, 1L, 4N	1R, 1N, 1Bi	2R
Pinprick	3Bi	1R, 2L, 5N	3R	1R, 1N
Proprioception	1R, 1Bi, 1N	1R, 7N	1R, 2N	2N
Vibration	2R, 1L	1R, 1L, 6N	2R, 1N	2N
CPSP	1L*			

Thg: thalamogeniculate; Pm: paramedian; Po: polar; R: right-sided, L: left-sided; Bi: bilateral; N: normal.

* Bilateral loss of tactile, pinprick and proprioceptive sensibility; vibration sense lost only over the left side.

Fitzek *et al.* (2001): Brainstem

Study (1 yr long) aimed at identifying clinical predictors and anatomical structures involved in pts with pain after dorso-lateral medullary infarction (MI). 5 lateral MI pts out of 58 pts with acute brainstem infarction plus 7 additional pts retrospectively identified. CPSP: 8/12 pts (67%). MRI identified lesions, principal trigeminal sensory nucleus intact

Clinical, MRI and QST findings

Pain site		Pts with pain			
		Ipsilateral face only (3 pts)	Ipsilateral face + contralateral limbs or trunk (3 pts)	Contralateral limbs or trunk only (2 pts)	Pts without pain (4 pts)
MRI evidence of partial	TST/N	3/3	3/3	1/2	4/4
or complete lesion of	STT	3/3	3/3	2/2	3/4
Acute neurological signs	TST/N affected	3/3[c]	1/3[b], 2/3[c]	1/2[a]	1/4[a], 2/4[b], 1/4[d]
	Non-affected	–	–	1/2[b]	–
	STT affected	3/3[c]	1/3[b], 2/3[c]	1/2[a]	1/3[a], 1/3[b], 1/3[d]
	Non-affected	–	–	1/2[b]	–
QST abnormal results	TST/N affected	3/3	3/3	0/2*	0/4*
	Non-affected	–	–	0/2	–
	STT affected	3/3	3/3	0/2*	0/3*
	Non-affected	–	–	–	0/1

(continued)

TABLE 2.12

Clinical, MRI and QST findings *(cont.)*

		Pts with pain		Pts without pain (4 pts)
		Pts with facial pain	Pts without facial pain	
Significantly raised thresholds (cheek ipsilateral to infarction) for	Touch	Yes		No
	Pain	Yes		No
	Cold	No (raised)		No
	Warm	No (raised)		No
	Cold pain	Yes		No
	Warm pain	Yes		No
Stimulus-response functions for pricking pain		Shifted downward		

* Sensory deficit resolved at time of QST.

a: ipsilateral impairment of facial pain and/or temperature sensation. b: contralateral impairment of pain and temperature sensation over trunk and limbs. c: a + b. d: no acute sensory signs of interest.

TST/N affected: lower or upper lesion.

TST/N: trigeminal spinal tract and/or nucleus; STT: spinothalamic tract.

Lesions comparison in pts facial pain (6) vs. pts without facial pain (6):

TST/N, Lower medulla: 5/6 vs. 1/6 ($p < 0.05$? More probably 0.316, Fisher exact test, NS)

TST/N, Upper medulla: 5/6 vs. 3/6

STT: 6/6

Pts with STT lesion and pain: 8/8

Authors' conclusion: Significant correlation between ipsilateral facial pain and (extent of) lower medullary lesions (including lesions of the spinal trigeminal tract and/or nucleus). None of the lesions involved the subnucleus caudalis, which contains most nociceptive neurons. Chronic facial pain in Wallenberg's syndrome is due to a peripheral type of lesion within the CNS.

Note: Authors' conclusions could be statistically flawed

Garcia-Larrea *et al.* (2002): Multiple levels, multiple types of lesions

Laser-evoked cortical potentials (LEPs) in CP pts. 64 consecutive pts (1997–2000). 42 CP pts (CNS lesion confirmed by clinical and imaging data). Other 10 pts eliminated for technical reasons or incomplete data. 12 pts with lateralized pain of non-organic origin (negative clinical and radiological study). Pain duration > 6 mos in both groups

Clinical assessment of somatosensory deficit

Sensibility tested	Standard clinical methods	Notes
2-point discrimination	Blunted needles	
Tactile hypoesthesia	Cotton balls	
Joint position sense	Movement of finger and toes, "searching hand"	
Graphesthesia ⎫ Stereognosis ⎭		Not systematically assessed
Thermal hypoesthesia	Hot/cold tubes; laser pulses of ascending/descending intensity	QST of hot/warm/cold thresholds performed in about 2/3 of cases
Abnormally provoked pain		Tested systematically
Static allodynia	Touch	
Dynamic allodynia	Rubbing the skin	
Hyperalgesia	Pinprick; supraliminal laser stimulation	Hyperalgesia to laser in 7 pts
Summation hyperpathia	Repeated stimulation	Temporal summation

Homologous normal territory as control

Results: On clinical examination all CP pts had decreased pain and temperature sensation over the affected area

Clinical examination

	Lesion site				
	Spinal	Brainstem	Thalamocortical	Total	
Spontaneous pain only	7/12 (58%)	4/10 (40%)	6/20 (30%)	17 (40.5%)	
Spontaneous pain + painful provoked dysesthesias (allodynia/hyperalgesia)	5/12 (42%)	6/10 (60%)	14/20 (70%)	25 (59.5%)	
Laser allodynia			1/20 (5%)	1 (2%)	7 (17%)
Laser hyperalgesia	1/12 (8%)	2/10 (20%)	2/20 (10%)	5 (12%)	
Laser summation hyperpathia			1/20 (5%)	1 (2%)	

Statistically significant difference in LEP amplitude and delay between affected and non-affected side

	Attenuated LEP	
	Baseline to peak	Peak to peak
Pts with spontaneous pain only*	Yes	Yes
Pts with spontaneous pain + painful provoked dysesthesias (allodynia/hyperalgesia)	Yes	Yes
Pts with pseudocentral non-organic pain	No	No

* LEPs were significantly more attenuated in this group of pts than in pts with allodynia/hyperesthesia, even after elimination of pts with laser induced hyperalgesia.

Statistically significant LEP enhancement between CP pts with hyperalgesia to CO_2 laser stimuli and non-organic pts

	Enhanced LEP	
	Baseline to peak	Peak to peak
Pts with spontaneous pain + painful provoked dysesthesias (allodynia/hyperalgesia)*	No	No
Pts with pseudocentral non-organic pain	No	Yes

* Occasionally (4/7 cases) ultra-late responses (>700 ms) to stimulation of the painful side in allodynic pts, with report of dull, painful, strongly unpleasant and poorly localized feeling.

LEPs were significantly attenuated after stimulation over the painful territory in pts with decreased pain/heat sensation and in pts with allodynia or hyperalgesia to laser pulses. Truly neuropathic hyperalgesia or allodynia were never associated to enhanced LEPs. In CP pts with exclusively spontaneous pain, LEPs attenuation was more pronounced than in pts with allodynia and hyperalgesia. Occasional ultra-late responses in allodynic pts (>700 msec) might reflect activation of a slow conducting medial pain system. Six non-organic pts described "hyperalgesia," always very well localized and rapidly disappearing. LEPs were never attenuated (but could be enhanced) in pts with non-organic pain. Enhanced LEPs were associated with hyperalgesia to laser stimuli only in non-organic pts

LEP attenuation was rather independent of the actual pain sensation triggered by the stimulus. In neuropathic cases, partial LEPs preservation might increase the probability of developing allodynia/hyperalgesia. The possible predictive value of this phenomenon remains to be demonstrated

Jensen _et al._ (2002): Brain

28 CP pts. QST. Spontaneous pain VAS: 6.4 (±1.9), evoked pain VAS: 4.1 (± 3.2)

Cold detection threshold and heat pain threshold respectively reduced and increased in all pts on the painful side vs. the normal one in all

Cold pain threshold, heat detection threshold and mechanical threshold did not differ between the two sides

No correlation found between spontaneous pain and cold detection or cold pain threshold

Weimar _et al._ (2002): Brain

119 post-stroke pts. 11 CPSP pts. Hemorrhagic stroke in 36% of CPSP pts vs. 8% of pts without CPSP

Higher incidence of CPSP in pts with hemorrhagic stroke, but mild pain in 3/4 pts

(continued)

TABLE 2.12 *(continued)*

1 pt with left MCA infarct reported recurrent pain in the right extremities from recurrent focal seizures (pain relief from effective antiepileptic treatment)

Pain site:

Hemibody: 1 pt (face spared)

Hemibody (patchy): 3 pts

Arm only: 1 pt

Leg only (foot): 1 pt

Arm + leg (torso spared): 5 pts

Willoch *et al.* (2004): Brain

PET study on changes in opioid receptor binding in CNS pain-processing structures

5 CPSP pts (3 ischemic 1 hemorrhagic strokes, 1 postoperative hemorrhage). Site of the lesion: 3 thalamocortical, 1 parietal, 1 midbrain lesions. All pts right-handed. Pain side/distribution: 3 pts: L hemibody (in 1 pt face spared), 2 pts: R hemibody

Pain quality:

Tormenting, dull and pulling, burning, squeezing and pressing, lacerating and burning, deep, dull, pressing and throbbing, pricking and lacerating

Temporal pattern:

Pt 1: continuous, fluctuating

Pt 2: initially fluctuating, then constant

Pt 3: continuous, almost absent at rest

Pt 4, 5: continuous

Aggravating factors (2/5 pts): movements and touch

Pain intensity (VAS): from 4 to 8/10 (mean: 5)

Neurological examination:

Hypesthesia: 1/5 pts

Hypalgesia: 4/5 pts

Dysesthesia: 4/5 pts

Paresthesia: 1/5 pts

Allodynia: 4/5 pts

Position sense impairment: 2/5 pts

Movement impairment/disorders: 5/5 pts

Cognitive impairment: 2/5 pts

Kong *et al.* (2004): Brain

Cross-sectional survey on the prevalence of chronic pain and the effect of pain on quality of life (QOL) 6 mos or more after a radiologically confirmed stroke. 107 pts out of 475 pts attending the outpatient clinic of a rehabilitation center, without significant cognitive and/or language deficits. Sensory impairment in 61 pts (57%). 13 CPSP (12%)

Comparison between 32 pts with musculoskeletal pain (MSP) and 13 pts with CPSP:

Months after stroke: MSP 15.5 CPSP 17.0 (difference not statistically significant, NS)

Sensory impairment: MSP 13/32 (41%) CPSP 11/13 (85%)

Pain on the average: MSP 3.3 CPSP 4.0 (NS)

Relief of pain by pain treatments (%): MSP 43.5 CPSP 42.5 (NS)

Interference with enjoyment of life: NS

Pain was more common in pts with a shorter post-stroke duration, but was not related to the nature of stroke (infarct or bleed), age, gender, presence of depression, and Modified Barthel Index score

Pts with CPSP show more sensory impairments, higher pain scores of the Brief Pain Inventory and lower scores on the vitality domain of the SF-36 than pts with MSP

Authors' conclusion: Pain is common in chronic stroke pts, and it does not appear to have a significant effect on pts' QOL (confirming Andersen *et al.*'s conclusion that CPSP had no significant effect on pt mood or participation in social activities)

Bowsher *et al.* (2004): Brain

2 CPSP pts out of 4 with small restricted cerebral cortical infarcts, sparing in all case SI (postcentral gyrus)

CPSP pts' findings (affected areas): mild spontaneous pain: absence of sharpness (pinprick) perception, impairment of warmth, cold, and heat pain perception

No CPSP pts' findings: absence of spontaneous pain, unimpaired sharpness (pinprick) perception, unimpaired warmth, cold, and heat pain perception

Perception of mechanical (skinfold pinch) pain: absent in all cases

Greater warm–cold difference in the affected regions in all subjects

Widar *et al.* (2004): Brain

Qualitative study aimed at describing pain, coping strategies, and experienced outcome of coping with long-term pain conditions after a stroke. Pt selection: people with cerebral infarct or hemorrhage (without other pain conditions or significant language deficits) registered in an inpatient register at a neurological clinic in a university hospital in Sweden. 356 people contacted, 65 non-responders, 245 no pain or other pain conditions

43/46 pts (3 drop-out) with CPSP, plus 28 non CPSP pts (nociceptive or tension-type headache)

Average pain duration: 20 mos

CPSP description:
Pain site:

entire hemibody, or arm, leg, or just hand or foot

Temporal qualities:

continuous or at least for a few hours daily

Pain qualities:

burning, cutting, dull, and/or numbness

Pain occurrence in connection with certain physical motions or static body positions, active or passive touch (including from temperate water), cold or windy conditions.

Pain-related problems:

incomprehensibility regarding pain cause, evolution and treatment, disturbed sleep, fatigue, diminished capacity in daily life, mood changes (depression, disheartening pain, irascibility), stress in relationships with family members.

Coping strategies:

Making the pain comprehensible (most common), efforts to avoid and to relieve pain (planning of activities, avoiding stressful activities or movements or events, changing body position, making physical exercise [avoiding overexertion]), taking or discontinuing (avoiding side effects for ineffective treatments) medications, communicating about pain, making comparisons (or imaging a worst scenario), distractions (leisure activities), enduring the pain or acceptance

Results of coping strategies:

Changing body position, making comparison, and enduring the pain were common in central or nociceptive pain, rest and relaxation in tension-type headache. Communicating pain give a feeling of perplexity and resignation. Consideration shown by others gave a feeling of satisfaction

(continued)

TABLE 2.12 *(continued)*

Greenspan *et al.* (2004): Brain strokes

Quantitative sensory testing in 13 consecutive pts (10 men, 3 women) with CPSP. MRI-confirmed CNS lesions

Clinical characteristics

Pain location	No. of pts				
	HE	HE-H	UE+LE	LE	PA
	2	3	4	1	3
VAS	≤5	6-7	8-9	10	Mean
	3	3	5	2	7.1 (2.0 SD)

HE-H: hemibody; HE: hemibody, sparing head; UE: upper extremity; LE: lower extremity;
PA: patchy. No statistically significant difference for pain and detection thresholds among pts grouped by
age, sex, side.

Psychophysical tests: thresholds assessed

innocuous warm and cold (contact Peltier stimulator, 7 cm^2 or 9 cm^2)

heat pain and cold pain (contact Peltier stimulator, 7 cm^2 or 9 cm^2, baseline temperature 35°C (heat) or 30°C (cold).
  Limits: 0–50°C)

tactile (Semmes–Wienstein monofilaments, dorsum of the hand or of the feet)

brushing allodynia (manual test, stiff brush)

Evaluation of thermal sensitivity: criterion of abnormal thresholds = mean ± 2 SD outside normative range. Thresholds as median values. Evaluation of laterality differences: normative data. In interpreting results of quantitative thermal sensory testing the side-to-side differences were considered more reliable, and a side-to-side difference greater than the 95% CI in the direction of decreased sensitivity on the affected side was interpreted as hypoesthsia. If the side-to-side differences were not significant, then the results were evaluated in terms of the absolute threshold. Statistical assessment of the results both within populations and individual pts

Sensory characteristics	No. of pts	Reduced	Normal	Hypoalgesia, hypoesthesia	Allodynia	Indeterminate[a]	Present	Absent
Cold threshold	13	11* (85%)	2 (15%)					
Cold pain threshold	13		2 (15%)	6 (46%)	3 (24%)[†]	2 (15%)		
Warm threshold	13	12‡ (92%)	1 (8%)					
Hot pain threshold	13		10 (77%)	1 (8%)	(2 borderline)	2 (15%)		
Non-painful tactile threshold	10§		5 (50%)	5 (50%)		3 (not tested)		
Tactile allodynia (brushing)	13						7 (54%)	6 (46%)¶

a: Side-to-side differences not significant and affected or unaffected threshold indeterminate at the greatest stimulus magnitude. Impossible to determine if the affected side was normal, hypo- or hyperalgesic

* Bilateral cold hypoesthesia with no laterality difference in 3 pts. Ipsilateral cold hypoesthesia (<<contralateral) in 3 other pts, with significant laterality difference.

† The most dramatic example of cold allodynia occurred in 1 of the 2 pts with normal cold detection threshold. The other 2 cases occurred in 2 pts with bilateral cold hypoesthesia with unilateral strokes contralateral to their allodynia and ongoing pain and the highest cold thresholds among pts with cold hyopesthesia.

‡ Bilateral warm hypoesthesia with no laterality difference in 2 pts (also with cold hypoesthesia). Ipsilateral warm hypoesthesia (<<contralateral) in 6 other pts, with significant laterality difference.

§ Ongoing pain rating not different between pts with normal tactile threshold and hypoesthesia.

¶ Brushes non-painful, monofilaments irritating in 1 pt. No difference by side or age. Higher incidence in men (not significant) and in pts with normal tactile thresholds vs. tactile hypoesthesia (5/5 vs. 1/5, $p < 0.05$).

Tactile allodynia occurred more in cases with spared tactile pathways. Thermal, mechanical and paresthetic descriptors of ongoing pain and pain rating did not differ between pts with normal and reduced tactile sensibility. The presence of tactile hypoesthesia did not correlate with the degree or quality of ongoing pain. All pts with insular lesions had tactile allodynia, but the incidence was not different from that occurring in other lesions

Cold allodynia: cold allodynia in 2/11 pts (or 0/8 pts). Cold allodynia is significantly related to the *absence* of cold hypoesthesia; cold hypoesthesia is neither necessary nor sufficient for cold allodynia. Despite the large prevalence of cold hypoesthesia in CP pts, cold allodynia is relatively an infrequent event. After statistical analysis it is also concluded that pts with cold hypoesthesia can have burning or hot or cold ongoing pain, but not necessarily. Two pts with insular lesions (50%) had cold allodynia, but the incidence was not different from that occurring in other lesions. The insular lesions however did not extend fully to the suggested cortical termination of VMpo (dorsal margin of the insula or adjacent parietal operculum)

Warm and heat pain: QST revealed predominantly warm hypoesthesia and normal heat pain sensibility. Two pts showed border line allodynia. Data do not fit the disinhibition hypothesis

Tactile hypesthesia: 50% of pts. Normal: 50% of pts. Tactile allodynia: to brushing: 54% of pts, to Von Frey hairs: 8%

Men showed a trend toward a higher incidence of brush allodynia. Tactile allodynia occurred significantly more often in cases with spared tactile pathways than those with normal tactile thresholds. Severity of pain was the same in both tactile normal and deficient groups

The presence of tactile hypesthesia did not correlate with the degree or quality of ongoing pain

Cold hypesthesia: in 85% of CPSP pts, some bilateral (either similar on both sides or with side prevalence)

Djaldetti *et al.* (2004): Parkinson's disease

36 pts with predominantly unilateral Parkinson's disease (PD), 15 PD pts with response fluctuations, 28 age-matched healthy control subjects

21 pts (8 women and 13 men) with hemi-PD and endogenous pain (initial symptom of the disease in 6 pts)

Pain variability by time of day, duration, and location

Pain quality: burning, itching, or tearing

Pain site: usually localized to the more affected side (difficult to pinpoint in some pts)

Mean VAS score: 48.9 ± 24.1 mm

Subjective pain assessment: VAS, Von Frey filaments (tactile thresholds), contact thermode for warm sensation (WS) and heat pain thresholds (HPTs)

	Pain side predominance			Symptoms side predominance
	Predominantly left-sided hemi-PD pts (15/21 pts)	Predominantly right-sided hemi-PD pts (6/21 pts)	PD pts with fluctuations (15 pts)	Hemi-PD pts without pain (15 pts)
Left	6	1	11	3
Right	1	1	4	12
Bilateral	8	4	Painful sensations (mostly bilateral) in 12 pts	
Mean VAS score (mm)	51.5 ± 25.8	46.6 ± 27.3	55.7 ± 21.43 mm	
Quantitative assessment of pain perception				
Tactile threshold	No difference between pts in both pt groups and control subjects nor between sides			
WS threshold	No difference between pts in both pt groups and control subjects nor between sides		No side differences between "on" and "off" periods	
HPTs	$42.6 \pm 3.0°C$		No side differences between "on" and "off" periods	$45.6 \pm 2.8°C$ ($p < 0.01$)
	PD pts with pain in the more affected side $41.4 \pm 2.6°C$	PD pts without pain in the more affected side $43.7 \pm 3.3°C$ ($p < 0.0001$)		

(continued)

TABLE 2.12 *(continued)*

The severity of subjective pain and HPTs on the affected side was correlated only with disease duration

Authors' conclusion: HPTs were lower in the PD pts compared with control subjects and lower in the PD pts with pain than without pain. In the pts with unilateral PD, HPTs were significantly lower on the more affected side compared with the less affected side. As endogenous pain in PD pts is accompanied by increased sensitivity to some painful stimuli, basal ganglia abnormality may involve pain encoding.

Bowsher (2005): Brain

9 CP pts (7 CPSP, 2 SCI) out of 34 pain pts. Study on dynamic mechanical allodynia in NP

Effects of repetitive stimulation at 3 Hz with a camel-hair paintbrush; refractory period tested by repetitive stimulation (intervals from 3 to 0.3 Hz).

Pain intensity evaluated by a VAS scale at the end of every stimulation period

Results:

(A) "Windup" in CP pts: <2/10 VAS points increase on repetitive stimulation in 2/7 CPSP and 1/2 SCI pts (not clinically significant in any case)

(B) Refractory period: response to a second (or third) allodynogenic stimulus delivered down to 1/3 s in every pt

Author's conclusion: There appear to be real differences in the response between CP and PNP pts with mechanical (tactile) allodynia and so the mechanisms of allodynia could be different.

Bowsher and Hagget (2005): Brain

Study on paradoxical burning sensation produced by cold stimulation in pts with NP

17 CPSP pts, 24 NP pts, 2 siblings with congenital indifference to pain

Results of quantitative thermal sensory perception threshold testing (response only to cold stimulation, pt description):
7/17 CPSP pts: no sensation at all down to 0°C (absence of cold sensation)
7/17 CPSP pts: "cold" sensation at threshold (which was below that on the mirror-image unaffected area)
3/17 CPSP pts: "burning" sensation

Authors' conclusion: Paradoxical burning sensation is produced by cold stimulation not only in CPSP but it seems to occur somewhat randomly in a variety of NP conditions.

necessitating an accurate neurological examination to detect them. Deep sensibility (articular, muscular, tendineal and osseous) was more profoundly and persistently affected. In many cases, patients could neither recognize vibration nor perceive active and passive movements, muscle power and strength; there was also a loss of joint position sense. Dejerine and Roussy noted in their patients the presence of allodynia, hyperesthesia and hyperalgesia/hyperpathia (described as excessive reaction to touch, cold or warm and pinprick). Head and Holmes (1911) later published an *unsurpassed* quantitative clinical analysis of sensory abnormalities in CP patients. Ever since, we know a wide spectrum of sensory abnormalities can be found among patients with CP. They range from a slightly raised threshold for one of the submodalities, to complete loss of all somatic sensibility in the painful region, or a very painful hyperesthesia. In some patients the abnormalities are subtle, but can often be detected by quantitative sensory tests (QST), as demonstrated by Head and Holmes.

A survey of the literature shows that the common feature of more than 95% of all CP patients is impaired temperature and pain (i.e., spinothalamic) sensibility at clinical or electrophysiological examination (Garcin 1937; Riddoch 1938; Tasker 2001); appreciation of pinprick and temperature is nearly always impaired, and there is almost always a raised threshold to innocuous thermal (both warm and cold) detection and to a lesser extent also to painful heat and pain. Some patients who have lost the ability to perceive cold and warm due to CNS lesions can nonetheless distinguish warm or cool objects by the distinctly different feelings they evoke (e.g., Kinnier Wilson 1927; Davison and Schick 1935). No unequivocal report of CP arising from lesions restricted to the lemniscal pathways has been published, and several patients (particularly in Wallenberg's syndrome) have normal thresholds for touch, vibration and kinesthesis (in such cases, the posterior columns may mediate evoked pains); instead, many cases of lesions restricted to the STT are on record (cordotomy, anterior spinal artery syndrome, medullary stroke). CP is independent of other neurological symptoms, including paresis, tremor, dystonia, speech disturbances, hemianopsia; only somatosensory abnormalities are always present, although these are far from uniform among patients (see also Gonzales *et al.* 2001). Pain distribution is usually well correlated with sensory abnormalities. The pain may also occur in patients with brain lesions who have recovered from clinically detectable sensory loss and persist in time; in this case, a crude sensory examination, weeks or months after the lesion, reveals no sensory deficit. Nonetheless, a lesion affecting the STT system "is a necessary but not sufficient condition" for the development of CP.

It is the experience of all groups doing research with CP that a few patients do not display thermoalgesic abnormalities (e.g. Garcin [1937]) reviewed cases in which there seemed to be only loss of epicritic sensibility and De Ajuriaguerra [1937] observed three patients without thermoalgesic deficits), even at QST. Examples include Boivie and Leijon (1991; 1 case), the series of Tasker *et al.* (1991; 2 cases, although one showed abnormalities of the late components of somatosensory evoked potentials), Shieff (1991; 4 cases), Gonzales and colleagues (1992; 1 patient), Bowsher (1996; 1 case – see other examples in Chapter 3, Section 4). Tasker and colleagues (1991) described a patient with pain associated with cord lesions that caused a preferential loss of touch, position and vibration with *almost* complete sparing of STT. Regev and colleagues (1983) reported a patient with a pontine hemorrhage producing no detectable somatosensory deficit, who developed transient spontaneous pain and allodynia to touch, pinprick and temperature. Sandyk (1985) reported a CP patient with a cortical parietal hematoma whose only somatosensory finding was allodynia induced by thermal (warm/cold) stimuli. However, in all those cases where no sensory loss was seen in the first place, imaging techniques suggest a central lesion appropriately located to damage the somatosensory system.

14. Sympathetic and other signs and symptoms

Signs of abnormal sympathetic nervous system activity within the region of disability (i.e., focal distribution) may sometimes be present: cooler and vasoconstricted skin in the painful area, edema, hypo/hyperhydrosis (rare), altered skin texture and color (mottled skin or livedo) (Garcin 1937; Riddoch 1938).

However, these signs are equally present in non-CP patients with CNS injury; decreased movement alone can cause autonomic changes. A cerebral lesion can cause trophic disturbances in contralateral limbs (Arseni and Boetz 1971), particularly the shoulder hand syndrome, even paroxysmally (Montgomery and King 1962). A common source of pain after stroke is *nociceptive pain localized to the shoulder* and resulting from paresis and changed muscular tone/posture and sensory loss. One fourth of stroke patients develop it within 2 weeks (Gamble *et al.* 2000).

Lance (1996) described the complaint of a *painful, burning, red ear* in a CP patient with a right sylvian infarction (F42, case 10). Some 6 weeks later she developed sharp pains "like a hot needle" in the left side of her head, which recurred with increasing frequency until it became a diffuse burning ache in the left side of her head and face, similar to the pain she experienced in her left shoulder and upper limb. When the burning pain exacerbated, onlookers commented that her left ear became red and might stay red all day. Sensory loss and weakness of her left arm persisted. Her pain was diminished to about one half of the previous severity by imipramine 125 mg daily. Three years after the accident, she developed left-sided migraine-like headaches associated with increased intensity of her burning pain.

Although there are no formal studies of the interaction of mood and pain state in CPSP, the experience of chronic pain can lead to depression, anxiety and sleep disturbance. As such, inquiries as to the length and quality of sleep as well as the patient's mood should be made.

SPECIAL CONSIDERATIONS

1. Sensory epilepsy

Epileptic pain is rare (0.3–2.8%: review of Scholz *et al.* 1999; 4.1%: Nair *et al.* 2001), although the exact frequency remains to be determined (amounting in the United States to no less than 15 000 patients, assuming an average pain prevalence of about 1%). Painful auras have been recognized as such for a long time (De Ajuriaguerra 1937). Ferré's textbook also reports instances of atrocious tearing pains during jacksonian fits, although De Ajuriaguerra noted that painful fits appeared to be less frequent than implied by Ferré, and this was in fact the general impression of the time. Rather, it was not clear whether the origin was thalamic or cortical (Garcin 1937). However, Penfield and Gage (1933) described the case of an epileptic woman in whom seizures were heralded by a sharp pain in the right lower quadrant of the abdomen, immediately followed by loss of consciousness. At operation, they found atrophy of a small convolution just posterior to SI and near the midline. Galvanic stimulation of this area reproduced her pain and this was confirmed in another patient (case 5) with postraumatic epilepsy and a normal cortex. They observed that "seizures beginning in the postcentral gyrus may be initiated by pain and discomfort in the opposite side of the body and without direct reference to the thalamus." Other cases too of pain and paresthesias in the same distribution had a march implying contralateral SI involvement (e.g., Young and Blume 1983). One epileptic patient had pain reproduced by neurosurgical stimulation of parietal BA5 (see in Scholz *et al.* 1999).

In the partial review of Scholz and colleagues (1999) of the literature, pain generally accompanied simple partial attacks, with or without a jacksonian march, and with no side prevalence, in both adults and children. Pain could involve the whole hemisoma (or sometimes the *whole body or limbs bilaterally*), a limb or hemiface, combinations of these, or also spread contralaterally; also described were visceral pain and throbbing, pricking or diffuse headache. The usual cause was a tumor (meningiomas, gliomas, metastases or abscesses) or rarely penetrating head trauma and stroke. In several cases, it was idiopathic.

Actually, during the attack, the patient may complain of unpleasant sensations — numbness, pins-and-needles, intensely unpleasant but difficult to define, burning, cramping, aching, gnawing, throbbing, stinging, electric shock-like, stabbing, "like a thousand bee-stings," "like a sharp knife" — besides true pain; these anomalous sensations are like those described by CP patients. In recent series, the parietal region (SI and SII) was the commonest — with exceptions — site for lesions responsible for the painful seizures; however, the site of the lesion may not always correlate with the site of the seizure during ictal pain, especially if the pain does not occur early in the ictal sequence. Bilateral EEG anomalies during painful fits are on record (Scholz *et al.* 1999).

Importantly, there is no objective sensory deficit (e.g., Retif *et al.* 1967); instead, it seems clear how the decreased inhibition accompanying a seizure interferes with pain control mechanisms in certain cortical areas. This might account for the apparent intensification of paresthetic or dysesthetic sensations to the point of becoming painful, in some patients.

2. Parkinson's disease (PD)

Pain as part of PD was recognized by Parkinson himself (Garcin 1937). According to Garcin, PD-associated pains

> siègent principalement aux membres, à la nuque et aux lombes, occupant surtout les articulations et les muscles sous forme de douleurs profondes parfois atroces ou survenant par crises d'élancements et de brûlures, surtout nocturnes. Elles sont souvent limitées au côté atteint dans les syndromes unilatéraux. Très souvent, ces douleurs précèdent les débuts apparents de la maladie ... Il est plus rare de les voir persister tout le long de la maladie.

> (principally affect the limbs, the nape and the loins, mostly at the level of joints and muscles as deep, sometimes atrocious, pains or shooting or burning painful paroxysms, mostly at night. They are often limited to the affected side in unilateral syndromes. Very often, these pains precede the onset of the disease ... more rarely they persist indefinitely.)

A current estimate is that one third to one half of patients suffer some form of pain. Sage (2004) classifies these into low-DOPA pain states (dystonic, pseudoradiculopathic, akathesic, genital, trigeminal neuralgia-like, abdominal, nonspecific, musculoskeletal and paresthetic, generally described as burning, tingling, numbness in distal limbs or groins), high-DOPA pain states (dystonic, choreic, paresthetic, which is generally described as burning in limbs or trunk) and others (oral, vaginal, joint, muscle tightness, headache, gastrointestinal, hemifacial dystonic, depression-associated).

Förster (1927) believed that the striopallidal system exerts an inhibitory action on the thalamus, possibly explaining CP apparently due to striatal lesions. However, stereotactic lesions of the globus pallidus for the treatment of extrapyramidal motor disorders never originated CP. Honey and colleagues (1999) improved one of two PD patients with poorly localized, bilateral, often burning dysesthesias with pallidotomy at 6 weeks postoperatively, but none at one year; instead, cramping and deep aching pains responded to pallidotomy, with most patients relieved or improved at 1 year. In a PET study of normal volunteers, Hagelberg and colleagues (2002) concluded that D2 receptor binding potential in the human, particularly in the striatum, may determine the individual cold pain response and the potential for central pain modulation: an individual with only few available D2 receptors in the forebrain is likely to have a high tonic level of pain suppression, combined with a low capacity to recruit more (dopaminergic) central pain inhibition by noxious conditioning stimulation. Hodge and King (1976) found that, following induction of sensory loss in humans, L-dopa increases pain and the area of denervation, while methyldopa does the opposite.

However, the central nature of at least some PD-associated pains has been called into question by Djaldetti and colleagues (2004). These authors found that: (1) PD patients ($n = 36$) have significantly lower heat pain thresholds than matched controls (while tactile and warm thresholds did not differ), (2) patients with painful PD have significantly lower heat pain thresholds than pain-free PD, (3) heat pain threshold is lowermost in the most affected limb and (4) there is no difference between ON and OFF phases. This study definitely rules out PD pain as a CP.

As regards *dystonia*, despite suggestions that part of the pain may be centrally mediated, the nature of the dysfunction is unknown and we feel not enough human evidence is available to advance the argument beyond speculation.

3. Iatrogenic lesions (Table 2.13)

Several neurosurgical operations can originate CP. These are briefly reviewed.

Hemispherectomy. In cases of infantile hemiplegia, CP is generally short-lived (weeks), being more persisting at long-term follow-up in cases operated on for cerebral tumors.

Mesencephalotomy. Unlike bulbar and spinal tractotomies, these also damage the epicritic pathways (medial lemnisci and tracts of Goll and Burdach); moreover, they invariably impinge on the midbrain reticular formation both in open and stereotactic operations. At midbrain level, the spinothalamic tract consists of only a small number of fibers (about 1500; Glees and Bailey 1951), since a large share stopped in the reticular formation, and the collaterals of the fibers severed at mesencephalic level may still convey pain impulses on the polysynaptic system of the brainstem. Mesencephalotomy also impinges on descending inhibitory systems centered on the periacqueductal gray.

Bulbar tractotomy. The low incidence of CP after bulbar tractotomies has been explained by the fact that the surgical incision interrupts both spinorcticular and

TABLE 2.13. Iatrogenic lesions originating central pain (selected studies)

Author(s)	Type of lesion	CP	Notes
1. Hemispherectomy*			
Dandy (1933)	Brain tumors (2 pts)	y	Allodynia in both
Bell and Karnosh (1949)		y	Transient (bar a trace) hyperpathia; allodynia
Obrador (1956)		y	As above
Laine and Gros (1956)		y	Transient hyperpathia and allodynia (movement) up to 1 week
Quarti and Terzian (1954)	6 cases	y	Transient hyperesthesia in the limbs in all (2 weeks)
Gardner et al. (1955)		y	Dysesthesias, thermal allodynia (long term)
Zuelch (1960) (see also Mueller et al. 1991)	13 cases	y	In the majority, transient (1 week in one)
2. Frontal lobotomies, topectomies, lobectomies			
Petit-Dutaillis et al. (1950)		n	Transient (2 mos) trigeminal paresthesias and overreaction to pain and thermal stimuli
3. Parietal cortectomy			
Lewin and Phillips (1952)	Cortectomy of the posterior lip of Rolando's fissure for amputation stump pain	y	
Tasker (1990)		n	Review: **no CP ever followed parietal cortectomies**
4. Destruction of thalamoparietal radiations			
Talairach et al. (1960)		n	
Riechert (1961)		n	
Cassinari et al. (1964)	Destruction with radioactive yttrium (2 pts)	y	Delayed (3 mos) in 1 brachial plexus avulsion pain, CP in regions not affected by the original pain

(continued)

TABLE 2.13 (continued)

Author(s)	Type of lesion	CP	Notes
5. Lesions of lenticular and caudate nuclei and adjacent areas			
Pagni (1977)		n	Review: no CP ever from "pure" lesions
6. Thalamotomies			
Hassler and Riechert (1959)	Vc	y	Delayed CP in 1/24 pts (phantom pain)
Mark et al. (1960)	Vc	y	Painful dysesthesias in 1/77 pts + numbness in 2
Bettag and Yoshida (1960)	Arcuate, CM, DM	y?	In 3/7 facial painful anesthesia pts (recurrence of the original pain or true CP?)
Obrador et al. (1961)	Vc, DM	y	Dysesthesia in 1 phantom pain pt
Urabe and Tsubokawa (1965)	Bilat CM	y	2/7 pts
Cassinari and Pagni (1969)	Vc, CM (1 pt, ^{90}γ); Vc-CM (2 pts); Vc-medial lemniscus at subthalamic level-CM (1 pt); CM (1 pt); CM first and Vc later (1 pt)	y	6/32 pts
Cassinari and Pagni (1969)		n	Review; stereotactic lesions of VL, VA, posterior lateral, dorsal median, centrum medianum, anterior, intralaminar, pulvinar and reticular nuclei sparing Vc and its basal part never cause CP
Nashold (1974)		n	Review; no CP after lesions confined exclusively to the medialis dorsalis, ventralis lateralis, anterior thalamic nuclei or pulvinar
Pagni (1977)		y	Review; CP follows thalamic surgery damaging or destroying Vc, when complete anesthesia is not obtained, immediately after lesioning
Tasker (1990)		y	CP follows always in a mild degree all stereotactic thalamotomies he performed; it never occurs after destructive lesions of the Vim and Vor nuclei to relieve motor disorders
7. Mesencephalotomies[†]			
Open lateral tractotomies			
Dogliotti (1938)		y	Almost immediate in 2/4 pts (another died)
Walker (1942a)		y	2/2 a few days to a few weeks later

Walker (1950)		y	Review
Schwarz (1950)		y	2/2
Drake and McKenzie (1953)	Lateral mesencephalotomy	y	3–14 days later in all 6 pts ("entirely new sensations"), touch sensibility only mildly affected
Bailey and colleagues (1954)	Lateral mesencephalotomy	y?	Hyperalgesia to pricking and touch allodynia in 1 cancer pt; no lemniscal deficits
Mikula et al. (1959)	Bilateral lateral mesencephalotomy	y	1 week later in 1 tabetic case; all over the body
Cassinari and Pagni (1969)		y	Review; lateral mesencephalotomies have the highest incidence of CP among all pain-relieving operations
Stereotactic mesencephalotomy			
Torvik (1959)	1. Destruction of STT/ML (complete) reticular formation + brachium inferior colic (partial) 2. Lesion of STT/ML extending to the most medial portion of the thalamus	y	1 of 2 (hyperpathia to painful stimuli and vibration allodynia); 1 pt died 14 days after the operation without CP
Roeder and Orthner (1961)		y	1 PNP case; 8 mos later, dynamic tactile allodynia in hemisoma
Wycis and Spegel (1962)	Lesion of the STT/QTT, a large part of the reticular substance at the level of the posterior colliculi	y	8/54; severe in 2 cases and transient in 1; mild transient sensory disturbances possible after ML lesions
Mazars and colleagues (1960)	Mesencephalic coagulations of the STT	n	86 cases
Voris and Whisler (1975)		y	6/52 cases
Nashold (1982)		y	Review; 70% after open mesencephalotomy, 5% after stereotactic mesencephalotomy
Frank and colleagues (1982)		y	2/14 cancer pain pts
Tasker and Dostrovsky (1989)		y	Review of 92 reports; 15–20% of pts submitted to mesencephalotomy develop dysesthesia

(continued)

105

TABLE 2.13 *(continued)*

Author(s)	Type of lesion	CP	Notes
8. Bulbar tractotomy			
Zuelch and Schmid (1953)		y	1 pt (burning hyperpathia to deep pressure)
Crawford and Knighton (1953)		y	1/8 pts
Crawford (1960)		y	2/4 pts (both neuropathic pains)
Cassinari and Pagni (1969)		y	Review of 63 mostly cancer pain cases; bulbar spinothalamic tractotomy only rarely gives rise to CP. This may depend on the surgical interruption of spinoreticular fibers intermingled with STT fibers, before reaching bulbar reticular formation; deep incisions injure reticular neurons. No injury to lemniscal fibers ensues with bulbar and spinal lesions
9. Bulbar trigeminal tractotomy (Sjöqvist's operation)			
Olivecrona (1947)	Tractotomy of the descending trigeminal root at obex level	n	
Le Beau et al. (1948)	Tractotomy of the descending trigeminal root at obex level	n	
Grant (1948)		y	2/6 pts
Hamby and colleagues (1948)		y	12/28 pts, very severe
Falconer (1949)		y	20 pts; disagreeable, but not bothering, sensations
Zuelch and Schmid (1953)	1 bilateral	y	2 pts; hyperpathia and allodynia
White and Sweet (1955)		y	Never immediate; > 65% of cases in 32 pts (many with cancer and tic), 2/35 unbearable, 18/35 milder; in some pts transient paresthesias. Paresthesias may increase or decrease with time
White (1962)	Tractotomy of the descending trigeminal root	y	Unpleasant paresthesias

Cassinari and Pagni (1969)		y	Review; never immediately, 1 week or later; 30% of cases, with wide range; usually paresthesia, rarely pain, generally not as intense as after Frazier's surgery
10. Pontine lesions			
Pagni (1977)		n	Review
11. Cordectomies			
Botterell et al. (1954)		y	Burning or dysesthetic sensations
Jefferson (1983)		y	Burning or dysesthetic sensations
12. Cordotomies[‡]			
Open technique			
Babtchine (1936)		y	A few cases out of 47
Dogliotti (1937)		y	Also in complete pain paths transection
Sasaki (1938)		y	7/19 pts; postoperative paresthesia
Sjöqvist (1950)		y	5/58 pts unpleasant sensation of heat or cold; 6/58 pts burning pain
Miserocchi (1951)		y	Heat allodynia? Troublesome paresthesias
Lapresle and Guiot (1953)		y	5/8 arthrosis pts; hyperpathia; at least in one case new pain exactly comparable to thalamic pain
Falconer (1953)	Cervical plus thoracic	y	Hyperalgesia plus hyperpathia; tactile allodynia in 4/6 phantom pains; "continuous sensation of pins-and-needles" in 1/6 phantom pain pts; burning pain
Zuelch and Schmid (1953)	Thoracic	y	Hyperpathia; tactile allodynia, hyperalgesia
White and Sweet (1955)		y	Icy cold sensations (in 1, >19 mos), paresthesias more severe after cervical cordotomies (>3 yrs); deep aching and shooting pains
Horrax and Lang (1957)		y	2/50 pts

(continued)

TABLE 2.13 (*continued*)

Author(s)	Type of lesion	CP	Notes
Grant and Wood (1958)		y	Dysesthesias in 8/105 C7–D3 incisions and in 4/98 C2–C5 incisions. Burning sensations below the level of analgesia; in only 4 hypalgesic zones involved. Spontaneous improvement in most of the cases; pain persisted over 10 years in one pt
Schwartz (1960)		y	Dysesthesias in 2/120 pts
Bohm (1960)		y	4/35 unilateral cervical cordotomies; 4/34 bilateral thoracic cordotomies (generally paresthesias-dysesthesias); in 1 pt a further higher cordotomy did not suppress burning paresthesia
Brihaye and Retif (1961)		y	1/109 pts; intense burning sensations in the analgesic territory 3 weeks later
Diemath et al. (1961)		y	1/121 pts (dysesthesia)
White and Sweet (1969)			3 severe and 9 mild dysesthesias out of 276 cancer pts. Delayed or very delayed. More likely to affect pts who lived longer (allowing analgesia to give way to hypalgesia); 3 severe and 6 mild dysesthesias out of 50 upper thoracic cordotomies and 1 severe and 3 mild dysesthesias out of 30 C1–2 cordotomies in non-cancer pts
			19% incidence in non-cancer-related pain. Generally long-lasting, commonly persisting until death of pt. Unlikely to be relieved by a new cordotomy
Percutaneous technique			
Rosomoff (1969)		y	Incidence: about 1%
Mansuy et al. (1976)		n	Cancer pain; average survival: 6 mos
Mazars (1976)		y	3%
Ganz and Mullen (1977)		y	High percentage of dysesthesia, with 1% of worrying burning dysesthesia after 1 yr
Kuhner (1981)		y	20%
Cowie and Hitchcock (1982)		y	Dysesthesia: 3/49 after unilateral cordotomy; 1/7 after bilateral cordotomy
Nathan and Smith (1972, 1984)		y	Dysesthesia: 1/41 after bilateral cordotomy; 3/79 after unilateral cordotomy

Reference		Description
Lipton (1989)	y	Severe dysesthesias in <2% of percutaneous cordotomies; higher incidence of not troublesome dysesthesias
La Huerta et al. (1994)	y	6% painful dysesthesias at/below lesion level in 181 cervical anterolateral cordotomies (developing, in one case, 200 days later)
Tasker and North (1997)	y	3.1% at discharge in 244 pts, persisting in 1.6%; burning or dysesthesias after a delay in all or part of the body rendered hypalgesic or analgesic
		Review: data in many series difficult to analyze

13. Posterior cordotomy

Reference		Description
Förster (1927)	y	Surgical interruption of the posterior columns in 2 pts with intramedullary tumor
Antonucci (1938)	y	Bilateral section of the tracts of Goll
		Hyperpathia and spontaneous pain likely due to other spinal tracts damage
		Numbness in one leg, one-night pain; complete disappearance of symptoms after about 3 weeks
Grant and Weinberger (1941)	?	Sjöqvist's operation
		Paresthesias attributed to the extension of the lesion to the ipsilateral cuneate nucleus
Pool (1946)	y	Incision at the C5–6 level impinging on lamina II and Lissauer's tract
		Allodynia; thermal hyperalgesia in large girdle area of torso (from incision level down to lower 3–10 dermatomes)
Browder and Gallagher (1948)	y	Pure dorsal column incision
		Intermittent burning type of pain in the stump of the arm (?)
White and Sweet (1955)	n	Lesions of nc cuneatus
Pagni (1977)	n	Review. No case among 43 pts

14. Commissural myelotomy

Reference		Description
Wertheimer and Lecuire (1953)	y	Girdle pains in 27/107 pts; dysesthesias-paresthesias in 28/107 pts (plus hyperalgesia). May be persistent
Sourek (1969)	y	Most of 24 pts, transiently
Broager (1974)	y	2 of 34 until death 3–6 mos later

TABLE 2.13 (continued)

Author(s)	Type of lesion	CP	Notes
Lippert et al. (1974)		y	Temporary paresthesias or dysesthesias in most pts, disappearing within a few days; long-lasting in 4/24 pts
Cook and Kawakami (1977)		y	12 of 24 pts developing immediate transient CP (max. 2 weeks)
King (1977)		y	In 9 pts, immediately after surgery, occasional dysesthesias, prominent or mild; no severe dysesthesias or hyperpathia in the long term
15. Section of the tract of Lissauer			
Hyndman (1942)		y	Mild tactile allodynia in 1/5 in analgesic areas
16. Dorsal root entry zone coagulation (DREZ)			
Nashold (1984)		y	CP does occur in some pts but the incidence is not high
Powers et al. (1984)		y	Dysesthesias
Sindou et al. (2001)		y	Sometimes perception of touch or pin-prick as dysesthesia or unpleasant sensation, but not pain. In the early period after surgery some pts developed dysesthesia
Falci et al. (2002)		y	4.7% (VAS 1–3)

* In cases of infantile hemiplegia, symptoms are generally short-lived (weeks); in tumoral resections, they last longer. Thalamus may be injured during surgery.

† At midbrain level, the STT consists of only 1500 fibers, since 90% stopped in the reticular formation in the brainstem; mesencephalic lesions may impinge on descending analgesia stations: this may relate to enhanced responsiveness to painful stimuli. Midbrain lesions invariably impinge on reticular formation.

‡ At times, after STT-tomies, a vivid girdle pain appears, on one or both sides, usually referred to the transitional area between the analgesic and normal skin on the side contralateral to the incision and accompanied by hyperesthesia; usually disappears in a few weeks; may be due to trauma to the exposed spinal roots.

NB: no CP after lesion of motor or extrapyramidal fibers.

spinothalamic fibers, before the former reach the nucleus gigantocellularis in the bulbar reticular formation. Also the reticular formation may be injured if the incision is too deep. No injury is normally caused to the lemniscal fibers.

Bulbar trigeminal tractotomy (Sjöqvist's operation). Trigeminal pain-relaying fibers give off collaterals which end in the other portions of the trigeminal complex sensory stations and in the reticular formation, and these are not involved in Sjöqvist's operation. A polysynaptic intranuclear pathway, similar to the supposed ascending polysynaptic pathway of spinal lamina II, transmits impulses from the caudal nucleus to the rostral portion and thence to the reticular formation (Stewart *et al.* 1964). Thus, if the bulbar trigeminal tractotomy interrupts only the descending tract of the trigeminus and not the nucleus with its intranuclear pathway, extratrigeminal impulses may still be transmitted, giving rise to sensory dysesthesias, while interruption of the nucleus too should block impulses ascending in the intranuclear pathway, making the occurrence of dysesthesias more unlikely.

Anterolateral cordotomy (open and percutaneous). The incidence ranges from 0 to more than 90% (Mazars 1976), being higher in patients undergoing cordotomy for the treatment of benign disease (e.g., 4% in cancer pain and 19% in non-cancer pain in White and Sweet 1969); this is accounted for by the latent period necessary for CP to arise. Symptoms are generally long-lasting, commonly persisting until the patient's death, relief by a new cordotomy being unlikely. A few without any postoperative CP are on record (e.g., Mansuy *et al.* 1976): this might also depend on short follow-up time (6 months). Mazars (1976) pointed out that a higher incidence in some series may depend on more extensive damage to the cord during surgery. Recent series can be as low as 1–3% or as high as 20% (reviewed in Tasker and North 1997).

Appearing a few days to many months after a successful operation, these are generally feelings of icy cold, burning dysesthesias or pain, sometimes with hyperpathia and hyperesthesia, generally referred to areas in which pain sensibility is recovering, but also to totally analgesic areas. They are often most pronounced in the original painful area for which the cordotomy was performed. CP can be distinguished from a relapse of the original pain: in the latter, the pinprick sensation deficit disappears in the painful area due to a retraction in the pinprick level, while in CP the pinprick level is retained and pinprick sensation is absent in the painful area. At times, following anterolateral cordotomies, a vivid *girdle pain* appears, which radiates to one or both sides, usually referred to the transitional area between the analgesic and normal skin on the side contralateral to the incision and accompanied by hyperesthesia. According to Sweet and Poletti (1989), girdle pain disappears usually in a few weeks, being due to temporary trauma to the exposed spinal roots.

Rarely, following anterolateral cordotomies, both mono- and bilateral (but also after vascular damage to the anterolateral quadrant), the patient perceives pain and temperature (but also non-painful) stimuli applied to analgesic or hypalgesic regions in a part of the affected or controlateral side of the body in which the sensibility is normal (*referred or reference of pain* when the pain is felt in a place apart from the spot where the noxious stimulation is applied; *mirror pain, allochiria, allachesthesia* when patients misperceive the location of a stimulus at the same point on the opposite side of the body), a phenomenon first described by Obersteiner (1881).

In cases of unilateral cordotomy, pain is usually referred to the symmetrical contra-lateral part of the body; in cases of bilateral anterolateral cordotomies (or vascular damage), giving rise to bilateral analgesia, it is referred to the ipsi or contralateral side above the analgesic zone. The patient reports that the pain slowly spreads, as stimulation is maintained, and arises from the interior, unlike the stimulus to the skin which is felt as external (Nagaro *et al.* 1993). However, referred pain is not CP, as a further cordotomy on the opposite side abolishes it (Chapter 8).

3 CENTRAL PAIN OF CORD ORIGIN

Central pain of cord origin is also known as below-level pain, remote pain, functionally limiting dysesthetic pain syndrome. Burning dysesthetic pain and central dysesthesia syndrome are general terms that have been used to describe CCP too.

1. Lesions causing CCP (Tables 3.1 and 3.2)

CP has been reported with virtually every type of disease or lesion affecting the spinal cord substance (dorsal horns), be it a complete or an incomplete lesion. Trauma/concussion (civilian gunshot wounds and automobile accidents in western countries) is the leading cause of CCP worlwide, but iatrogenic lesions dismayingly follow suit. CP, although only one of the many chronic pains observed after SCI (Table 3.3), is by far the most severe and disabling, and in many patients may limit their functional ability and daily activities.

2. Incidence and prevalence (Table 3.4)

Literature series are not comparable, because pain terms used are not homogeneous and research methods vary widely (e.g. subjective self-reports versus objective study); moreover, CCP can be "simulated" by other concurrent pains, making it difficult to tease out, and in most series there is no agreement on what "true CP" is. Thus, quoted estimates of CCP in the literature range from a few to almost all. Burke (1973) even reported different incidences of pain among paraplegics in different societies, which he blamed on some aspects of patient management. Prospective studies with enough power have not been published, but Siddal and colleagues (1999) found that almost 20% of their SCI patients developed below-level pain at 6 months and Bonica (1991), in reviewing a total of 2465 SCI patients in the literature, found that no less than 25% had CP. CP is next in order of frequency among SCI pains after end-zone pain; however, in the 41-patient series (36 ASIA A) of Falci *et al.* (2002), below-level pain was the predominant pain, occurring in 31 (end-zone in 8, simultaneously in 2). In the United States and the EU, there are about 600 000 SCI patients and 150 000 may be suffering CP; worldwide, 2.5 million spinal cord injured patients are estimated to exist.

Injuries that result in severe damage or disruption of the spinal cord and its adjacent tissues (e.g., gunshot wounds) as well as those with large intraspinal

TABLE 3.1. Causes of cord central pain (compiled from a complete survey of the literature and personal observations)

(1) Spinal trauma with fracture and/or dislocations producing complete or partial transection or concussion of the spinal cord

(2) Ischemic/hemorrhagic (e.g., aortic dissection, systemic hypotension, atherosclerosis/thromboembolism/infarcts, hematomyelia*/subarachnoid hemorrhage due to AVMs[†], cavernomas, dural fistula, traumatic/nontraumatic/iatrogenic cervical anterior spinal cord syndrome, etc.)

(3) Rheumatological and degenerative disorders (e.g., myelopathy due to cervical spinal stenosis-spondylosis and cervical discal hernia, ankylosing spondylitis with conus lesions, Paget's disease, rheumatoid arthritis, posterior longitudinal ligament ossification)

(4) Intra- and extramedullary tumors[‡]

(5) Congenital and developmental (nontumoral cysts, syringomyelia, dysraphism, diastematomyelia, spina bifida, myelomeningocele, etc.)

(6) Inflammatory-infective (multiple sclerosis: transverse myelitis, viral (e.g., herpes zoster, cytomegalovirus, HIV, poliovirus), bacterial (e.g., mycobacteria/Pott's disease, luetic gumma[¶]), fungal (e.g., cryptococcus) or parasitic infections/abscesses (e.g., toxoplasma, schistosoma) or infective transverse myelitis)

(7) Degenerative CNS disorders

(8) Toxic (antiblastic agents, radiation, etc.)

(9) Genetic and metabolic

(10) Iatrogenic (cordotomy, aortic repair surgery, surgery for spinal angiomas/fistulas/hernias/spondylosis/intra- and extramedullary tumors, spinal fusion surgery, myelography, anticoagulant therapy with epidural/subdural hematomas)

---

* Sudden at-level pain, sometimes followed by below-level pain.
[†]Initially produce at-level pain, then commonly below-level pain.
[‡]Cervical-thoracic extramedullary tumors generally produce long-lasting at-level pain and shorter-lasting below-level pain more often involving the lower limbs. Pain or dysesthesias can be the only (or initial) symptom for a long time. Intramedullary tumors generate less frequent, below-level (short-lived) pain/(long-lived) dysesthesias, often in both legs and at-level ("armor-like" constrictive band).
[¶]The pathological process in tabes dorsalis, which can originate CP, is known not to be confined to the posterior columns (Vierck 1973).

TABLE 3.2. Distribution of causes of CCP

	Series A* (%)	Series B[†] (%)	
Trauma	65	75.3	(gunshot — closed trauma)
Tumors	6	6.2	(ependymoma, meningioma, schwannoma, etc.)
Inflammatory	9	5	(MS, etc.)
Infective		3.6	
Skeletal	2	2.5	(cervical stenosis, etc.)
Vascular/ischemic	2	1.2	
Congenital (or uncertain [A])	4	1.2	(syrinx, etc.)
Iatrogenic	12	10	(surgery for cervical disk (2.5% in B), radiotherapy others, etc.)

* Tasker et al. (1992) (127 CCP patients seen between 1961 and 1989), Canada.
[†]Rogano et al. (2003) (81 patients seen prospectively), Brazil.

TABLE 3.3. IASP classification of SCI pains (adapted from Siddall *et al*. 2001)

Nociceptive

(1) Musculoskeletal (mechanical and lesional pain). Dull, aching, movement-related, eased by rest, responsive to opioids and NSAIDs. Located in musculoskeletal structures. Bone, joint, disk, ligament, muscle and soft tissue trauma and inflammation (e.g., strain in latissimus dorsi in a C7 "complete" quadriplegic); mechanical instability, muscle spasms, secondary overuse syndromes. It may add to and compound certain end-zone pains. Muscle pain is caused by stress consequent to mechanical deformity due to immobility or overuse of shoulders, arms and back, when innervated, for balance and mobility purposes, but also to secondary changes following fractures and fixation, mechanical instability, and osteoporosis. Muscle spasms may sometimes produce discomfort and cramping pain in the legs and abdominal muscles. Pain is referred at injury level or right above it (including spasm-related). Especially when acute, it usually recedes with treatment.

(2) Visceral pain. Dull, cramping. Located in abdominal region with preserved innervation. Renal calculus, bowel dysfunction, sphincter dysfunction, etc. Also includes dysreflexic headache. It usually presents in high-thoracic and cervical SCI (quadriplegic) patients, despite varying degrees of sensory anesthesia and/or paralysis, as chronic cramping pain or discomfort/fullness centered mostly in the periumbilical/ hypogastric and pelvic areas. It is both spontaneous and provoked by a full urinary bladder, fecal impaction of the colon and rectum and other conditions that distend hollow viscera. It may be associated with nausea, flushing of the face, headache, piloerection and sweating. It may present in the absence of any abdominal organ dysfunction. Visceral sensation is conveyed via the dorsal columns. Some visceral pain can actually be CP.

Neuropathic pain

(1) Above-level pain (in the region of sensory preservation). Compressive mononeuropathies (carpal tunnel syndrome) present in up to half of paraplegics, often due to wheelchair propelling; complex regional pain syndrome observed as arm pain and swelling in quadriplegics and rarely in incomplete paraplegics, mostly bilaterally.

(2) Below-level pain. CCP (see text).

(3) At-level pain (also known as transitional zone, radicular/root, girdle, segmental, end-zone, junctional, boundary zone pain). Occurs at or just above the level of the sensory loss, in the cutaneous transition zone from the area of analgesia to areas of normal sensation (i.e., hypesthetic) and extends for 1–2 dermatomes and often more caudad (5–6 dermatomes) into the anesthetic zone; often it is not strictly dermatomal (radiculometameric), can be uni- or bilateral (asymmetrically more than not), and can be observed at all levels, perhaps with some preponderance, often in clinically complete injuries. It is generally described as dull, aching (sometimes burning) with superimposed paroxysms of throbbing, stabbing, electric shock-like or cramping pain lasting from one to several minutes. Allodynia and hyperalgesia are frequent: touching/stroking the skin in the painful dermatomes, which may also present as a very narrow band of hyperalgesia, often activates the pain itself, causing it to radiate into the lower parts of the body, especially the legs. Trigger spots can also be found on the surface of the skin, in the hypesthetic, painful areas, but sometimes as far as 6 dermatomes above the level of spinal trauma. When these spots are touched, the pain is aggravated. Visceral stimulation (e.g., full bladder) can also trigger it. When pain due to T8–L2 vertebral lesion is referred to the legs, many patients present with muscular spasms of ana- or hypoesthetic paraplegic legs, and pain is spasm-related. At-level pain is usually due to direct injury to the dorsal roots at or near the site of trauma, but also Lissauer's tract and posterior horns, or even local arachnoiditis/scarring with entrapment (occasional worsening by arm/leg movement suggests traction on these roots). One-third of SCI patients have it, making it the most common type of pain in association with paraplegia (Nashold 1991; Beric 1999). A subset of these pains is cauda equina pain (damage from T12 caudad), and involves the legs, feet, perineum, genitals, buttocks and rectum. It is generally very severe; usually burning, it may often be seen with dysesthesias and neuralgic pain in the thighs, calves or feet. Double lesion syndrome (DLS), seen more frequently in patients with complete cervical or upper

(continued)

Table 3.3 *(continued)*

thoracic lesions (perhaps 20%), is essentially a cauda equina/root dysfunction that modifies leg spasticity and bladder behavior due to upper cord damage: the pain is most often sharp, pricking and electric shock-like, with occasional burning, as well as aching and dull. Although usually stabilizing within several months, or several years, it remains constant, with minimal fluctuation. Most patients eventually adapt to it. It generally asymmetrically involves the leg, groin, thigh or foot, often in association with the perineum, rectum and genitals (Beric 1999). It is not CP. L5−S1 avulsion injuries of the conus (with myelocele at the L5/S1 foramen) are typically due to severe pelvic fracture (which may also cause pelvic plexus injuries). The pain is typically confined to the leg and associated with varying degrees of weakness. Progressive posttraumatic myelomalacic myelopathy too may lead to transitional zone pain.

Despite past claims, there is no evidence for *"psychogenic pain"* in the setting of spinal cord injury.

hemorrhages are more prone to produce pain than a compression lesion produced by simple fracture dislocation (Nashold 1991; Tasker 2001). CCP after trauma at levels higher than T10 has historically been considered rarer and of lesser intensity in almost all series (e.g., Davis and Martin 1947; Freeman and Heimburger 1947), as conocaudal injury adds a peripheral component due to nerve and/or nerve root damage (Nashold 1991). For instance, Davis and Martin reported very severe CP in 8/77 cervical lesions, 73/288 thoracic lesions and 45/106 lumbar lesions; previous series indicating the contrary (e.g., Holmes 1919) were written off as small in size and with short follow-up. However, a review of data clearly shows that CCP is equally represented at cervical, thoracic and lumbar levels and with similar intensity; what appears to differ is the frequency of superimposed paroxysms, higher in conocaudal injury. Also, quadriplegics may suffer more pain than paraplegics. Neither vertebral level nor completeness of lesion affect the incidence of steady CCP, although steady (usually burning) perineal pain occurs more frequently with complete lesions; intermittent pain occurs equally in complete and incomplete lesions at all spinal levels, but most frequently with lesions at T10−L2 level (57%) (Tasker *et al.* 1992). Since intermittent pain is the most painful component of CCP, this may go some way to explaining the reported lower frequency of CCP at cervicodorsal levels.

3. Age of onset and sex distribution
Patients with traumatic CCP are generally males (about 75%) and under the age of 40 (about 60%), reflecting younger males' susceptibility to trauma. No data are available for other lesions.

4. Time to pain onset
Similar to BCP, CCP can also start immediately or even years after insult, although sometimes it may be difficult to ascertain it amidst several other pains. In the consecutive series of Rogano and colleagues (2003) of 81 CCP (64.2% incomplete, 35.8% complete) patients, 43.2% of the patients developed CCP within the first week, 21% at 1−4 weeks and 35.8% after 4 weeks (mean: 110.4 weeks): thus, onset is within a month in almost two-thirds. In the series of Tasker and colleagues (1992), traumatic CCP was delayed in about 80% of cases, in two-thirds within 1 year of

TABLE 3.4. Incidence and prevalence

Author	Pathology	No. of patients	Patients with CP (%)
Beric et al. (1988)	Spinal cord injury	243	Chronic SCI patients. CP in 13/243 patients (5.3%)
Milhorat et al. (1996)	Syringomyelia	137	Retrospective review. *Segmental dysesthesia* (burning pain, hyperesthesia, pins and needles sensations and throphic changes): 51/137 patients (37%); burning pain: 43 (31.4%); hyperesthesia: 41 (29.9%); pins and needles: 37 (27.0%); stretching or pressure of skin: 17 (12.4%)
Stormer et al. (1997)	Spinal cord injury	901	Multicenter study. Pain and/or dysesthesia in 591 patients (66%). Pain alone in 50% of patients; painful dysesthesia in 11%; distressing dysesthesia without pain in 5%. Below-lesion pain: 278 patients (47%) Transitional and/or below-lesion pain: 508 patients (86%)
Siddall et al. (1999)	Spinal cord injury	100	Prospective longitudinal study. *Prevalence of neuropathic pain at 6 months*: at-level pain, 36%; below-level pain, 19%
Finnerup et al. (2001)	Spinal cord injury	330	Postal survey in a community-based sample of SCI patients. 330/436 responses. Pain or unpleasant sensations in 254 (77%). Below- and/or at-level pain/dysesthesia in 221 (67%)

trauma. The SCI patients of Falci and colleagues (2002) (T10–L1: 35; T4–T9: 6) experienced pain immediately in 63% of cases, within 2 months in 84%, within 6 months in 95% and within 1 year of injury in all cases. In contrast, one-third of the patients of Nashold (1991) developed it up to 6 years later. About one-third of patients with a delay of up to 1 year and more than half with a delay of more than 1 year harbored a posttraumatic syrinx in the series of Tasker and colleagues (1992). In these cases, the syrinx rather than the original injury seems responsible for the pain. Thus, late onset of pain (and always facial pain) must raise suspicions of a syrinx. Like CPSP, CCP usually appears with some functional recovery in more severe cases (Beric 1999).

5. Level of lesion

In two representative series (A: Tasker *et al.* 1992; B: Rogano *et al.* 2003) for a total of 208 patients, CCP was caused by cervical lesions in 42% (A) and 28.4% (B) of the cases, thoracic in 21% (A: down to T9) and 44.4% (B: up to T11?) and conocaudal in 37% (A: T10−L2) and 27.2% (B). In sum, conocaudal lesions are not the most frequent lesions causing CCP, and that is also our experience (Canavero and Bonicalzi 2004a) and that of others (see Beric 1999).

6. Distribution of pain

Pain may involve the entire body region below the level of injury (*diffuse pain*), but usually is more intense in the sacral dermatomes, buttocks and genitalia, and the feet (Friedman and Nashold 1986), never following a dermatomal distribution. Pain is usually diffusely and symmetrically (although not at all times during follow-up) referred to the parts of the body whose sensation is affected by the cord lesion; however, a quarter complains of localized pain within a much larger area of sensory alteration, some having a pain sharply localized to a small body part, usually the saddle area. Tasker and colleagues (1992) found, in patients with complete lesions, that steady pain occurred as a band at the upper level of cord damage in about 7% of cases, diffusely below that level in less than 20%, patchily below the level in about 60% and in the perineum in 15%; in those with incomplete lesions, the pain occurred diffusely below the level of cord dysfunction in two-thirds of cases, patchily in three-quarters and as a band at the upper level in less than 20%. Patients with facial pain (about 4%) all had incomplete lesions and a syrinx. Intermittent pain tended to run around the trunk at the level of the cord lesion in complete cases, and shoot up and down the body and/or the legs in incomplete lesions. While pain generally starts from the level of injury and caudad, there may be a free area from the zone of injury to the area of dysesthesias. In a series, the most common locations included the legs (84%), posterior trunk (63%), anterior trunk (42%) and arms (16%; 100% in quadriplegics) (see Beric 1999).

The bizarre distribution of CCP is demonstrated by Jefferson (1983), who broke down his paraplegia pain patients into three groups:

1) Six patients had an area of pain on the front of, or just above, the knees (a "blob" of about same size as, or marginally bigger than, the patella), symmetrically or with side prevalence. Invariably there were also pains occupying the front of the thighs or else the front of the shins. One had pain on the tops of his feet and some (very localized) pain on the back of his calves (the only patient with a significant proportion of the pain occupying the posterior aspect of the leg in the first two groups). Only one patient complained of pain involving the pelvis (rectum and vagina).

2) Three patients described pain occupying the anterior aspect of the thighs. In two of them the pain was symmetrical and there was no pain felt in any other part of the body. In the third patient, the pain occupied a large part of the front of the right thigh, extending upwards almost to the groin and downwards to the middle of the patella. There was less severe pain in a similar distribution on the left, together with an area of pronounced hyperesthesia in the skin overlying the medial aspect of the left knee. Additionally, there was slight pain behind the right knee.

3) The third group (6 patients) had fairly widespread pain, extending from the groin to the feet. Unlike groups (1) and (2), the pain spread downwards from iliac crests or groins and in half the patients it also involved the backs of the legs. Two patients had diffuse pain down the fronts of the thighs, knees and shins and in one of them the pain extended round the hips symmetrically into the lateral part of the buttocks. Three of the patients felt pain as extensively on the back of the legs as on the front, in two with involvement of the feet. One of these patients additionally described an episodic sensation which was likened to "an explosion" in the rectum. One patient had leg pains and pain involving the lower abdomen, the genitalia and the buttocks. Two patients with no involvement of mid-thighs, knees or shins had pains in areas that would be covered by bathing trunks (i.e., top of thighs, lower abdomen, buttocks plus anus and rectum either on the anterior or the posterior aspect). One of these patients also had isolated pains around the heels and ankles. Of the three patients who had lesions involving the D10 vertebra the pains were distributed either throughout the leg or legs or else in a "bathing trunks" distribution.

Like BCP, CCP can be felt superficially or — perhaps more frequently — deeply. In Brown-Sequard's syndrome (hemisection of the cord), on the lesion side, intense pain spreading to the paralyzed, but not analgesic, limbs may be felt suddenly at the moment of injury, fading away in a few days or weeks: this is not CP (Garcin 1937; Riddoch 1938). Below-level CP is observed in the contralateral hemisoma with respect to the lesion (end-zone pain is observed ipsilateral to hemisection).

In some cases, pain is felt contralaterally after stimulation of the affected hypoesthetic areas (allochiria).

7. Quality

There are different pains present in different patients and also different pains present in the same patient at different times or simultaneously. Sometimes, characteristics change as they appear or disappear. Like BCP, there is no one quality prevailing in all studies and CCP may be described with many terms by patients. However, the steady component may be more often burning, but also aching, cutting, piercing, radiating, tight, stinging, compressive or distractive; it may be dysesthetic (generally tingling but also cold). Intermittent pain is generally described as shooting or coming in electric shocks. Aching pain may prevail at neck—shoulder—back levels, especially in tetraplegics, and burning elsewhere (Widerstrom-Noga et al. 2001). In the series of Falci and colleagues (2002) (41 patients; T10—L1: 35; T4—T9: 6; at-level pain: 30.9%; below-level pain: 69.1%), the pain was most frequently described as burning (91%) or sharp/stabbing (61%), but also as cramping/pressure (38%), stinging/pins and needles (23%), electrical/shooting (12%), aching (12%), cold/freezing (2%), vibrating (2%). If pain occurred at and below level, the pain was different in character. In the series of Rogano and colleagues (2003) (81 patients, complete SCI in 35.8%, incomplete in 64.2%), pain was burning in 86%, shock-like in 39%, throbbing in 14.8%, pricking in 13.5% and aching in 11.2%.

In the series of Garcia-Larrea and colleagues (2003) of 32 SC incomplete injury cases (no midline pain or complete injuries) (proximal to DRG) (MS 9, trauma 7, tumor 5, syrinx 5, spondylotic myelopathy 4, zoster myelitis 2), 22 had spontaneous continuous burning pain (68.7%), 17 crushing pain (53.1%) and 19 paresthesias (59.3%); 5 had spontaneous intermittent/paroxysmal cramping pain (15.6%) or 17 electric discharge-like pains (53.1%). Seven also had mechanical pain. Davidoff and Roth (1991) had 19 SCI patients; pain qualities were cutting (63%), burning (58%), piercing (47%), radiating (47%), tight (37%), cruel (37%), nagging (37%). SCI and syringomyelia pain may have a prominent dysesthetic element, e.g., "pins and needles" and stretching or pressure of the skin. Dysesthesias may be particularly common in incomplete spinal lesions (Davidoff *et al.* 1987b; Beric *et al.* 1988).

8. Intensity
The intensity of the pain varies from mild, unpleasant tingling to one of the most agonizing torments known to humans. When more components of pain are present, the intermittent will be the more severe. The steady component is generally fluctuating during the day and from day to day, also in bursts of activity and cyclically (namely, every other day or even every other week) (Falci *et al.* 2002) and is not always so harassing as to induce the patient to ask for medical help. Pain may be more intense in the legs (Widerstrom-Noga *et al.* 2001). Generally speaking, CCP is always very intense. In the series of Garcia-Larrea and colleagues (2003) of 32 SC incomplete injury cases, CP was never scored less than 7. In the series of Rogano and colleagues (2003), mean VAS score was 9.4, with pain more severe with gunshot injuries ($p < 0.001$). A higher level of education may be reflected in more perceived pain. SCI CP may or may not be perceived as worse than motor deficits (Nepomuceno *et al.* 1979; Davidoff *et al.* 1987).

9. Components
CCP consists of three components (Tasker *et al.* 1992): a steady, spontaneous pain (almost all), an intermittent, spontaneous pain (about one-third, singly found in 1% of patients) and evoked pain (about one-half, singly in 3%). So, for instance, a single patient may complain of episodic lightning pains down a leg, superimposed on a continuous background of burning pain. Intermittent pain is particularly common in patients with T10−L1 injuries, whether complete or incomplete (57%), and often shooting down one or both legs: 69% of Tasker's CCP patients with intermittent pain had thoracolumbar lesions. The steady, intermittent and evoked components are often associated in a single patient. The type of pain has no rapport with the causative lesion (Tasker *et al.* 1992).

10. Evoked pains
Evoked pain does not depend on the vertebral level nor on the completeness of the spinal lesion and exclusively occurs in areas of incompletely or clinically undetectable sensory loss or as a band at the upper margin of complete sensory loss; it can be elicited throughout the entire area of hypoestesia or only in part of it, by one or several modalities of sensory stimulation (Tasker *et al.* 1992). Trigger points can be identified even distant from areas of sensory deficit. In rare instances, evoked pain affects skin with clinically normal sensation (hyperesthesia). Overall, evoked pains

TABLE 3.5. Clinical features (representative series; Defrin *et al.* 2001)

15 SCI pts with below-level pain

Quality of pain:
  burning: 73%
  electric shock-like: 53%
  pressing: 27%
  cutting: 20%
  shooting: 18%

Pain was described as deep by 93% of pts (superficial by 7%)
Pain localization (tested areas):
  tight: 55%
  shin: 83%
  foot: 100%

Onset of pain: from several days to 8 years after the injury (within 1 mo: 46%; within 2 mos: 59%; within 6 mos: 93%).
Pain increased with the years in 73% of pts, ameliorated in 6% and remained unchanged in 20%.

Factors affecting pain sensation:
  external or internal factors exacerbated pain in 94% of pts:
  environmental temperature change: 70%
  illness (fever, infection): 50%
  changes in the fullness of GI or urinary system: 27%
  mental state: 26%

Ameliorating factors in 30% of pts:
  warming the room or limb: 61%
  evacuation of the bladder or stomach: 46%
  sport activity or work: 30%
  alcohol consumption: 23%
  posture change: 15%
  medication (CBZ, clonazepam, baclofen and dypirone): 84%

may be less frequent in SCI than in other CPs (Beric 1999). Tasker and colleagues (1992) observed evoked pain in about 40% of patients with complete lesions and in about 50% of those with incomplete lesions. The Danish group (Finnerup *et al.* 2003a) found that 60% of their patients had allodynia (30% tactile, 26% cold, 14% warm), while Garcia-Larrea and colleagues (2003) observed it in 7/32 CCP cases (21.5%); the SCI patients of Falci and colleagues (2002) rarely showed allodynia (7% touch allodynia).

CCP can be worsened by the same factors as BCP, as well as skin sores and infections. Factors such as secondary gain or drug-seeking behavior will significantly affect the severity and chronicity of the pain.

Table 3.5 gives summary data in a representative series.

11. Somatosensory deficits (Table 3.6)

In CCP, like BCP, temperature and pain sensation is uniformly absent or impaired, unlike touch and vibration sensation (Beric 1999). All patients have involvement of the STT, with very few exceptions, although STT damage can be present without CCP (Beric 1999; Eide *et al.* 1996; Defrin *et al.* 2001; Finnerup *et al.* 2003).

TABLE 3.6. Somatosensory findings in selected series

Eide *et al.* (1996). Spinal cord injury

Sixteen SCI pts. Somatosensory testing carried out within a normal skin area above the lesion level, within a non-painful skin area with impaired sensory perception and within a painful skin area with impaired sensory perception.

Threshold temperatures for warm, cold heat and heat pain determined by a Thermotester; thresholds for tactile sensation assessed by Von Frey hairs; two-point discrimination tested with a compass; vibration tested with a tuning fork; light touch examined by means of a cotton wool; joint position tested conventionally. Allodynia tested by applying an electric toothbrush and wind-up-like pain evoked by repeatedly pricking the skin. Below-level pain in (presumably) 6/16 pts. In 10 pts (presumably) there was at-level pain. Results not broken down according to the level of pain.

Authors' conclusion: Threshold values for detection of thermal (heat, cold, heat pain, cold pain) and tactile stimulation significantly changed in denervated skin areas, without significant differences between painful and non-painful denervated areas. Sensibility for touch, vibration, joint position and two-point discrimination not significantly differing between denervated painful and non-painful areas. Allodynia and wind-up-like pain significantly more common in painful than non-painful denervated areas.

Bouhassira *et al.* (2000). Syringomyelia

Twenty-one consecutive pts (7 women, 14 men; mean age 39 yrs; median duration of symptoms 6 yrs) with clinical and radiologic (MRI) evidence of syringomyelia. Painful syringomyelia in 10 pts (48%). No statistical difference for age, mean duration and etiology of syrinx between pts with and without pain. No analgesic at evaluation.
Mean VAS at evaluation: 4.7. Pain commonly described as burning, often associated with paroxysmal lancinating pain. Area of maximal pain confined within the area of maximal thermal deficit in 8/10 pts; in 2 pts with unilateral deficit, pain was localized on the "normal" side, where no thermal or mechanical deficits were evident.

Clinical examination

Sense	Assessed by means of:	Notes
Touch	Cotton swab	
Graphesthesia		
Joint position		Detection of movement direction
Stereognosis		
Vibration	Vibrameter	
Pinprick	Pinwheel	
Thermal sensibility extension	Thermo–rollers (40 and 25°C)	
Thermal detection thresholds (warm and cold)	Thermotest (0–50.5°C)	
Thermal pain thresholds	Thermotest (5–48°C)	
Detection of pain threshold to mechanical stimuli	Von Frey hairs	After threshold determination, application of pseudorandom suprathreshold stimuli. Pain quantified on a VAS
Tactile (dynamic) allodynia	Brush	Repetitive brushing (3 times)

QST performed in the area of maximal thermal deficit and in a normal area for all pts. In pts with pain measurements were performed in both the area of maximal spontaneous pain and an adjacent lesioned but not painful area.

Neurologic functions	Statistically significant difference between			Differences between pts with	
	Pain pts (n = 10) and pain-free pts (n = 11)	Maximal pain area and non-painful adjacent area	"Pure" pain*	"Pure" pain (n = 5)*	"Hyperalgesia" (n = 5)†
Warm detection threshold	No	No	No	46.6°C	35.5°C
Cold detection threshold	No	No	No	13.2°C	29°C
Heat pain threshold	No	No			Reduced (2)
Cold pain threshold	No	No			Reduced (3)
Cold detection threshold		No			
Mechanical deficits	No				
Mechanical detection threshold		No	No		
Mechanical pain threshold		No			Reduced (3)
Vibration deficits	No			Yes‡	
Extension of mechanical deficits	No				
Extension of vibration deficits	No				
Impaired graphesthesia	No	No		Yes‡	No (4)
Impaired detection of movement direction	No	No		Yes‡	
Impaired detection of joint position	No			Yes‡	
Tactile thresholds	No				No (4)

* "Pure" spontaneous ongoing pain located within an area of profound thermal deficit. Stimulus–response curves not significantly different in that area and adjacent non-painful areas.

† Pattern of stimulus–response curves to thermal and mechanical stimuli suggestive of hyperalgesia. Less severe sensory deficits. In some pts reduced pain thresholds, suggestive of allodynia (in 2 pts there was a second allodynic/hyperalgesic area not coexisting with that of spontaneous pain but located in the border area).

‡ Symptoms suggestive of dorsal column lesion.

CP symptoms commonly confined within the area of maximal thermal deficit. Deficits magnitude between painful and adjacent non-painful lesioned area and between pain and pain-free pts not different. Two groups of pts, with different sensory deficits. Lesion of the STT is a necessary, but probably not sufficient condition to account for CP

(continued)

TABLE 3.6 (continued)

Defrin et al. (2001). Spinal cord injury

Characterization of chronic pain (mean duration 14.9 yrs, range 2.35 yrs) and somatosensory function in SCI subjects. Pts with

  incomplete SCI and chronic below-level pain (= CP): 15 (mean age: 38.9 ± 9.2 yrs)
  incomplete SCI without chronic pain: 7 (mean age: 37.6 ± 9.1 yrs)
  healthy volunteers: 18 (mean age: 35.6 ± 7.4 yrs)

Lesion level: restricted to lumbar and thoracic segments (L3–T4). Hand considered intact area above lesion. All pain pts complained of pain in the legs. 60% of SCI-CP pts injured in the T12–L1 region. Pts without pain had injuries distributed equally along L3–T4 ($p < 0.01$).

Neurological examination:

Three test sessions. Sensory testing was conducted below the level of injury. Testing regions (standardized areas): mid-thigh, middle of the lateral shin, center of the dorsal aspect of foot. No test in these areas if the pt refused to allow further testing (very painful/sensitive area). Testing was also conducted in all areas from which pain originates. Pts with lumbar lesion were tested only in distal areas. Reference area: dorsal surface of the hand. Pain rating: VAS (0–10).

Sensory examination

Sensibility	Test method	Notes
Spinothalamic function		
Warmth	Computerized thermal	Warmth, cold, cold pain and heat pain
Cold	stimulator	thresholds measured with the method of
Heat pain		limits (cut-off values: warmth 45°C, cold
Cold pain		15°C, thermal pain 53°C)
Dorsal column function		
Fine touch	Piece of cotton fabric	Closed eyes
Graphesthesia		Identification of 2 digits (numbers 2 and 3) and
		geometric shape (circle and square) traced on the
		skin. Intact dorsal column specifically required
Stimulus movement	Finger movement on the skin	Report of movement, direction and velocity.
on the skin	(10 cm/4 s and 10 cm/1 s)	Intact dorsal column specifically required
Allodynia		
Static allodynia	Single application of a	
	Von Frey hair	
Dynamic allodynia	Dragging of the Von Frey hair	
	along the limb	
Mechanical wind-up pain	Consecutive application of a	Two different rates: 1 stimulus every 3 s
	Von Frey hair	and 1 stimulus every 10 s
Hyperpathia	Heating of the skin	

A 4-point rank order scale was constructed for all normal sensations tested. Statistical analysis performed between groups.

Threshold values for warmth, cold and heat pain and qualitative evaluation of tactile sensibilities were stable across testing sessions. SCI pts both with and without CP had a mixture of skin areas with normal and abnormal sensation below the lesion level.

Mean thresholds (SD) for sensation

	Warm	Cold	Heat pain	p
SCI with CP	42.4 (3.5)	15.3 (8.8)	48.8 (4.3)	
SCI without CP	42.8 (3.0)	14.3 (6.9)	48.6 (4.2)	
Normal subjects	35.9 (2.0)	28.5 (1.8)	42.4 (2.4)	<0.01[*]

	Warm	Cold	Heat pain	p
SCI pts with CP				
Painful skin areas	43.9 (2.7)	17 (4.5)	49.5 (4.1)	
Painless skin areas[†]	36.2 (2.4)	26.9 (4.0)	42.0 (3.5)	<0.001

* SCI versus normal. No differences between SCI groups.
† Thresholds almost identical to those of normal subjects.

Patients both with and without CP showed significant impairment in thermal sensibilities without significant difference. Pain appeared only in regions with thermal sensibility impairment and, in the same pt, pain was perceived in all areas with impaired thermal sensibility. In CP - but not in pain-free - pts, a much more severe impairment of thermal sensibility was seen in the feet compared to the shins and thighs ($p < 0.05$).

Test areas with preserved thermal and tactile sensation in pts with and without CP

	58 test areas	38 test areas	
Sensation	SCI-CP pts, N (%)	Pain-free SCI pts, N (%)	p
Warmth	17 (29)	18 (47)	ns
Cold	19 (32)	16 (42)	ns
Heat pain	17 (29)*	12 (32)[†]	ns
Touch	47 (81)	33 (87)	ns
Graphesthesia	25 (43)	19 (50)	ns
Speed of movement	26 (45)	21 (55)	ns

* In 20/29 regions thermal noxious stimulation ($48.1 \pm 2.9°C$) produced pricking pain without thermal characteristics and followed by explosive hyperpathic pain, also lacking thermal characteristics.
† Loss of thermal sensation and pricking pain only in 5/38 regions, with hyperpathic response.

Pts with CP tended to have a more severe impairment of spinothalamic function. Dorsal column function appeared identical in both groups. Anterolateral cord function was more severely impaired than dorsal column function ($p < 0.01$).

		No. of SCI pts			
Abnormal sensations		CP	Pain-free	p*	Mean VAS (range)
Allodynia[†]		12/15 (80%)	0/7 (0%)	<0.001	5.6 (2.4-9.3)
	Mechanical dynamic	12/12 (100%)			
	Mechanical static	1/12 (8%)			
Wind-up pain[‡]		11/15 (73%)	1/7 (14%)	<0.001	
Hyperpathic[§]		13/15 (87%)	2/7 (29%)	<0.01	8.6 (3.7-10)

* Chi-square test. According to authors: 0, 21. Recalculated with Fisher exact test: 0.03–0.26.
† Incidence: foot, 81%; shin, 66%; thigh, 25%. Normal thermal thresholds only in 3% of allodynic areas. No difference between thermal thresholds in allodynic areas and non-allodynic painful areas. Tactile sensibility more spared in allodynic areas ($p < 0.05$). Thermal sensibility more impaired than tactile sensibility ($p < 0.05$). Intense pain from touch of fabric or bed sheet in some pts.
‡ Elicited only at stimulation rate of 1/3 s and only in 42% of painful areas.
§ Elicited only in 44% of painful areas. Thermal thresholds in these regions were elevated when compared to non-hyperpathic regions. Heat pain thresholds were, in contrast, reduced. No difference in cold thresholds or dorsal column function.

Abnormal sensations were elicited almost exclusively in pts with spontaneous pain and only in (spontaneously) painful regions. Only 48% of allodynic areas were also hyperpathic and only 61% of hyperpathic areas were also allodynic. Non-hyperpathic allodynic areas had completely impaired spinothalamic function, which may account for the lack of hyperpathia.

Damage to ascending anterolateral conduction system, and not the dorsal columns, necessary but not sufficient condition for the development of CP. Pain-free areas do not show spinothalamic impairment in CP pts. No relationship between the degree of imbalance in somatosensory transmission and intensity of chronic pain.

(continued)

TABLE 3.6 *(continued)*

Finnerup *et al.* (2003). Spinal cord injury

Comparison of clinical examination, quantitative sensory testing (QST) and somatosensory evoked potentials (SEPs) in 3 similar groups of 20 SCI pts with spontaneous pain (below-level pain, at least 2 dermatome segments below the lesion level) or dysesthesia, 20 SCI pts without pain and 20 non-injured subjects. Pain onset within 6 months in 13 pts. Lower lesion level above T10 in all SCI pts (MRI confirmed, injury above the conus medullaris). Mean duration of pain 14 yrs. No analgesic allowed during the study. Pain assessment: VAS/NRS. SEPs were determined in 14 pain and 12 pain-free pts (posterior tibial nerve stimulation). Responses scored as normal, decreased and absent.

Clinical examination

Sense	Assessment (carried out 10 cm below the dominant knee) by means of:	Notes
Tactile sensitivity	Von Frey hairs (Semmes-Weinstein monofilaments)	Single stimuli. Detection within 3 s
Touch localization	Cotton wool	Detection within 2 s
Slowly moving stimulus	Cotton wool	Ability to determine the stimulus and its direction
Vibration	Electronic vibrameter	Tested on the anterior surface of the tibia. 120 Hz, application pressure kept stable. Mean of 3 measurements as threshold
Thermal	Thermotest (0–50.5°C)	Warm and cold detection thresholds, heat and cold pain thresholds and heat pain tolerance recorded using the method of limits. Average of 5 measurements
Pressure pain	Hand-held electronic pressure algometer	Assessed over the anterior tibial muscle
Skinfold pinch pain	Forceps coupled to an algometer	Tested above the knee
Evoked pain		Studied below the level of injury, in the area of maximal pain, and at injury level. Border zone mapped for brush, pinprick and cold
Brush-evoked pain	Small brush	
Cold allodynia	Thermo roll (20–22°C)	
Pinprick hyperalgesia	Von Frey hair	Repetitive tapping

Neurologic functions

	SCI with pain	N	D	I	A	P	NA	SCI without pain	N	D	I	A	P	NA	P*
Spontaneous below-level pain	20/20							0							
Dysesthesia	19/20							†							
Spontaneous at-level pain	5/20							0							
Pain restricted to an area with impaired pinprick or touch sensibility	19/20							0							
Allodynia	8/20							0							
Evoked below-level pain					16	4						20			
Evoked at-level sensations‡					10	10						17	3		
Evoked at-level pain¶					13	7						13	7		

SCI with pain	N	D	I	A	P	NA	SCI without pain	N	D	I	A	P	NA	P*
Thresholds detection														
Vibration	1	4	2	13				1[b]	5		13[b]		1	ns
Tactile (single stimulus)	1	5		14				1[b]	6		13[b]			ns
Pinprick			3	17					1		19[b]			
Cold (0–30°C)		2		18[b]				1[b]			19[b]			ns
Cold pain														ns
Warm (30–50.5°C)	1	1		18[b]							20			ns
Heat pain														ns
Heat pain tolerance														ns
Pressure pain	2[b]			14	4				1		16[b]	3[b]		ns
Pressure pain tolerance														ns
Skinfold pinch pain	2[b]			12	6			1[b]			16[b]	3[b]		ns
Skinfold pinch pain tolerance														ns
Tactile pain														ns
SEP	1	3		10	6				4		8	8		

N: normal; D: decreased; I: increased; A: absent; P: present; NA: not accessible (not done).
* P: statistically significant difference between pain and pain-free SCI pts.
† Pts in the pain-free SCI group had non-painful sensations described as pricking, tingling, taut, warm or throbbing.
‡ Pain/dysesthesia from brush or cold; pinprick hyperalgesia.
¶ Pain from repetitive pinprick.
ᵃ Non-consensual; ᵇ consensual.

Median pain intensity score: 5 (on a 0–10 NRS). The area of pain generally represented a fraction of the area with sensory abnormalities.

Pain described as: pricking, tingling, burning or scalding, freezing, taut.

Mechanical and thermal detection and pain thresholds and SEPs were similarly reduced in pts with or without pain.

At-level brush- or cold-evoked pain, dysesthesia or pinprick hyperalgesia were more frequent in pts with pain than in those without pain, but the intensity of pain evoked by repeated at-level pinprick did not differ between the 2 groups.

There was a significant correlation between intensity of at-level brush-evoked dysesthesia and below-level spontaneous pain.

The lesion of the spinothalamic tract alone cannot account for CP in SCI. Neuronal hyperexcitability at injury or higher level may be an important mechanism for pain below injury level.

Attal et al. (2004). Syringomyelia

Sixteen consecutive pts (4 women, 12 men; mean age 36.9 (±10.2) yrs; mean duration of symptoms 5.2 yrs, range 6 months on 14 yrs) with clinical and radiologic (MRI) evidence of syringomyelia associated with Chiari type I malformation ($n = 11$) or spinal cord trauma with syringomyelia above the injury ($n = 5$).

Pts with neuropathic pain at the sensory level: 8/16 (50%)

Mean pain duration: 3.9 (± 3.2) yrs

Pain intensity (baseline):

continuous ongoing pain at rest: about 45/100 mm (VAS)
pain aggravated by strain: about 65/100 mm (VAS)
(numerical values not reported, data inferred from Fig. 4)
Clinical examination and QST performed as previously reported in Bouhassira et al. (2000).

(continued)

TABLE 3.6 *(continued)*

Overall results:

thermal and mechanical (pinprick) deficits in 16/16 pts
anesthesia to heat in 6/16 pts
anesthesia to cold in 8/16 pts
vibration deficits or fine tactile impairment in 11/16 pts
vibration deficits in the feet in 7/11 pts with Chiari malformation.

Pts presumably at least in part already reported in Attal *et al.* (1999) and Bouhassira *et al.* (2000).

In a minority of patients, the initially documented sensory loss may fade, even though pain subsequently develops. Some studies failed to demonstrate any differences in STT and lemniscal function between patients with CP and pain-free patients or between painful and nonpainful denervated areas (Eide *et al.* 1996; Finnerup *et al.* 2003). Tasker and colleagues (1992) described a patient with trauma-related CCP, who had a normal appreciation of temperature and pinprick. Yet, the patient was not studied with electrophysiological methods.

12. Sympathetic and other signs and symptoms

Similar comments as made for BCP apply to CCP. Sometimes (> 20%), following total spinal cord transection, after the phase of spinal shock, the patient complains of *phantom sensations* referred to the legs, and these are very similar to amputees' sensations, being painful, uncomfortable and unpleasant, but not disabling. They appear early, almost immediately after SCI and vanish soon after SCI (rarely they linger on for months) (e.g., Davis and Martin 1947; see Beric 1999). Unlike amputees, telescoping or shrinkage of the involved body parts occurs only rarely in paraplegics and the length or posture of the phantom do not change; in addition, they are less vivid. Paraplegics describe sensations projected from the surface, but few postural sensations, with both voluntary and involuntary movements of the phantoms. Phantom sensations must be distinguished from phantom pain. CP appears when phantom sensations fade.

13. Course

Although in some cases it lasts only a few months, if paraplegia pain persists for longer than 6–8 months after the injury (the majority), it will become a long-term problem. Unlike BCP which usually tends not to change significantly, except in degree, over time, CCP may change markedly, even dramatically, over the years: it may increase in severity for several years and even change in distribution and quality, sometimes dramatically. The patients of Davis and Martin (1947) complained of hot burning suddenly turning into "streams of fire" or pressure of a knife being burned in the tissue, twisted around rapidly and finally withdrawn. Some patients follow an aggressive course with intensity escalation, a few having an abatement of pain after a few years which becomes nondisabling (Beric 1999; Tasker 2001a). In Davis and Martin's (1947) series, 40 of 217 patients still experienced pain in the long term.

SPECIAL CONSIDERATIONS

1. Syringomyelia

Syringomyelia (in the spinal cord) and syringobulbia (in the lower brainstem) are rare diseases. The lesion is a cystic cavity filled with CSF-like fluid, varying from a small lesion in the dorsal part of the spinal cord over a couple of segments to huge cavities extending from the most caudal part of the cord into the medulla oblongata (Milhorat *et al.* 1996 and references therein). The largest cavities leave only a thin layer of spinal cord tissue undamaged at the maximally cavitated regions; gray matter necrosis and wallerian degeneration are usually seen. Cavities are thought to arise in the center of the cord, which is where STT fibers cross the midline to reach their position in the ventrolaterally located STT. A lesion with this location will affect the sensibility to temperature and pain, i.e., a dissociated sensory loss will appear. Syrinxes may be associated with Chiari I malformation, cervical disk disease/ spondylosis, basilar impression and communicating hydrocephalus; they may also be posttraumatic and be caused by spinal cord hematomas.

Spontaneous pain and subjective sensory disturbances may often precede by many years any other sign of this slowly progressing disease. The complaint is especially common with posttraumatic syringomyelia. Pain is generally segmental, involving one arm (seldom both), neck, shoulder and hemithorax, i.e., in the distribution of the suspended dissociated sensory loss (Garcin 1968). Facial pain is frequently reported with syringobulbia. Below-level pain (e.g., leg, generally singly) is rare, and can be observed when the syrinx enlarges. Segmental pain is attributed to lesions of the dorsal horns or of spinothalamic fibers crossing the midline. Sensations range from an unbearable dysesthetic crawling to acute, severe, violent, lancinating (but also burning, aching and pressing) pain; warmth and cold are often felt as painful, and radiation may be present (Riddoch 1938). At first they are unilateral and intermittent, occurring in attacks; later they become bilateral and continuous (likely due to skewed unilateral encroachment with greater pain-inducing damage), and may persist even when analgesia and thermanesthesia in the affected dermatomes are complete. One series (Ducreux *et al.* 2006) showed that 27 out of 31 patients suffered CP in the arm, 12 with additional pain in the neck or in the thorax, and another 5 in both the thorax and the leg. CP extended over 2–10 dermatomes, unilaterally in 24. Spontaneous pain occurred on its own in 11 and was associated with evoked pain in 20 (allodynia to brush 12, heat 5, and cold 11). Pain was described as burning in 23, deep (pressure, squeezing) in 14, paroxysmal (electric shocks, stabbing) in 19; paresthesias and/or dysesthesias (tingling, pins-and-needles) were reported in 24.

Painful dysesthesias (burning pain, pins-and-needles, stretching-pressure of the skin, in most cases hyperesthesias) occur in $\leq40\%$ of syringomyelia patients (see references in Milhorat *et al.* 1996) and may be more frequent in females (39 versus 12 males in the series of Milhorat *et al.* 1996). In that series, MRI demonstrated extension of the syrinx into the dorsolateral quadrant of the spinal cord on the same side and at the level of pain in 43/51 (84%) cases. In 42/51 cases, the dermatomal pattern of pain overlapped with a segment of analgesia–anesthesia. Obvious trophic changes were seen in 15/51 patients (29%).

Quantitative sensory testing (QST) shows that all patients with syrinx have abnormal temperature and pain sensibility, mostly pronounced with total loss of temperature sensibility. Patients in advanced stages also have impairment of lemniscal sensibility. For instance, Attal and colleagues (2004) performed QST before and after surgery (3 and 9 months) in patients with cervical and dorsolumbar syrinxes, most suffering pain. Thermoalgesic, but not lemniscal, deficits were found in all. Spontaneous pain was generally located within an area of thermal defict, but its intensity was not correlated with the magnitude of the deficit. Surgery induced a significant decrease of the deficits (tactile more than thermal), but those on pain were variable and not correlated with the effects on thermal sensibility.

Nashold (1991), in his series of paraplegics with pain, found a spinal cyst in 60% of the patients, generally extending from the site of the spinal trauma rostrally, involving multiple segments of the normal spinal cord. In a few patients, at operation, two separate cysts that extended above and below the site of the trauma were found, but they were not interconnected.

Paraplegics who suffer from a traumatic syringomyelia often develop pain extending above injury level, even many years after injury (15 in one of the patients of Durward et al. 1982), probably due to the slow enlargement of the spinal cyst and the subsequent pressure on the normal spinal cord above the level of the trauma; up to two-thirds of paraplegics with pain of delayed onset exhibit a syringomyelia. The pain is generally sharp or aching, electrical and burning in character, being often located in the dermatomes adjacent to the injury level, but may expand to involve higher dermatomes. The paraplegic is often aware that his or her sensory level has risen, and, if a spinal cyst encroaches on the cervical spinal cord, motor deficits can occur in the arms. This pain may be activated along with diffuse visceral pain by infections of the urinary tract or by constipation. Continuous escalation in pain is the natural course. Shunting is generally ineffective in reversing the pain in a significant number of cases (Dworkin and Staats 1985; Milhorat et al. 1996; Kramer and Levine 1997).

Type I Chiari malformations can originate a central cord syndrome with symptoms including pain (frequently "burning"), often diffuse, but also restricted to a few dermatomes, most often in the cervical region and arms, plus dissociated and posterior column sensory loss, due to tonsillar herniation or the associated syrinx (Meadows et al. 2001; Bejjani and Cockerham 2001).

2. Multiple sclerosis (MS)

CP as a symptom of MS has been recognized since the nineteenth century (De Ajuraguerra 1937). Plaques of demyelination are most frequently found in the spinal cord, particularly in the dorsal columns, in the brainstem and periventricularly in the forebrain. Yet, despite the difficulty in determining the exact location of the lesions that result in CP, due to widespread dissemination in the CNS, nonetheless, the topographical distribution of the symptoms and signs in MS appear to indicate that many, perhaps the majority, of the MS lesions that cause CP are spinal.

The largest (1672 patients from 26 centers) and best conducted study to date found a prevalence of CP of 18.1% (Solaro et al. 2004); trigeminal neuralgia, found in 2%, and Lhermitte's sign (9%) are also considered part of the CP spectrum. All previous studies showed major flaws, making them unreliable or "not sufficient to evaluate the prevalence of CP versus nociceptive pain" (Svendsen *et al.* 2005; see global discussion in Solaro *et al.* 2004). CP is correlated with increasing age, EDSS, disease duration, but not sex. Some patients with MS have CP for a limited period during relapses (days to months); others have chronic CP. Since the worldwide prevalence is estimated nearly 3 million, we expect that about 500 000 patients suffer CP.

MS CP is generally dysesthetic, but also tingling, pins-and-needles, pricking, cold or warm. Like all CPs several other qualities, singly or in combination, may be present, particularly burning and aching; a pressing belt-like (girdle) pain at the level of the upper border of the lesion may also be seen.

CP, when maximal, was generally described as tingling (59%), tiring (52%), taut (45%), burning, dull and grueling (41% each) in one study (Svendsen *et al.* 2005). Intensity is often high. Pruritus is also part of the spectrum (Canavero *et al.* 1997). During relapses, it can affect any part of the body, in different combinations at different levels; in chronic stages, a great majority of those affected have pain in the lower extremities, about one-third in the arm, and one-fifth in the trunk, partially or totally, unilaterally (one-quarter) or bilaterally (three-quarters), hemipain being uncommon. In MS patients it is not possible to relate the time of the onset of pain to the time of development of the demyelinating lesions, because the latter cannot be determined with certainty. However, some patients experience CP before other symptoms, others complain of pain along with other symptoms and signs. It tends to be worst at night and to affect less disabled patients. The pain tends to be constant, but can be intermittent, deep more than superficial or both, and can radiate (Svendsen *et al.* 2005).

As for other CPs, there is no correlation between pain and nonsensory signs. Not infrequently, patients have signs of involvement of the posterior column-lemniscal rather than spinothalamic dysfunction (Moulin *et al.* 1988), which can be less prominent than, for example, in CPSP (Portenoy *et al.* 1988). Osterberg *et al.* (1994) found decreased innocuous temperature – heat and cold (90%), pinprick (60%) and noxious temperature (80%) (plus 82% and 72% for vibration and touch); only two patients had no spinothalamic impairment at QST (note that there is a duplicate paper from this group [Osterberg *et al.* 2005] with differing data from the same study population). A recent study that employed QST found STT involvement in all CP cases (Svendsen *et al.* 2005): all CP patients had signs of STT dysfunction with decreased or increased sensation to pinprick and/or temperature sense at maximal pain site. MS patients with pain had decreased sensibility to touch, temperature and vibration versus healthy subjects, but no differences between patients with and without pain were detected in detection thresholds evaluated by QST, although patients with pain tended to have higher vibration and tactile detection thresholds. Results from bedside testing and QST differed: a higher frequency of pain patients had decreased sensation to touch, vibration/joint position and warmth compared with pain-free subjects at bedside examination. However, even on QST, there was a tendency of lower tactile pain threshold in the pain group and pressure pain detection threshold was lower and cold allodynia as well as temporal summation were more frequent in the pain group.

Contrary to some belief, allodynia is found in MS patients: generally it consists of anomalous sensations as one passes a hand over the affected area or worsening of pain or dysesthesias during movement. CP can also develop or worsen during a rise of temperature (exercise, sunbathing), so-called Uhthoff's sign. In one study (Svendsen *et al.* 2005), aggravating factors were cold in 12 patients, warmth in 5, same position for a long time in 11, body movement including walking in 6, physical strain in 6, touch (clothes, etc.) in 9, tiredness in 4, stress in 2 and loud noise in 1. Alleviating factors were physiotherapy/massage/extension in 12 cases, analgesics in 11, rest in 5, warmth in 4, cold in 4, change of position in 4 and body movements in 3. Touch allodynia was most commonly reported in CP patients: these more often had cold and/or mechanical allodynia than patients with musculoskeletal pain (a statistically significant difference). The frequency of temporal summation tended to be higher in CP patients.

In MS, facial pain is at first usually identical to tic douloureux, with plaques involving the trigeminal root entry zone. Later, with involvement of the descending root, pain becomes continuous and disagreeable and paresthesias appear.

In MS (as well as cervical spondylotic chronic myelopathies and extramedullary tumors, both cervical and of the foramen magnum), an uncomfortable, not truly painful, sensation, closely resembling that produced by an electric current, can be elicited by the active or passive flexion of the head, and radiating from the cervical to the coccigeal region and to the four limbs, so-called Lhermitte's sign (Lhermitte *et al.* 1927; Garcin 1968).

3. Spinal epilepsy

Tonic-clonic fits sometimes accompanied by paroxysmal burning, lancinating or even electric shock-like pain in the legs, glutei or pelvis, both ipsi and contralateral to the fits, have been described for extramedullary tumors, multiple sclerosis and transverse myelitis (McAlhany and Netsky 1955; Ekbom *et al.* 1968; Harrington and Bone 1981). Nathanson (1962) reported a patient with an extramedullary meningioma at T1 presenting with paroxysms of severe burning pain, lasting about twenty seconds in the left buttock and leg, with stiffening of the entire limb (the thigh slowly flexed on the hip as the leg partially extended). Pagni and Regolo (1987) reported the case of a woman who presented tonic-clonic spasms followed by clonic jerks in the left limb, along with pain in the glutei and in the anterior aspect of the leg: an anterior meningioma at T10 was found. In both cases, the attacks ceased within a few days of tumor removal. Miró and colleagues (1988) described paroxysmal pelvic pain, occurring 1–3 times a day, as a symptom of MS. Pagni and Canavero (1993) reported a woman with paroxysms of pelvic pain resembling tic douloureux: the pain, which was at first itching and burning, became electric shock-like as the frequency of the attacks, which always lasted a few seconds, increased in time. MRI disclosed a dorsal extramedullary meningioma at T6–7. Carbamazepine – and, later, surgery – abolished the attacks.

The dorsal columns are known to convey visceral nociception (Willis and Westlund 2004). In spinal cases, focal demyelination induced by compression can induce hyperexcitable foci in the cord fibers and these foci may both discharge spontaneously and be triggered by mechanical distortion of the cord (Pagni and Canavero 1993). Such fibers convey nociception, making these patients instances of CP.

4 DIAGNOSING CENTRAL PAIN

CP is pain due to a CNS lesion along the spinothalamoparietal path. Thus, an appropriate lesion must be demonstrated in such a location. At the same time, the presence of PNP, which may mimic CP (e.g., diabetic polyneuropathy in stroke patients), but also nociceptive musculoskeletal pains, must be excluded. A common source of diagnostic uncertainty is that symptoms of CPSP regularly occur after a significant passage of time from the precipitating event, calling for careful interviewing.

CP is a somatosensory symptom. Nonsensory symptoms and signs do occur in many patients with CP, because they are a direct consequence of the lesions, which are seldom restricted to somatosensory structures, but these may be lacking completely.

CP is independent of nonsensory abnormalities, namely in muscle function, coordination, vision, hearing, vestibular functions and higher cortical functions, and these may be present at the moment of examination or have subsided. In addition, the degree of pain and sensory abnormalities may not be necessarily correlated with the severity of other neurologic disabilities (Riddoch 1938; Garcin 1968; Tasker 2001). The distribution of these abnormalities will overlap or contain the perceived location of the pain.

Mental status is usually normal and CP patients are no more depressed or anxious than other chronic pain patients; psychiatric consultation is unnecessary. The psychological evaluation is usually done with the Minnesota Personality Inventory (MMPI), and other more detailed psychological tests (Hamilton, Beck, etc.) as indicated; elevation on the scales of depression, hysteria and somatization is important in sorting out the dysfunctional state.

Only the accompanying neurologic symptoms and signs help distinguish the different subtypes of CP, caused by cord, brainstem or brain damage: pain and dysesthesias have the same characteristics whatever the level or etiology. Similar symptoms can be caused not only by diseases affecting primarily the CNS, but also by lesions neighboring the neuraxis (e.g., extramedullary tumors) and damaging the nervous tissue only secondarily. Sometimes pain is the presenting symptom and remains an isolated finding for a long time, as occurs in syringomyelia, and exceptionally other diseases (e.g., spinal cord tumors).

By adhering to the following ladder, diagnosis of CP will be secured in practically all patients. Particularly in spinal cord lesion cases, CP can be missed among other accompanying pains or be misidentified for nociceptive pain tout court. CP appears in many disguises and therefore requires a meticulous diagnostic workup.

STEP 1. A comprehensive bedside examination should be performed, above all probing of somatosensory functions with cotton (touch sensation), an ice cube and a warm vial (temperature sensation) and a pin (pain sensation). Quantitative sensory testing (QST) may be indicated when sensory loss is not readily demonstrated, although bedside testing and QST may not totally overlap (see a review of techniques in Dotson 1997). The best way to get a history from a CP patient is to ask about all possible pain qualities, rather than leaving it up to the patient, who will usually not get past the burning dysesthesia and lancinating pains. Body distribution and any summations or gradients should be included in the description. Painstaking and repetitious questioning is required. Experience and subtlety are required for evaluation. A pain drawing filled out by the patient helps delineate the distribution of spontaneous pain (a pain diary assesses intensity fluctuations and, later, response to therapy). Sensory testing should start in an unaffected area and compared to testing in the affected area, moving outward until skin that responds normally to stimuli is found (and vice versa when testing for evoked pains, in order to minimize the patient's exposure to painful stimuli). Description of pain (quality, intensity, etc.) is usually assessed with Huskisson's numerical rating scale (0: no pain; 10: worst imaginable pain) and/or visual analog scale (NRS/VAS) and the McGill Pain Questionnaire (MPQ), a multidimensional inventory of pain, the Sternbach Pain and Intensity Profile, the Zhung Pain and Distress Scale, and others (Elliott et al. 2003). Magnitude of CP may be inferred indirectly by self-reports or interference with social, vocational and daily life activities. CP can also be inferred from observable behavior, including facial grimace, and abnormal movement or posture. Afferent function may on occasion be assessed by differential blocks implemented by either mechanical pressure (direct nerve compression or tourniquet ischemia) or injection of local anesthetics. Mechanical methods block fibers in order of size (Aβ, mechanical, first; Aδ, cooling and first pain perception, second; C, warming and second pain perception, last) with recovery in the reverse order. These sequences are reversed for local anesthetic blocks. Such blocks help dissect the type of fibers subserving evoked pains, as each recognizes different mechanisms.

STEP 2. MRI of the brain and cord is the neuroimaging technique of choice in all patients: it should reveal a CNS lesion that is consistent with the findings on neurologic examination. However, it cannot be relied upon exclusively in differentiating between complete and incomplete cord lesions.

STEP 3. When there is no clear-cut lesion visible on MRI and/or QST, cutaneous stimulation of Aδ fibers with pulses from an infrared or argon (or more tissue damaging CO_2) laser, which are selectively sensitive to abnormalities along the STT activated by noxious and thermal stimuli, will usually reveal a late potential recorded from the vertex at a peak negative wave latency of approximately 250 ms followed by a peak positivity of about 320 ms (LEPs). A dissociation between LEP reduction and increased pain sensation is possible (Casey *et al.* 1996; Wu *et al.* 1999). Ordinary somatosensory evoked potentials (SSEPs) evoked by electrical stimulation of the median and tibial/sural nerves assess Aβ dorsal column-lemniscal (touch-vibration) mechanoreceptive fibers: these may impaired in CP, but, as discussed, are not the prime mover; however, the N150-P260 component of the SSEPs may be a good correlate of subjectively experienced pain (Treede and Bromm 1991). If LEPs are not available, the latency of the flexion reflex (RIII reflex) in patients with CP (particularly CCP) should be investigated: this is dependent on activation of nociceptor afferents. Lesions in the CNS leading to decreased pain sensibility result in a delay (prolongation) of this reflex following electrical stimulation of the sural nerve (Dehen *et al.* 1983; Weiller *et al.* 1989). Some patients will show no sign of impairment at the time of examination; of course, this does not exclude that they had this initially.

STEP 4. In doubtful cases or in order to assess therapeutic response, SPECT/PET may be indicated as well as pharmacological dissection with subhypnotic propofol IV challenge (see Chapters 5 and 6). The propofol test is particularly useful in differentiating CP from (unresponsive) PNP and nociceptive pain in the cord trauma setting, but also the classic nociceptive shoulder pain of stroke patients.

EMG, thermography and regional blocks (Kingery 1997; Bonicalzi and Canavero 1999) have no place in the diagnostic approach to CP. However, abnormal lumbar SEPs in an incomplete quadriplegic or high paraplegic may provide clues as to a DLS, in those who present with leg or perineal segmental pain, while cauda equina versus conus medullaris pains can be differentiated by lumbosacral SEPs and videourodynamics (Beric 1999).

Some orienting clinical features of CP include (Garcin 1937, 1968; Pagni 1977):

a)   Pain from injury to the posterior horn of the spinal cord and Lissauer's tract is on the same side of the lesion and corresponds to the affected or neighboring metameres. Bilateral girdle pain is typical in cases of intramedullary tumors or syringomyelia. CP after thoracic lesions can be confused with DLS, which is usually sacral and lumbosacral, especially if at-level pain is also present. Under these circumstances, the pain can mimic CP, as it appears to cover the entire area below lesion level (Beric 1999).

b)   Pain from injury to the anterolateral funiculus of the cord is referred to the opposite side of the body below the lesion.

c)   Dysesthesias from injury to the posterior column or to the nuclei of Goll and Burdach are on the same side, below the lesion, and may be uni- or bilateral. Usually, they are of short duration. Lhermitte's sign is considered to be due to mechanical excitation of the posterior columns: it is observed not only in MS, but also in other myelopathies.

d)   Pain and dysesthesia due to vascular bulbar lesion (Wallenberg's syndrome) usually have a crossed distribution: to the face on the lesion side and to the limbs and trunk on the contralateral side. Bulbar lesions can give rise to

TABLE 4.1. Examination protocol for central pain (IASP)

DEFINITION: Pain caused by lesion or dysfunction in the central nervous system

DATE OF THIS REPORT:

HISTORICAL INFORMATION:

(1) Is pain the major or primary complaint? If not, indicate the alternative (e.g., weakness)

(2) Nature of primary neurologic disability
    (a) Primary diagnosis (e.g., stroke, tumor, etc.)
    (b) Location of disability (e.g., left hemiparesis)

(3) Date of onset of neurologic signs/symptoms
    Date of onset of pain

(4) Description of pain
    (a) Location:
        Body area — preferably use pain drawing
        Superficial (skin) and/or deep (muscle, viscera)
        Radiation or referral
    (b) Intensity (1–10 or VAS categorical scaling)
        Most common intensity: at maximum; at minimum
    (c) Temporal features
        Steady, unchanging
        Fluctuates over (minutes, hours, days, weeks)
        Paroxysmal features (shooting pain, tic-like)
    (d) Quality
        Thermal (burning, freezing, etc.)
        Mechanical (pressure, cramping, etc.)
        Chemical (stinging, etc.)
    (e) Factors increasing the pain (cold, emotions, etc.)
    (f) Factors decreasing the pain (rest, drugs, etc.)

(5) Neurological symptoms besides pain
    (a) Motor (paresis, ataxia, involuntary movements)
    (b) Sensory (hypo-, hyperesthesia, paresthesia, dysesthesia, numbness, overreaction)
    (c) Others (speech, visual, cognitive, mood, etc.)

EXAMINATION:

(1) Neurological disease — results of CT, MRI, SPECT, PET, CSF assays,
    neurophysiological examinations, etc.

(2) Major neurologic finding (e.g., spastic paraparesis)

(3) Sensory examination
    Preferably use sensory chart with the dermatomes. Indicate if modalities
    listed have normal, increased or decreased threshold, and paresthesias and
    dysesthesias are evoked
    (a) Vibratory sense (tuning fork, biothesiometer or vibrameter)
    (b) Tactile (cotton wool, hair movement — include von Frey if possible, nylon filaments)
    (c) Skin direction sense, graphesthesis
    (d) Kinesthesia (joint movements)
    (e) Temperature (specify how tested, e.g., Thermotest apparatus)
        Cold (noxious and innocuous); warm (noxious and innocuous)
    (f) Pinprick
    (g) Deep pain (specify how tested)
    (h) Allodynia
        To mechanical stimuli
        To cold
        To heat
    (i) Hyperpathia (specify how tested)
    (j) Other abnormalities like radiation, summation, prolonged after-sensation

bilateral facial pain if the lesion impinges on the descending root of the trigeminus of one side and on the crossed quintothalamic fibers, coming from the other side. In pontine lesions pain has a hemiplegic distribution, that is, also includes the face contralateral to the lesion. There have been cases of bulbopontine lesions that obey no rule in which the pains affected the lower limbs and one side of the face.

e) Pain following mesencephalopontine lesions occurs on the side of the body contralateral to the lesion, with hemiplegic distribution.

f) Pain and dysesthesia due to thalamic lesions have a hemiplegic distribution and affect the side of the body contralateral to the injured thalamus. Extension and distribution are variable, but generally pain is referred to the extremities and face; in some cases a peculiar cheirooral distribution of sensory disturbances is observed (Garcin and Lapresle 1954).

g) As in thalamic lesions, pain due to cortical or subcortical lesions is referred to the contralateral distal parts (face, hands and feet), that is, to the regions with the most extensive cortical and thalamic representation. Immediate onset limb CP with ipsilateral hemiballismus-hemichorea may be typical of an anterior parietal artery stroke (Rossetti *et al.* 2003).

In sum, lesion level and site can be clinically diagnosed only in cases of posterior horn lesion (girdle pain) and bulbar lesions (crossed sensory syndrome). Except in certain particular cases, such as the cheirooral distribution of sensory disturbances as in thalamic lesions, it is practically impossible, on the basis of the topography and clinical characteristics of pain alone, to distinguish between cortical, subcortical and thalamic lesions. Bilateral pain and dysesthesia referred to the limbs, although usually pointing to a spinal cord lesion, may be exceptionally observed after unilateral brain lesions (see Chapter 8).

5   DRUG THERAPY

At the beginning of the twenty-first century, a vast array of interventions is available to help patients; unfortunately the full gamut of treatments is poorly appreciated by medical professionals and, worse yet, pain therapists, and is ill-applied. CP remains one of the most ill-diagnosed and ill-treated entities among chronic pain syndromes, as proved by recent literature concerning patients submitted to, among others, gabapentin, carbamazepine, baclofen, opioids, tramadol, behavioral therapy and psychotherapy (Helmchen *et al.* 2002) or phenytoin, carbamazepine, valproate, baclofen, fluoxetine and trazodone (Fukuhara *et al.* 1999), all ineffective or only poorly effective agents.

Up to now, trial-and-error has been the norm in the treatment of CP. As months or years go by, the typical CP patient finds no or unsatisfactory relief from the handful of drugs the average pain therapist knows and administers. Many patients often end up intoxicated or develop important side effects, with addiction to opioids and benzodiazepines. Useless surgical procedures can also be attempted, usually without lasting relief. Even moderate enduring pain after any treatment can still be crippling and in time can "relapse" as the patient forgets about the previous level of suffering.

The goal of treatment is the abolition of all pain, permanently. Here, we will attempt to make the treatment of CP less empirical and more evidence-based. An important caveat should be borne in mind: time is not an option. CP slowly "erodes" patients' will, incapacitating the vast majority, sapping their resources, and must be treated aggressively, just like "a cancer of the soul." The best results for many patients will come from combination therapy in the very first place. Polypharmacy, by whatever route, should be the norm, rather than not, eventually combined with neuroaugmentative therapies.

Although many would object to prepackaged strategies for CP as a whole, we believe otherwise: pathophysiological evidence (Chapters 7 and 8) strongly suggests a common substratum to all CPs. In addition, *pharmacologic dissection* helps guide therapy in the single patient, driving us away from tradition toward a more scientifically based approach.

There are basically two tiers of therapies available for CP: pharmacologic (oral and parenteral) and neuromodulative (electrical and chemical). Other approaches will be discussed for the sake of completeness.

ORAL AND PARENTERAL DRUG THERAPY (Tables 5.1–5.4)

"There seems little doubt that neurosurgical procedures will be replaced to a large extent by drugs, at present unknown." (**A. E. Walker, 1950**)

1. General comments

Common to all studies is the short follow-up (generally weeks or months, versus an absolute optimum of 5 years or more), rarely undertaken by independent observers, and the small size, raising the possibility of type II errors (false negatives). To evaluate properly response, the following indications have been suggested: for moderate pain, a 20% reduction on a 0–10 scale is minimal improvement, 35% reduction is much improved and 45% reduction is very much improved; for severe pain, decreases on a numerical scale (NRS) have to be larger to obtain similar degrees of pain relief. In other words, the change in pain intensity that is meaningful to patients increases as the severity of their baseline pain increases (Cepeda *et al.* 2003; see also Mamie *et al.* 2000). Instead, analgesic use as a measure of outcome is probably of poor value, as it may be complicated by dependency and coexistent nociceptive pains. Last, but not least, in most studies, sensory and affective effects are not analyzed separately.

As noted above, valuable time should not be wasted trying all possible effective drugs and the clinician should focus on those with the best chances of success, over a defined timeline (see Table 6.8). CCP is often refractory to this tier and thermal allodynia is considered more resistant than spontaneous and tactile allodynia. Thus, if these fail, neuromodulation should be rapidly undertaken.

a. GABA drugs. The only such drug assessed in a formal RCT is IV *propofol* (Canavero and Bonicalzi 2004), a strongly hydrophobic IV anesthetic agent structurally unrelated to other anesthetic agents. Tasker (2001, and references therein) previously reported that IV infusions of 136 mg (mean) of sodium pentothal, a GABAergic agonist, reduced brain CP in 73% of his patients (versus none with 15 to 18 mg of morphine). In our studies, propofol effectively controlled CP at 0.2 mg/kg (one-tenth of the narcotic ED95 in humans), 5 times as effectively as pentothal at equipotent doses for CP (discussed in Canavero *et al.* 1995). Convergent evidence shows a specific effect of propofol for CP, but not PNP, migraine or nociceptive pains, at the doses reported above (discussed and referenced in Canavero *et al.* 1995, Canavero and Bonicalzi 2004). Unlike morphine and lidocaine, which are effective in allaying mechanical allodynia-hyperalgesia, but not cold allodynia-hyperalgesia (Section 5.1.e), our data suggest that, in CP, GABA modulation can allay both. Propofol analgesia shows a clear-cut post-effect: after several hours of infusion, analgesia can last for up to 24 hours (or more with longer duration of infusion). Propofol modulates GABA neurotransmission in different

TABLE 5.1. Controlled studies of oral drugs

Authors		Drug(s)	Final daily dose (mg)	No. of patients	Study design	Rating	Outcome	Notes	Authors' conclusions
Davidoff et al. (1987)	SCI	Trazodone HCl	150	18	Randomized, double-blind, parallel, placebo controlled (8 wks)	Pain relief	Trazodone effects did not significantly differ from placebo	At- or below-level pain	NNT: 9 (95% CI: 1.8–∞)
Leijin and Boivie (1989)	CPSP	Carbamazepine	CBZ: 800	15	Randomized, double-blind, crossover (3 × 4 wks, + 2 × 1 wk washout), placebo controlled	Daily pain intensity: verbal scale. Post treatment global ratings. Comprehensive psychological rating scale	5/14 improved on CBZ 10/15 improved on AMY 1/15 improved on placebo	Double dummy (identical active or placebo). 80% men. Stepped increase to final dose of CBZ (starting at 100 mg 2 × day) and AMY (starting at 12.5 mg 2 × day). No follow-up. 1 drop out	AMY, but not CBZ, produced a statistically significant reduction of pain vs. placebo, CBZ only from 3rd week. NNT CBZ: 3.4 (95% CI: 1.7–105). NNT AMY: 1.7 (95% CI: 1.1–3.0). Higher plasma levels correlated with better analgesia. NB: not confirmed in other studies
		Amitriptyline	AMY: 25 (morning) 50 (evening)						
Drewes et al. (1994)	SCI	Valproate	VAL: up to 2400	20	Double-blind, placebo controlled, crossover (2 × 3 wks, 2 wks washout)	Pain relief: McGill Pain Questionnaire. Present pain (rating scale 1–5)	6/20 improved on VAL 4/20 improved on placebo	Low-quality study (see Wiffen et al. Cochrane review, 2004). VAL: stepped increase starting at 600 mg 2 × day. Dose increased	No significant analgesic effect for VAL. NNT VAL: 10 (95% CI: 2.7–∞)

								according to serum levels. 1 dropout. Blind status not clear (serum level measured)	
McQuay *et al.* (1994)	CPSP	Dextro-methorphan	DEX: up to 81	9	Randomized, double-blind, placebo controlled, crossover. Integral *n*-of-1 design (2 × 10 day periods)	Pain relief, pain intensity, mood, sleep, global rating	0/9 improved on DEX 0/9 improved on placebo	19 pts with chronic pain. 1st treatment period: DEX 13.5 mg 3 × day; 2nd treatment period: DEX 27 mg 3 × day. No long-term clinical benefit	No significant analgesic effect
Vestergaard *et al.* (1996)	CPSP	Citalopram	CIT: 10–40	9/4	Randomized, double-blind, parallel, placebo controlled		No dichotomous data	SSRI	No significant analgesic effect
Chiou-Tan *et al.* (1999)	SCI	Mexiletine	MEX: 450	11	Randomized, double-blind, placebo controlled, crossover (1 wk washout, 2 × 4 wks)	Pain relief: VAS, McGill Pain Questionnaire	No dichotomous data	SCI dysesthetic at- or below-level pain. 15 pts enrolled, 11 completed the study	No significant analgesic effect at this low dose
Haines and Gaines (1999)	CP	Ketamine	Up to 100 PO	2 BCP; 3 CCP (1 MS)	*N* of 1 randomized, controlled	Daily pain diary; VAS; Likert scale	No effect during the unblended "run-in" period in any CP pt		Intolerable side effects in the whole group

(continued)

TABLE 5.1 (continued)

Authors		Drug(s)	Final daily dose (mg)	No. of patients	Study design	Rating	Outcome	Notes	Authors' conclusions
Vestergaard et al. (2001)	CPSP	Lamotrigine	LAM: 200	30	Randomized, double-blind, placebo controlled, crossover (2 × 8 wks, 2 wks washout)	Pain relief: Likert scale. Global pain score. Stimulus evoked pain. Primary end point: median pain score during the last wk of treatment	12/30 improved on LAM 3/30 improved on placebo	Stepped increased to final dose of LAM (25 mg 1st–2nd wk, 50 mg 3rd–4th wk, 100 mg 5th–6th wk, 200 mg 7th–8th wk). Median pain score: LAM 200 mg; 5; placebo; 7. Significant reduction of cold allodynia. 1 pt withdrawn because of LAM adverse events. ITT analysis (200 mg of LAM)	No significant effects at lower doses. LAM reduced pain score approximately 30% (meaningful reduction for CPSP pts). LAM is a moderately effective treatment for CPSP: NNT LAM: n.a.
Heiskanen et al. (2002)	CPSP	Dextro-methorphan	DEX: 100. Administration followed (4 h) by intravenous infusion of morphine 15 mg	2	Randomized, double-blind, crossover, placebo controlled	Pain relief: VASpi, MPQ, QST	DEX had no effect on morphine analgesia. 8 pts responded to morphine after placebo	Mixed population of 20 pts with chronic pain. DEX or placebo given 4 h prior to an IV morphine administration (15 mg)	Results not broken down according to pain type
Finnerup et al. (2002)	SCI	Lamotrigine	LAM: up to 400	30	Randomized, double-blind, crossover, placebo	Pain relief: change in median pain	Categorical slight to complete pain relief (secondary outcome	At or below-level pain. Slow LAM increase. 22 pts completed the	No statistically significant effect of LAM in the total

Study	Pain	Drug (dose)	Design	Outcome measures	Dichotomous data	Results/Comments
			controlled (1 wk baseline period, 2 × 9 wks, 2 wks washout)	score from baseline	measure): 10/22 on LAM, 5/22 on placebo	study. LAM more effective in pts with brush-evoked allodynia and wind-up like pain (7/7 pain relief vs. 1/14 without). 3 pts withdrawn because of adverse events. ITT analysis (200 mg LAM) — sample. In 7/8 pts with incomplete cord lesions LAM was more effective than placebo on at- or below-level pain. NNT LAM (incomplete lesions, 50% pain relief): 12 (2−∞)
Cardenas et al. (2002)	SCI	Amitriptyline Benztropine besilate (active placebo). AMI: 10-125 Benztropine 0.5. (84) SCI pain: 26. Transition zone pain: 6	Randomized, double-blind, placebo controlled (6 wks)	Pain relief: average pain intensity (NRS, 0−10). MPQ, BPI, FMI, SWLS, CHART	No dichotomous data	84 pts. 44 pts AMI, 40 placebo. Aim of the study: whether AMI is efficacious in relieving chronic pain in pts with SCI. ITT analysis and study completers analysis — No significant differences between AMI and placebo in pain intensity (also with regression analysis for different types of pain) or pain-related disability. SWLS > in placebo group. Certain subgroups of pts may benefit. 18% of pts chose to continue AMI, but 5% chose to continue placebo. No significant difference in AMI-placebo side effects. No CP in some pts.

(continued)

TABLE 5.1 (continued)

Authors		Drug(s)	Final daily dose (mg)	No. of patients	Study design	Rating	Outcome	Notes	Authors' conclusions
Lampl et al. (2002)	CPSP	Amitriptyline extended release Placebo	AMI: 75	19 20	Randomized, double-blind, placebo controlled (1 yr)	Aim of the study: to investigate, under controlled conditions, the effectiveness of AMI for the prophylactic treatment of pts with acute thalamic stroke in preventing CPSP	Primary end point: occurrence of CPSP within 1 yr	All pts had lesions in the ventroposterior thalamic region. AMI was slowly titrated from 10 to 75 mg in extended release. CPSP in AMI group: 4/18 pts; CPSP in placebo group: 3/19 pts	The placebo group showed a pain rate of 21% within 1 yr, compared with 17% in those under prophylactic treatment with AMI. Prophylactic treatment with AMI did not show any statistically significant beneficial effect to prevent the development of CPSP
Tai et al. (2002)	SCI	Gabapentin	GAB: 1800	7	Prospective, randomized, double-blind, placebo controlled, cross-over (2 × 4 wks, 2 wks washout)	Pain relief: NPS	GAB = placebo among pain descriptors with the exception of "unpleasant feeling"	Results limited by the small sample size and low maximum dosage of GAB	Nonsignificant trend to benefit on unpleasant feeling, pain intensity, and burning sensation only
Harden et al. (2002)	SCI	Topiramate	TOP: 800 (titrated over 10 wks)	9 (+5)	Parallel, randomized, placebo controlled study	Pain relief: VAS and descriptor scale	TOP = PLA (below 800 mg). TOP > PLA on descriptor scale but not VAS scale in final 2 wks only at 800 mg	Many side effects at 800 mg	

144

Study	Pain type	Drug	Dosage	Patients	Study design	Outcome measures	Results	Comments
Rowbotham et al. (2003)	CP	Levorphanol	LEV: 0.15 or 0.75 to a maximum of 21 capsules/day. Low strength: mean daily dosage: 2.7. High strength: mean daily dosage: 8.9	23. CPSP: 10; SCI: 5; MS: 8. CPSP:5; SCI: 2; MS: 4. CPSP: 5; SCI: 3; MS: 4	Randomized, double-blind, dose-response (8 wks)	Pain relief: VAS (0–10 cm). Primary outcome: mean pain rating	% reduction from base line. (A) Low strength: CPSP: 6; SCI: 13; MS: 9. (B) High strength: CPSP: 16; SCI: 30; MS: 63	Pts who completed the study: 15. CPSP: 3/10 (mean pain reduction: 20%). SCI: 4/5 (mean pain reduction: 22%). MS: 8/8 (% mean pain reduction: 27%). Low strength (% mean pain reduction): CPSP: 14; SCI: 13; MS: 9. High-strength (% mean pain reduction): CPSP: 23; SCI: 31; MS: 63	Capsules intake titrated by the pt. 7 of 10 pts with CPSP did not complete the study (reasons not described). 27% of pts withdrew. Few pts will benefit from opioids. SCI pain may have included CP. MS pain may have included dysesthetic pain
Morley et al. (2003)	NP	Methadone	MET: 10 or 20	19. CPSP: 2. Transverse myelitis: 1	Randomized, double-blind, placebo controlled	Pain relief (maximum pain intensity, average pain intensity and pain relief): VAS	Average pain intensity MET vs. placebo (VAS). MET 10 mg: CPSP 1: 59 vs. 65.8; CPSP 2: 33.4 vs. 46.4; cord: 47.8 vs. 42.8. MET 20 mg: CPSP1: 66.9 vs. 66.6; CPSP 2: 26.6 vs. 47; cord: not tested	All pts poor responders to traditional analgesic regimen. 20 mg daily dose resulted in statistically significant pain improvement. The analgesic effects extended over 48 hours. Daily dose of 10 mg failed to reach statistical significance.

(continued)

TABLE 5.1 (continued)

Authors		Drug(s)	Final daily dose (mg)	No. of patients	Study design	Rating	Outcome	Notes	Authors' conclusions
Wade et al. (2004)	MS SCI	Plant-derived cannabis medicinal extracts (CME)	1:1 CBD:THC, 2.5−120	24. MS: 18; SCI: 4	Consecutive series of double-blind, randomized, placebo-controlled single-patient crossover trials (2 wks)	Patients recorded symptom, well-being and intoxication scores on a daily basis: VAS + observer rating (at 2 wks)	Pain relief associated with both THC and CBD was significantly superior to placebo	Self-administered sublingual spray. Dose titration against symptom relief or unwanted effects	CME can improve neurogenic symptoms unresponsive to standard treatments
Svendsen et al. (2004)	MS CP	Dronabinol	DRO. Maximum daily dosage: 10	24	Randomized, double-blind, placebo controlled, crossover (2 × 3 wks, 15−21 days; 2 wks, 19−57 days; washout)	Median spontaneous pain intensity (numerical rating scale) in the last week of treatment. QST	Median spontaneous pain intensity significantly lower with dronabinol than placebo. Median pain relief score: VAS 3 vs. 0		DRO has a modest analgesia on MS CP. NNT for 50% pain relief: 3.5 (95% CI: 1.9−24.8)
Levendoglu et al. (2004)	SCI	Gabapentin	GAB. Maximum daily dosage: 3.6 g (gradually titrated dosage)	20	Prospective, randomized, double-blind, placebo controlled, crossover (18 wks; 4 wks medication/ placebo titration, 4 wks stable	Pain relief: NPS, VAS (0−100), LQ	GAB reduced the intensity and the frequency of pain, and improved the quality of life. Neuropathic pain descriptors not relieved: itchy,	Complete SCI at the thoracic and lumbar level. Neuropathic pain for more than 6 months. All patients completed the study. Mean	

Study	Condition	Drug	Dose	N	Design	Outcome measure	Results	Comments	Conclusion
			effective dose: 2235 mg. Dysesthetic pain included. Below-level pain not specifically mentioned		maximum tolerated dose, 4 wks crossover medication/ placebo titration, 4 wks stable maximum tolerated dose		sensitive, dull and cold		
Carlsson et al. (2004)	SCI	Dextro-methorphan	DEX: 270	2	Randomized, double-blind, placebo controlled, crossover (2 separate administrations)	Pain relief: VAS (0–100)	No effect in 1 pt, 69% VAS reduction in 1 pt	Study population: 15 pts with neuropathic pain of traumatic origin. Most patients experienced adverse effects, none of which was considered severe	A single high dose of DEX has an analgesic effect (up to 30% pain reduction vs. placebo) in patients with neuropathic pain of traumatic origin
Notcutt et al. (2004)	MS pain	Cannabis extract	Wide range of dosing	16	Randomized, placebo controlled		Benefit at no fixed dose	Side effects comparable to psychoactive drugs	

(continued)

147

TABLE 5.1 (continued)

Authors		Drug(s)	Final daily dose (mg)	No. of patients	Study design	Rating	Outcome	Notes	Authors' conclusions
Rog et al. (2005)	MS	Whole-plant cannabis-based medicine (CBM; delta-9-tetrahydro-cannabinol: cannabidiol [THC:CBD])	THC 2.7 CBD 2.5 (each spray). Gradual self-titration to a max. 48 spray/day	66	Randomized, double-blind, placebo controlled, parallel group (5 wks: 1 wk run-in, 4 wk treatment)	Daily pain and sleep disturbance (11-point numerical rating scale). Neuropathic Pain Scale (NPS). Cognitive function, mood, MS-related disability, Patient's Global Impression of Change	Trial completed by 64 pts (97%): 32 CBM pts (2 withdrawn), 32 placebo pts. ITT analysis. Results at week 4 (mean change): pain intensity: CBM: −2.7 (95% CI: −3.4 to −2.0). PLA: −1.4 (95% CI: −2.0 to −0.8), $p = 0.005$). Sleep disturbance: CBM: −2.5 (95% CI: −3.4 to −1.7). PLA: −0.8 (95% CI: −1.5 to −0.1), $p = 0.003$)	Inclusion criteria: pts with spontaneous or evoked dysesthetic pain (burning, aching, pricking, stabbing, and squeezing) and pts with painful tonic spasms. CBM generally well tolerated (1 pt withdrawn because of adverse effects; but more pts on CBM than PLA reported dizziness, dry mouth, and somnolence)	CBM delivered via an oromucosal spray, as adjunctive analgesic treatment. Mean number of daily sprays: CBM 9.6 ± 6 (range 2−25) placebo: 19.1 ± 12.9 (range 1−47). THC:CBD ratio approximately 1:1 (other cannabis-based compounds <10%). CBM was superior to placebo in reducing the mean intensity of pain and sleep disturbance. PIGC: no difference between the proportion of pts rating themselves as "much" or "very much improved" in the CBM group (9/34) vs. PLA group (4/32). Cognitive side effects: limited to long-term memory storage

TABLE 5.2. Controlled studies of parenteral drugs

Authors		Drug(s)	Dosage	No. of patients	Study design	Rating	Outcome	Notes	Authors' conclusions
Portenoy et al. (1986)	CP and others	Oral opioids		3 SCI, 1 syrinx, 1 spinal AVM, 2 CPSP				Results not broken down according to type	
Arner and Meyerson (1988)	CP and others	Morphine IV	15 mg	CCP (1 pt)	Randomized, single-blind, placebo controlled trial		Ineffective	Acute boluses. SCS and PVG DBS: ineffective	
Portenoy et al. (1990)	CP	Morphine		2	Controlled trial			Some benefit	
Kupers et al. (1991)	CP and others	Morphine	0.3 mg/kg IV	CPSP: 4; SCI: 2	Double-blind, placebo controlled crossover study	Affective and sensory dimensions of pain sensation: 101-point rating scale	Statistically significant reduction of pain affect rating (from 62 to 43). Pain sensory rating not affected, with trend toward increasing		
Bainton et al. (1992)	CPSP	Naloxone	NAL: up to 8 mg 20 in 20 mL vehicle	20	Randomized, double-blind, crossover, placebo controlled	Pain relief: VAS, verbal pain scores	Transient pain relief: 3/20 with NAL, 4/20 with saline, 4/20 with both	Pain scores obtained immediately before and after NAL or saline injection. Subjective ratings followed for 2 wks	IV NAL ineffective on CPSP

(continued)

TABLE 5.2 *(continued)*

Authors		Drug(s)	Dosage	No. of patients	Study design	Rating	Outcome	Notes	Authors' conclusions
Hansebout et al. (1993)	SCI	4-aminopyridine (4-AP)	Escalating total dose from 18.0 to 33.5 mg (IV, 2 separated (2 wks) infusions over 2 h)	8	Randomized, double-blind, crossover	Neurological motor and sensory evaluation	Significant temporary neurologic improvement, including reduction in chronic pain, in 5/6 pts with incomplete SCI. No effect was detected in 2 pts with complete and 1 severe incomplete SCI	Effects persisted up to 48 h after infusion	
Backonja et al. (1994)	CP	Ketamine	0.25 mg/kg (IV bolus over 5 min)	6; CPSP: 2	Randomized, double-blind, placebo controlled, crossover	Pain rating scale 0–10	Pain relief in CPSP pts. Ketamine: pt D: 50% (ongoing pain); pt F: 100% pain relief (ongoing, allodynia, hyperalgesia). Placebo: pt D: 0%, pt F: modest		Pain relief lasting 2–3 hours. Ketamine affected the evoked pain and associated after-sensation more than ongoing constant pain. Allodynia, hyperalgesia and after-sensation improved. Side effects during single-dose injections mild and well tolerated

Reference	Diagnosis	Drug	n	Design	Outcome			
Canavero et al. (1995)	CP	Propofol	CPSP: 8; SCI: 8	Double-blind, placebo controlled, crossover	Pain relief: VAS (0–10)	Effect lasting no more than 20 min (generally 10 min)	Continuous (6–24 h) IV infusion in propofol-responsive pts. Temporarily effective with hours-long post-effect	Pain and allodynia abolition in propofol-responsive pts. Propofol did not reduce non-CP, nor did placebo
Eide et al. (1995)	SCI	Ketamine (KET)	9	Randomized, double-blind, crossover	Continuous and evoked pain relief	KET = ALF > PLA	Neither ketamine nor alfentanil significantly changed thresholds for the sensation of heat pain. No clear differential effects on at- and below-level pains	Both continuous and evoked pains were markedly reduced by ketamine and by alfentanil. Bothersome dizziness in one patient
		Alfentanil (ALF)	7 μg/kg (IV bolus, +0.6 μg/kg/min for 17–20 min) (3 infusions, 2 h apart)			ALF = KET > PLA		
Hamamci et al. (1996)	?	Calcitonin	26	Placebo controlled	Pain score	Pain score of the calcitonin group was significantly lower than that of the control group	Post-stroke pts with hemiplegia and "RSD." 4 wks study. 26 pts received calcitonin, 16 saline	Uncertain diagnosis. CPSP in some pts?

Note: Propofol dosing — 0.2 mg/kg (single IV bolus); 0.3 mg/kg/h (continuous IV infusion). Ketamine dosing — 60 μg/kg (IV bolus, +6 μg/kg/min for 17–20 min). Calcitonin dosing — 1 × 100 IU/day (IM).

(continued)

TABLE 5.2 (continued)

Authors		Drug(s)	Dosage	No. of patients	Study design	Rating	Outcome	Notes	Authors' conclusions
Dellemijn and Vanneste (1997)	CP	Fentanyl	FEN: 5 μg/kg/h (mean dose: 873 μg)	3	Randomized, double-blind, active placebo controlled, crossover (drugs infused at a constant rate for a maximum of 5 h)	Pain relief: rating scales (including unpleasant-ness)	Maximum relief of pain intensity was better with FEN than with DIA (66% (95% CI 53–80) vs. 23% (12–35)) or with saline (50% (36–63) vs. 12% (4–20)). FEN responders: 1/3. Placebo responders: 0/3	Mixed population of 53 pts with neuropathic pain. DIA as active placebo. Saline as inert placebo. 2 consecutive double-blind infusions: FEN + DIA and FEN + saline	DIA had no clinically significant effect on pain intensity and pain unpleasantness. The beneficial effect of FEN was independent of the type of neuropathic pain and the degree of sedation. FEN therapy produced equal relief of pain intensity and pain unpleasantness. DIA and saline did not reduce either pain index. Side effects more common with FEN than with DIA or saline. No severe side effects. The clinical characteristics of neuropathic pain do not predict response to opioids
		Diazepam	DIA: 0.2 μg/kg/h (mean dose: 52.1 mg)						
Mailis et al. (1997)	SCI	Amobarbital	4–7 mg/kg (IV infusion, 7–10 min, max. dose 500 mg or 50 mg/kg)	1	Placebo controlled	Pain relief: VAS. Sensory testing	VAS reduction from about 6 to about 4. Dramatic reduction of allodynia. Substantial reduction of hyperalgesia	17 NP pts. 1 pt with C4 myelopathy (AVM)	No benefit on deep pain. Sympathetic block responder

Study	Condition	Drug	N	Design	Outcome measures	Results	Comments	
Potter et al. (1998)	SCI	Fampridine-SR (sustained release 4-aminopyridine) 12.5 and 17.5 mg bid (PO, 2-wks) treatment period, +1 wk washout	26	Randomized double-blind dose-titration crossover	Patient satisfaction, sensory scores, motor scores	No statistically significant benefits on measures of pain	Incomplete SCI in all pts	
Attal et al. (2000)	CP	Lidocaine 5 mg/kg (IV infusion over 30 min)	CPSP: 6; SCI: 10 (syrinx: 5; SCI: 3; spondylotic myelopathy: 2)	Randomized, double-blind, placebo — PLA (saline) controlled, crossover	Pain relief: VAS (0–10), global assessment, QST	Pain relief >50%: 11/16 with lidocaine; 6/16 with PLA. 3 had no benefit or worse pain vs. 8 with PLA. 2 pts had more relief with PLA. Burning totally/partially relieved in 6 vs. 2 (PLA), paresthesias abolished in 8/11 vs. 2/11. In 5 pts (62%), allodynia reduced ≥50% by lidocaine (vs. 1 by PLA), in 4 by 100% for up to 1 hour postinjection (never with PLA)	Post-study follow-up: 12 pts took oral mexiletine (400–800 mg/day) for 4–12 wks. 30–50% relief in 3 pts (2 lidocaine responders, 1 placebo responder). No improvement in 8 pts (6 lidocaine responders). Intolerable side effects from long-term mexiletine. Difference between lidocaine and PLA: moderate. In 7 pts refractory to all previous treatments, spontaneous pain responded less to lidocaine	Significant greater pain relief starting 15 min postinjection and lasting up to 30 min after the end. With lidocaine, significant brush-induced allodynia and static mechanical hyperalgesia reduction. No effect on thermal evoked pains. In 2 pts, 30–50% relief for 2–10 days. NNT: 5 (SCI pts). Side effects in two thirds of patients

(continued)

TABLE 5.2 (continued)

Authors	CP	Drug(s)	Dosage	No. of patients	Study design	Rating	Outcome	Notes	Authors' conclusions
Attal et al. (2002)	CP	Morphine	16 mg IV (mean dosage, range 9–30)	15. SCI: 9; CPSP: 6	Randomized, double-blind, placebo – PLA (saline) controlled, crossover	Pain relief: VAS (1–100), QST	No significant difference in pain reduction between morphine and placebo. 3 pts 100% relieved at the end of injection (vs. 1 with PLA), 2 for > 2 h, 1 pt worsened by morphine. 1 syrinx pt with prominent mechanical allodynia 100% relieved	Morphine effect correlated with decreased responses to suprathreshold thermal stimuli (general antinociceptive activity). Following the completion of the study all pts began to take sustained oral morphine (mean dosage: 93 mg; range 60–140 mg) in a long-term study on efficacy and side effects	Morphine significantly reduced brush-induced allodynia but had *no effect on static mechanical and thermal evoked pains*. Ongoing pain was not significantly reduced, but 7 pts (46%) responded to morphine. The effects of IV morphine correlated with those of oral morphine at 1 month. Oral morphine was effective only in 3 (2 SCI, 1 CPSP)/14 pts (1 lost to follow-up) at 12–18 months with 50–75% relief, starting from week 1 and peaking at week 4. Morphine PO less tolerated than IV

Study		Drug	Dose	N	Outcome measure	Design	Results	
Kalman et al. (2002)	MS	Morphine	Up to 1 mg/kg over 20 min, continuous IV infusion	14	Pain relief: VAS	Single-blind, placebo (saline) controlled. Followed by naloxone	4 pts were opioid responders (no pain relief from placebo, >50% pain reduction with morphine and >25% pain increase with naloxone). Effective dose: 43, 47, 50 and 25 mg	Morphine is effective only in a minority of pts (29%) and only at high doses. Same results reported by these authors in discussion for CPSP
Canavero and Bonicalzi (2004)	CP	Propofol	0.2 mg/kg (single IV bolus)	44. CPSP: 23; SCI: 21	Pain relief: VAS (0–10); NVS (0–4)	Randomized, double-blind, placebo controlled, crossover	Pain relief (spontaneous pain intensity reduction >30% or allodynia reduction >50%): 24/44 pts with propofol, 6/44 pts with placebo	Propofol was significantly superior to the placebo in reducing the intensity of spontaneous ongoing pain (for up to 1 h after the injection) and of both mechanical and cold allodynia. In a few cases, only the evoked components were abolished. Study aimed at validating IV subhypnotic propofol as a diagnostic test for CP

(continued)

TABLE 5.2 *(continued)*

Authors	Drug(s)	Dosage	No. of patients	Study design	Rating	Outcome	Notes	Authors' conclusions
Kvarnstrom et al. (2004) SCI	Ketamine	0.4 mg/kg (IV infusion over 40 min)	10	Randomized, double-blind, three-period, three-treatment, placebo controlled, crossover	Pain relief: VAS. QST, traditional sensory tests	Positive response (50% reduction in VAS score during infusion): 5/10 pts with ketamine, 1/10 pts with lidocaine, 0/10 pts with placebo. Temperature thresholds: no changes. Sensibility: no changes	Primary objective of the study: to examine the analgesic effect of ketamine and lidocaine on SCI below-level pain. Secondary objective: to assess sensory abnormalities to identify responders. Sensory assessments do not predict response to treatment	Ketamine, but not lidocaine, showed a significant analgesic effect in SCI-CP. Pain relief not associated with altered temperature thresholds or other changes of sensory function. Lidocaine and particularly ketamine were associated with frequent side-effects
	Lidocaine	2.5 mg/kg (IV infusion over 40 min)						
Finnerup et al. (2005) SCI	Lidocaine	5 mg/kg (IV infusion over 30 min)	24	Randomized, double-blind, placebo controlled, crossover	Pain relief: VAS. QST	Neuropathic at-level and below-level spontaneous pain: 1: significantly reduced in all patients	26 pts with NP at or below level enrolled, 2 dropped out before any treatment. Evoked pain in 12 pts.	SCI at and below level pain is reduced by IV lidocaine irrespective of the presence or absence of evoked pain.

$(p < 0.01)$ 2: significantly reduced in 12 pts with evoked pain $(p < 0.01)$ 3: significantly reduced in 12 pts without evoked pain $(p < 0.048)$ No difference in number of pts with pain reduction ≥33% between the patients with $(n = 6)$ and without $(n = 5)$ evoked pain. At-level brush-evoked dysesthesia significantly reduced. Median pain reduction: about 35%. NNT for 50% pain relief: 3

No evoked pain in 12 pts. Adverse effects: IV lidocaine, 19 pts; placebo, 1. No correlation between maximal plasma concentration and maximal pain relief or pain intensity. No significant decrease in cold allodynia, pinprick hyperalgesia, or pain evoked by repetitive pinprick

Lidocaine is usually not suited for long-term treatment

(continued)

TABLE 5.2 (continued)

Authors	Drug(s)	Dosage	No. of patients	Study design	Rating	Outcome	Notes	Authors' conclusions
Vranken et al. CP (2005)	S(+)-ketamine	50 or 75 mg daily (transdermal iontophoretic administration)	33 (CPSP, 8; MS, 1; thalamic PD, 1; lesion, 3; brainstem lesion, 4; SC lesion, 16)	Randomized, double-blind, placebo controlled	Pain intensity: VAS. Health status (PDI, EQ-5D). Quality of life (SF-36). Safety assessment	No statistically significant differences in VAS between ketamine (both dosages) and placebo. *Pre- vs. post-treatment VAS scores:* Placebo group: 7.1 vs. 6.4 Ketamine 50 mg: 7.3 vs 6.2 Ketamine 75 mg:	1 week trial. Appropriate dose from an open-label preliminary study. Sample size and power calculated pre-study (with 33 pts, power 0.8 for estimated VAS differences). Only mild and spontaneously resolving adverse events without	Iontophoretic administration of S(+)-ketamine was no more effective than placebo in reducing pain scores, but daily administration of 75 mg of S(+)-ketamine improved health status and quality of life

7.3 vs 5.7

No improvement in health status or quality of life from ketamine 50 mg. Significant improvement in PDI, EQ-5D and SF-36 (except for role-physical functioning and general health perception) from ketamine 75 mg

differences between ketamine and placebo groups.

TABLE 5.3. Uncontrolled studies: oral drugs

Authors	Pain type/ no. of pts	Drug(s)	Dosage	Study design	Rating	Outcome and notes	Authors' conclusions
Fine (1967)	Epileptic pain (poststroke): 5	Phenytoin, phenobarbital				All relieved	Paroxysmal pain
Albert (1969)	MS CP: 6	Carbamazepine	600 mg			4 definite reliefs	Paroxysmal and burning pain responsive
Espir and Millac (1970)	MS (pain in limbs) 7;	Carbamazepine				No data for true CP	Paroxysmal pains responsive (placebo ineffective)
Gibson and White (1970)	SCI pain: 2	Carbamazepine		Case reports		Partial to very good relief at 4–8 months (never 100%)	Effect on lancinating, pulsatile pain; burning at low level remains
Cantor (1972)	CPSP: 2	Phenytoin		Case reports		Partial benefit at 150 mg in both, in 1 pt at 1 yr	
Mladinich (1974)	CP: brainstem	Phenytoin				Benefit	
Agnew and Goldberg (1976)	CPSP: 8. Plus 2 other non-CP pain pts	Phenytoin	Full dosage	Case series	Charts for pain estimation	Incomplete data. Marked improvement: 3. Minimal improvement: 2. Unchanged: 2. Pain worsened: 3	Return of pain on stopping phenytoin in improved pts
Heilporn et al. (1978)	SCI CP (diffuse pain): 11	Melitracen (150 mg PO), flupenthixol (3 mg PO die) plus TENS				8 pts benefited	
Gimenez-Roldan and Martin (1981)	Tabetic pain. 6	Carbamazepine		Case series		IV penicillin versus carbamazepine. 1/6 pain relief with penicillin, 5/5 pain relief with CBZ	

Reference	Patients	Treatment	Dose	Study type	Outcome	Results	Comments
Clifford and Trotter (1984)	MS burning pain in legs, nonburning dysesthesia: 11	Tricyclics		Case series		100% relief in 8, partial in 3 (in one baclofen PO led to 100% relief); nonburning dysesthesia: relieved	1 pt relieved by PO baclofen; 1 relieved only by phenol spinal block
Schott and Loh (1984)	CPSP: 5	Physostigmine, piridostigmine				2 long-term reliefs	
Bowsher et al. (1987)	Tabetic pain	Valproate				Effect on lightning pain	
Tourian (1987)	CPSP: 10	Doxepin (75–200 mg die) plus propanolol 82 mg die)				About 50% long-lasting relief	Propanolol potentiates doxepin
Moulin et al. (1988)	MS pains	Amitriptyline, imipramine, carbamazepine	Up to 100 mg	Case series		Poor results for true CP	One-third of patients had no thermoalgesic impairment
Portenoy et al. (1988)	MS CP: 3	Opioids; tricyclics (amitriptyline, imipramine)		Case series		Partial relief from PO opioids; high dose imipramine in 1 but not another; amitriptyline highly effective in 1	Drugs ineffective in 2 cases: doxepin, CBZ, PHT, clonazepam, valproate, tryptophan, fluphenazine. TENS useless in 2/2; cognitive behavioral therapy useless in 1/1
Hampf and Bowsher (1989)	CPSP	Distigmine plus AD					
Awerbuch and Sandyk (1990)	CPSP: 9	Mexiletine	Up to 10 mg/kg/day; 4 wk period	Case series	Pain relief: 5 point scale	Days 1–3: 150 mg; days 4–6: 300 mg. At least moderate relief in 8/9 pts	Mexiletine may be a safe and effective agent in the management

(continued)

TABLE 5.3 *(continued)*

Authors	Pain type/ no. of pts	Drug(s)	Dosage	Study design	Rating	Outcome and notes	Authors' conclusions
							of thalamic pain and possibly other paroxysmal pain syndromes of central origin
Michel et al. (1990)	CPSP: 3	Fluvoxamine	NR	Case series		1 partial pain relief, 1 scarce effect, 1 no effect	
	CPSP: 5	Clonazepam	NR			Partial pain relief in 2 pts, scarce effect in 2, no effect in 1	
Maurer et al. (1990)	CP: 1	Delta-9 THC (5 mg) plus codeine (50 mg)				More effective than placebo on painful dysesthesias	
Tourian (1991)	CP: number not available	Baclofen PO (80 mg) with/ without clonidine (0.4–1 mg die)				Relief in some pts	
Sanford et al. (1992)	SCI CP: 1	Amitriptyline, carbamazepine	150 mg die, 400 mg die			Some relief with AMI, substantial relief of burning and paroxysmal pains by adding CBZ at 3 yrs	Effect only by combining both drugs, not singly
Fenollosa et al. (1993)	SCI (postal survey of 380 pts, 38% of whom responded)	Amitriptyline + clonazepam + NSAIDs or amitriptyline + clonazepam + 5-OH-tryptophane + TENS, or amitriptyline + clonazepam + SCS, or morphine (continuous IT administration)	NR	Case series review	Pain relief	"Satisfactory relief" in 35% of the pts who responded	Morphine used by intrathecal route is very safe and useful in selected pts

Study	Patients	Drug	Dose	Study type	Outcome measure	Results	Comments
Edmondson et al. (1993)	CP: 4	Mexiletine PO		Case series		Previous effective lidocaine infusion. Two have continued taking the drug and reported excellent relief at 12 months; two had intolerable side effects	
De Salles and Bittar (1994)	CPSP: 1	Carbamazepine				Partial relief	
Bowsher (1994)	CP: number not specified	Mexiletine PO				Effective in several pts	
Zachariah et al. (1994)	SCI: 3 pts	Divalproex sodium				Relief in 2	1 dropped out
Canavero and Bonicalzi (1996)	CPSP: 3; CCP: 1	Lamotrigine	From 50 mg/day PO to 200 mg 3×/day	Placebo controlled in 2 pt	Patient self-reports and pain scores	Pain relapse after switching to placebo or drug discontinuation in 3 pts. Amitriptyline added in 1 pt with additional analgesia	
Sist et al. (1997)		Gabapentin				Mixed pain population, including CP pts; GBP effective	
Houtchens et al. (1997)	MS: 25	Gabapentin	300–2400 mg die	Case series		Best response on throbbing pain/needles, least effect on dull aching pain	
Zylicz (1997)	CPSP: 1	Methadone	From 5 mg 2×/day to 30 mg/day (gradual increase)	Case report	Pain relief: pt report	Previous trial with IV morphine, from 2.5 to 6 mg/h, continuous infusion	
Wood and Sloan (1997)	CP	Ketamine		Case report		Effective	
McGowan et al. (1997)	CP (brainstem): 16	Amitriptyline		Case series		2 pts: 100% relief; 14 pts: partial relief	Effective. Amitriptyline, dexamethasone, CBZ, paracetamol ineffective
Carrieri et al. (1998)	CPSP: 1	Lamotrigine	100 mg 2×/day	Case report		Pain relapse on stopping lamotrigine	Prompt relapse upon weaning

(continued)

TABLE 5.3 (continued)

Authors	Drug(s)	Pain type/ no. of pts	Dosage	Study design	Rating	Outcome and notes	Authors' conclusions
McCleane (1998a)	Lamotrigine	CPSP	25 mg/day up to 200 mg/day	Placebo controlled, double blind (2×8 wks, 2 wks washout)	Pain relief	31 pts. 22 pts completed the study. 3 adverse events. Effective	
McCleane (1998b)	Lamotrigine	MS: 1	50 mg/day up to 200 mg/day	Case report		100% relief; relapse upon cessation; again 100% control, but discontinuation for rash	Tramadol not effective. Carbamazepine partially effective
Attal et al. (1998)	Gabapentin	CP: 7; CPSP: 2	Up to 2400 mg/day		Spontaneous ongoing pain: VAS (1–100). Paroxysmal pain: number of daily attacks	Mixed pain population, including CP pts. Gabapentin starting dosage: 600 mg. Study duration: 6 wks. Spontaneous ongoing pain and daily attack number: significant decrease at 6 wks. Significant reduction of brush-induced and cold allodynia	Results not broken down according to pain type
Merren (1998)	Gabapentin		Up to 2700 mg/day	Case series		Mixed pain population, including centrally mediated pain	Best responses occurred in patients with peripherally mediated pain
Ness et al. (1998) Also includes case report on Pain 1998	Gabapentin	Cord CP (SCI/MS): 6	900 mg/day or more (according to pain relief)	Case report	Pain relief: VAS	No benefit in 3 pts. Long-term benefit (reduction of pain score of at least 3) after 6 months: 3. True CP not very responsive	
Mercadante (1998)	Gabapentin	SCI: 3	Up to 2400 mg/day		Pain relief: VAS	Previous medications or surgical treatments ineffective. Tramadol in 1 pt	

Reference	Population	Treatment	Dose	Study type	Outcome measure	Results	Conclusion
Cianchetti et al. (1999)	MS: 21; 15 with burning paresthesias	Lamotrigine	25 mg/day increased slowly to a maximum of 400 mg/day	Case series	Pain relief: pts report, verbal scale	Marked improvement in 3, moderate improvement in 5 (of 15 MS CP pts). Globally, 13 of 21 100% improved, 11 with sustained benefit at >1 yr	Lamotrigine is effective in controlling painful paroxysmal phenomena in MS pts
Enarson et al. (1999)	Mixed pain population, including CP: 21	Ketamine	Starting dose 100 mg/day, titrated upward. Median final dose: 220 mg/day	Case series review		Titration upward by 40 mg/day until efficacy was reached, or until side effects became limiting. Intolerable side effects: 9 pts. No effect: 4 pts. Equivocal responses: 4 pts. Long-term treatment in 4 pts (100–500 mg/day)	Demographic data not shown. More effective if pain <5 yrs
Fisher and Hagen (1999)	SCI: 1	Ketamine	10 mg 3tid, titrated upward up to 25 mg 3tid	Case report	Pain relief: VAS (0–10)	IV followed by SC ketamine as starting treatment. Haloperidol added. Pain relief from 5/10 (8/10 at night) to 3/10	
Sakurai and Kanazawa (1999)	MS CP: 14	Lidocaine, mexiletine	Lidocaine infusion: 6–8.8 mg/kg/h over 30 min, then 2-2.8; Mex: 300–400 mg/day	Case series		Effective in most. Placebo not or scarcely effective	Almost complete abolition of painful tonic seizures. Lidocaine > mexiletine, although both effective. In 1 pt, no benefit from CBZ (400 mg).

(continued)

TABLE 5.3 *(continued)*

Authors	Pain type/ no. of pts	Drug(s)	Dosage	Study design	Rating	Outcome and notes	Authors' conclusions
							valproate (800 mg) and clonazepam (2.5 mg). Truncal more resistant than limb dysesthesias
Van Bastelaere and De Laat (1999)	SCI CP: 1	Lamotrigine	600 mg/day	Case report		Pain abolition	3600 mg/day morphine ineffective
Kapadia and Harden (2000)	SCI CP: 1	Gabapentin Doxepin	1800 mg/die 100 mg	Case report	Pain relief: VAS, MPQ	Good control	Opioids, CBZ, tricyclic antidepressants and TENS ineffective
Vick and Lamer (2001)	CPSP: 1	Ketamine IV Ketamine PO	0.2 mg/kg bolus 50 mg	Case report	Pain relief: VAS	Marked relief Relief (VAS 3) at 9 months	CBZ, PHT, GBP, amantadine, IV lidocaine, opioids, TCA ineffective
D'Aleo et al. (2001)	MS CP	Topiramate	200–550 mg/day	Case series		Three reliefs (none 100%); 1 dropped out	
Shimodozono et al. (2002)	CPSP: 31	Fluvoxamine	25–125 mg/day	Open label	Pain relief: VAS (1–10)	After 2 to 4 wks significant VAS decrease from 7.7 to 6	Significant effect only if stroke <1 yr
Canavero et al. (2002)	CPSP: 3. Syringomyelia: 1; cord lesions: 3; BCP 1, CCP 1 CPSP 1, CCP 1 plus other 2 CP	Topiramate Amantadine Dextrometorphan	Up to 600 mg/day Up to 100 mg/day 100–1000 mg/day		Pain relief: VAS	No effect. Pain worsened in 3 pts Pain worsened 2 moderate reliefs, 20% benefit	

166

Study	Patient population	Drug	Dose	Study design	Outcome measure	Results	Comments
Canavero et al. (2002)	CPSP: 3. Syringomyelia: 1; SCI: 2	Reboxetine	Up to 10 mg/day	Single-blind, prospective	Pain relief: VAS	Pain reduction. >50% (cut-off limit for analgesia): 1 pt (treatment disclosure); <50%: 2 pts; none: 3 pts	Reboxetine (selective noradrenaline re-uptake inhibitor) does not appear to exert major analgesic effects in CP
Bowsher (2002)	CPSP: 64	Amitriptyline				Modestly significant correlation between onset of therapy and efficacy (>50%); 89% of those beginning treatment within 6 months of onset achieved target benefit vs. 42% starting it >1 yr from onset	
Chen et al. (2002)	CPSP: 1	Gabapentin				Significant pain relief and function improvement within 2 wks	
Putzke et al. (2002)	SCI: 27	Gabapentin	1800–3600 mg/day (in 2 cases <900 mg)	Case series follow-up	Pain relief: pain rating scale	6 discontinued. 21 had ≥2 VAS points reduction at 6 months. 3 years later, 10 of 14 responders still benefited. Below lesion pain: 8 responders, 4 non responders	Below-lesion CP: 8 benefits, 4 failures. Rectal-perineal CP: 4 benefits, 2 failures. Complete SCI: 3 benefits, 2 failures. Incomplete SCI: 11 benefits, 5 failures.

(continued)

TABLE 5.3 (continued)

Authors	Pain type/no. of pts	Drug(s)	Dosage	Study design	Rating	Outcome and notes	Authors' conclusions
							Burning pain: 9 benefits, 4 failures. Nonburning pain: 5 benefits, 3 failures
Takano et al. (2002)	CPSP: 2	Amantadine	50–150 mg die			May have responded: no details	Previous response to IV ketamine
Ahn et al. (2003)	SCI: 31	Gabapentin	1800 mg/day or maximum tolerated dose	Case series	VAS	Comparison among pts with different duration of symptoms (less or more than 6 months)	Gabapentin may be effective in SCI pts whose duration of symptoms is less than 6 months. Pts with duration of symptoms >6 months showed a significant but lesser decrease
Takahashi et al. (2004)	CPSP: 2 (both of immediate onset)	Zonisamide	200 mg/day	Case report		Pt 1: "pain well controlled" (follow-up 5 months). Pt 2: VAS reduction from 7 to 2 (follow-up 1 yr)	No side effects
Attal et al. (2004)	CPSP: 1; SCI: 4	Dronabinol	2.5 mg bid up to 25 mg/day (maximum dosage)	Case series	Pain relief: VAS. MPQ. Number of painful attacks	Consecutive pts. Side effects in all. No significant effect on ongoing pain and evoked pains	
Sakai et al. (2004)	MS: 1	Ketamine	20 mg increased to 40 mg/day PO	Placebo controlled	Pain relief: VAS	Effective on severe pain and allodynia. Pain reduction from IV lidocaine (3 mg/kg) and oral mexiletine (300 mg/day)	

168

Study	Population	Treatment	Dose	Study type	Pain intensity	Primary end-point: global pain relief. Pain relief in CP pts:			Good outcome of therapy with IMI or GAB is not predicted neither by definite evidence of nervous system lesion nor by the presence of abnormal sensory phenomena. Study's results do not support a mechanism-based approach in classifying and treating pain
							IMI	GAB	
Rasmussen et al. (2004)	Brain CP: 6; spinal CP: 10	Imipramine (IMI) or gabapentin (GAB)	IMI: ≥50 mg/day. GAB: up to 2.4 g/day	Case series	Numeric Pain Rating Scale. Pain relief: 4-point scale (0–25%, 26–50%, 51–75%, or 76–100% global pain relief)	0–25%	0 BCP, 2 SCP	0 BCP, 2 SCP	
						26–50%	1BCP, 4 SCP	0 BCP, 2 SCP	
						51–75%	3 BCP, 0 SCP	2 BCP, 0 SCP	
						76–100%	0 BCP, 0 SCP	0 BCP, 0 SCP	
Henkel and Bengel (2005)	Wallenberg: 1	Gabapentin and amitriptyline	NA	Case report	VAS	Marked reduction of pain			Opioids ineffective. Iatrogenic streptococcal meningoen-cephalitis following cervical myelography
Seghier et al. (2005)	CPSP: 1	Amitriptyline, gabapentin	75 mg/day, 2400 mg/day	Case report	VAS	40% pain reduction			
Montes et al. (2005)	CPSP: 1	Carbamazepine	NA	Case report	VAS	Initial response, but rapid relapse			
		Gabapentin, lamotrigine, oxcarbazepine, amitriptyline, bromazepam,				No effect			

(continued)

TABLE 5.3 (continued)

Authors	Pain type/ no. of pts	Drug(s)	Dosage	Study design	Rating	Outcome and notes	Authors' conclusions
		paracetamol-codeine, IV morphine IV ketamine				Increased burning	
Canavero and Bonicalzi (2005)	BCP: 9; CCP: 7	Mexiletine-gabapentin	Up to 1000 mg/day (Mex). Up to 3600 mg/day (GBP)	Case series	VAS	68.75% of pts had ≥50% reduction, 1 less than that, 1 made worse, 2 intolerant	3 stopped due to side effects after initial benefit. 50% of patients had at least 50% relief up to 7 yrs

TABLE 5.4. Uncontrolled studies: parenteral drugs

Authors	Drug(s)	Route/dosage	Pain type; no. of patients	Study design	Outcome	Other details
Di Biagio (1959)	Atophanyl	IV	CP: 2	Placebo controlled	Great relief in 1, 0% in another	Some control attempted, partially single blind. Pain relief evaluated by a 10 point scale. Several days between morphine and pentobarbital test. Morphine followed by naloxone 0.8 mg. "Morphine saturation test method" as per Hosobuchi.
Plotkin (1982)	Morphine	IV 1.5 mg/min up to 30 mg	Thalamic pain: 1; SCI: 3	Case series	No response to morphine Results not broken down according to pain.	
	Pentobarbital	IV 25 mg/min				Pentobarbital administered until the pt is on the point of unconsciousness, at which time pain should totally disappear if central
Boas et al. (1982)	Lidocaine	IV 3 mg/kg (infusion 240 mg)	CP, thalamic: 1		90% relief (transient)	1.5–2 mg/kg enough for CP
Tasker (1984)	Pentothal	IV 50–225 mg (average: 136 mg)	BCP/CCP	Case series	73% responded to therapy	CP is not dependent on opiate mechanism; 55% of CCP cases responded to morphine, but only the evoked pains and less frequently lancinating pains, *rarely steady pain*
	Morphine (some also fentanyl)	IV 15–18 mg	BCP/CCP		0%	

(continued)

TABLE 5.4 (continued)

Authors	Drug(s)	Route/dosage	Pain type; no. of patients	Study design	Outcome	Other details
Edwards et al. (1985)	Lidocaine	IV	CP		Benefit	
Budd (1985)	Naloxone	20–50 mg IV	CP		Benefit	
Bowsher (1988)	Naloxone	IV 0.8 mg	Cordotomized pts with mirror pain		Increased pain in one third and induced it in one not suffering it	
Backonja and Gombar (1992)	Lidocaine	IV. Single infusion	BCP: 6; CCP: 2	Case series	3 BCP benefited over 8–20 weeks; partial relief in 2 SCI cases	
Edmonson et al. (1993)	Lidocaine	IV. Initial bolus: 50–100 mg + continuous infusion for 48 h	CPSP: 4	Case series	All patients reported some relief within the first 12 h of infusion. Subsequent oral mexiletine trial: 2 pts had excellent relief at 1 yr, 2 stopped because of intolerable side effects	
Galer et al. (1993)	Lidocaine	5 mg/kg/h for 60–90 min IV	CP: 13	Retrospective series	1 excellent relief, 3 partial reliefs, 9 0% reliefs	
Nagaro et al. (1995)	Lidocaine	IV. 1.5 mg/kg in 1 min	CP and PNP	Case series	Pain score measured by visual analog scale (VAS, 0–10), 5, 15 and 35 min after the infusion decreased to less than 50% of pre-infusion value in more than 75% of cases of thalamic pain	SCI pain relatively refractory
Migita et al. (1995)	Thyamilal, morphine	Doses as per Yamamoto et al. (1997)	CP: 2	Case report	Pt 1: barbiturate and morphine ineffective. Pt 2: barbiturate effective, morphine ineffective	Study on TMS

Study	Drug	Condition	Study type	Dose	Comments
Yamamoto et al. (1997)	Morphine, then naloxone	CPSP: 39 (thalamic 25, extrathalamic 14, brainstem 0)	Case series	IV 3 mg every 5 min up to 18 mg	Study evaluating the effect of IV morphine (day 1), IV thiamylal (day 2) and IV ketamine (day 3). A few pts fell asleep with barbiturate. Threshold of significance: ≥40%. No differences between thalamic and suprathalamic cases. All ketamine responsive cases except 1 also sensitive to thiamylal, but 4 cases resistant to ketamine responded to thiamylal.	1 thalamic and 1 suprathalamic pts (of 3 sensitive to IV morphine) relieved at long term by oral morphine 30–120 mg die All pts refractory to imipramine (75 mg), maprotiline (60 mg), bromazepam (12 mg), ibuprofen (600 mg) Pain worsened by ketamine in 2 pts
	Thiamylal			IV 50 mg every 5 min up to 250 mg		
	Ketamine	CPSP: 23		IV 5 mg every 5 min up to 25 mg.		
Kumar et al. (1997)	Morphine	CPSP: 5; CCP: 3	Case series of DBS	25 mg IV	0% relief in all	
Koyama et al. (1998)	Amobarbital	CPSP: 1	Case report	IV. 50 mg	IV (but not PO) AMO was effective in reducing CP, although similar plasma concentration levels were reached PO and IV	CP after loss of his left upper extremity. IV AMO was followed by 300–400 mg/day AMO PO

(continued)

TABLE 5.4 (continued)

Authors	Drug(s)	Route/dosage	Pain type; no. of patients	Study design	Outcome	Other details
Canavero and Bonicalzi 1998	Propofol	IV, 0.2 mg/kg	CCP: 1	Review with case report	IT midazolam effective; propofol effective; baclofen and other agents not as effective	All drugs proposed as diagnostic test
	Lidocaine	IV, 3–5 mg/kg in 30 min				
	Ketamine	IV, 60 µg/kg + 6 µg/kg/min				
	Midazolam	IT, 1–2.5 mg				
	Baclofen	IT, 50 µg				
	Fentanyl	IV, 50 µg				
	Alfentanil	IV, 0.6 µg/kg + 6 µg/kg/min				
	Clonidine	IT				
Wajma et al. (2000)	Thiopental	IV (approximately 1 mg/kg)	SCI: 1	Case report	IM butorphanol, saline and atropine sulfate as placebo, IT morphine HCL, mexiletine, IV lidocaine ineffective. IV thiopental, fentanyl, butorphanol, ketamine, midazolam, droperidol, sevoflurane-oxygen anesthesia quite effective	Original CP decreased after 16 subarachnoid blocks with local anesthetic. IV thiopental was the most effective treatment in CP. CP worsened by spinal anesthesia
Trentin and Visentin (2000)	Lidocaine	4 mg/kg IV over 30 min	CP: 16	Case series	44% responded; after 45 min, LIDO = PLA	Later good response to mexiletine PO, but not amitriptyline
Chatterjee et al. (2002)	Herbal cannabis	1 "joint" daily	CPSP: 1	Case report	Complete pain relief and marked improvement in dystonia from	Right hemiplegic painful dystonia (left-sided idiopathic

Reference	Drug	Route/Dose	Condition	Study type	Effect	Comments
					smoked cannabis (3 months follow-up)	caudate atrophy). 3 temporarily successful thalamotomies performed. Partial response to morphine plus buproprion and amitriptyline (VAS reduction from 9/10 to 4/10)
Willoch et al. (2004)	Morphine	PO	CPSP: 2		Poorly effective	
Cahana et al. (2004)	Lidocaine	IV, 5 mg/kg (in 150 mL of saline) over 30 min without a bolus. 2 daily cycles for 5 days at a 6 month interval	CP (postinfective pontine lesion): 1	Case report	Persistent spontaneous pain and frequency of pain attacks reduction was observed immediately, 1, 3 and 7 days and 1, 2, and 3 months after treatment in all body areas, but the chin	Persistent pain relief after repeated IV lidocaine infusions. PET study. Thalamic hypoperfusion renormalized. CP unresponsive to amitriptyline, nortriptyline, carbamazepine, oxcarbazepine, gabapentin, valproate, lamotrigine, baclofen and clonazepam
Cohen and DeJesus (2004)	Ketamine	PCA device (2.7 mg/h basal; same dose on demand)	CCP (syrinx): 1	Case report	One year later, pain dramatically decreased, opioids significantly reduced	Previous high dose opioids ineffective
Nuti et al. (2005)	Morphine	IV test	CP: 7 pts	Case series	No significant effect	

ways from barbiturates and benzodiazepines, although IT midazolam, but not oral benzodiazepines, reduces CP in propofol-responsive patients (Canavero and Bonicalzi 1998, 2004). Most importantly, propofol at doses effective for CP has an exclusive GABA A action, without appreciable effects on other transmitters/ modulators and ion channels (see complete references in Canavero and Bonicalzi 2004). PET studies reveal that propofol at subhypnotic doses first targets the cortex, then the thalamus; it is thus possible that subhypnotic propofol allays CP by renormalizing a specific derangement at cortical level (discussed and referenced in Canavero and Bonicalzi 1998, 2004; see also Hofbauer *et al.* 2004). Propofol also renormalizes brain deactivations seen in CP patients (see Chapter 7). Occasional worsening might depend on drug increasing ongoing overinhibition at CNS sites.

Barbiturates can reduce CP, but their pharmacodynamic profile goes beyond simple GABA agonism and may even reduce (like halothane, a volatile anesthetic with a GABA A profile) descending inhibition, favoring long-term increases in nociception (Sandkuehler 1996). Thiopental is administered IV at 50 mg boluses up to 225 mg and thiamylal at 50 mg IV every 5 minutes up to 250 mg: when effective, relief appears after 5—8 minutes and lasts several minutes (Migita *et al.* 1995; Mailis *et al.* 1997; Yamamoto *et al.* 1997; Koyama *et al.* 1998). There is no experience in treating CP paroxysms with IV boluses of *midazolam* (3—5 mg), but this deserves consideration. *Oral benzodiazepines* have no effect on CP, with the possible exception of clonazepam on painful paroxysms. Benzodiazepines enhance GABA A-mediated inhibition within thalamic reticular nucleus and thereby suppress GABA B-mediated inhibition in relay neurons (Huguenard and Prince 1997). *Baclofen*, a GABA-B agonist, has relieved CP via the IT route (Chapter 6), but no meaningful analgesia is generally seen at orally tolerated doses (<60 mg die).

On the basis of these studies, we distinguish two classes of CP: GABA responsive (Class A) and GABA refractory (Class B) (Canavero and Bonicalzi 2004). GABA responsiveness (Class A) marks patients who stand the best chances of relief from neuromodulation (Chapter 6). There may also be a differential of responsiveness between disruptive and compressive CP-related lesions, with the former less responsive than the latter (unpublished observations), but this awaits confirmation.

Several other oral drugs display GABA agonism (Moshè 2000) and may reduce CP. *Gabapentin* increases GABA levels in the human brain via a poorly characterized, non-GABA receptor-mediated mechanism, with highest affinity for locations in the outer layers of the frontoparietal (and other) cortices. This drug has relieved some patients (particularly evoked pains in one series); however, in our extensive experience, no more than 5% of CP patients are relieved in monotherapy at 2400—3600 mg and, in line with other investigators (Ness *et al.* 2002), "gabapentin does not have proven utility as a monotherapy in the experience of…(SCI) patients." Even in a recent randomized, controlled study which also included nine CP patients, relief greater than 50% was seen in only 21% of patients versus 14% on placebo over 8 weeks (Serpell *et al.* 2002). Despite a reputation for tolerability, actually gabapentin has an incidence of major side effects no different from carbamazepine (Wiffen *et al.* 2000) and in SCI pain, clomipramine seems to be more effective — although less well tolerated — than gabapentin (55% versus 48% of patients) (Reboiledo *et al.* 2002). Progabide, a GABA A agonist, awaits to be tested.

We saw no major effect with *vigabatrin*, an irreversible GABA transaminase blocker, which diffusely increases GABA levels. Thus, drugs such as vigabatrin and perhaps *tiagabine* (a selective GABA reuptake blocker) and *pregabalin*, but also *topiramate*, might not be the appropriate choice, as GABA is excessively increased unselectively throughout the brain (unlike lamotrigine and gabapentin); *anesthetic gases* (GABA A agonists) also do not relieve CP. In the human brain, vigabatrin/tiagabine increase GABA 300%, topiramate 200%, lamotrigine/valproate/gabapentin (*c.* 1200 mg) 150% (Verhoeff *et al.* 1999); after single doses, cerebral GABA rises 70% acutely (hours) with topiramate, 48% with gabapentin and 0% with lamotrigine; with target dose reached at 4 weeks, these increases are, respectively, 46, 25 and 25% (Kuzniecky *et al.* 2002). GABA is rapidly reuptaken by neurons and glia, but with some drugs the excess cannot be eliminated. If confirmed, this would be in line with the observation that there are only a few specific brain regions in which augmentation of GABA function is anticonvulsant (Gale 1992): enhanced GABA transmission can either reduce or *increase* brain excitability depending on the brain region in which this happens. Moreover, only GABA elevation associated with nerve terminals, but not with metabolic compartments, can lead to enhanced GABA transmission. Differences among drugs may also depend on electrophysiological factors, e.g., enhancement of the frequency of opening rather than the open channel duration of the receptor. Spike-wave discharges are blocked by GABA A agonists such as benzodiazepines or T-type Ca^{2+} blockers and are worsened by direct activation of GABA currents, for instance by phenobarbital (also a non-T calcium, sodium and AMPA blocker), a drug ineffective for CP. Also, GABA B activation results in more hyperpolarization than does GABA A activation. However, the neuronal conductance increase and thus the decrease in neuronal input resistance is much greater with GABA A than B; accordingly, GABA A inhibits more by clamping the membrane at a subthreshold level and thus shunting EPSPs, while GABA B inhibits more by hyperpolarizing the membrane. Unlike GABA B (voltage subtractor), the GABA A response is much more nonlinear (voltage multiplicator) and GABA A response is faster than B (Shepherd 2004). Finally, we do not expect neurosteroids (e.g., ganaxolone) or gamma hydroxybutyrate, naturally present substances in the brain with GABA effects, to have major effects in CP.

b. Antiglutamatergic agents.

b. Antiglutamatergic agents. The glutamate NMDA receptor subtype is widely believed to play a pivotal role in pain transmission along with the AMPA subtype. Although extensive animal experimentation concluded for a major role in the mechanisms of neuropathic pain, actually, agents that antagonize the NMDA receptor have basically no place in the long-term treatment of CP: their side effect profile is unfavorable, particularly for ketamine, and the achieved benefit is no greater than other better-tolerated drugs. Even patients with different chronic pains selected for oral treatment after IV ketamine challenge (e.g., 0.4 mg/kg IM) do not uniformly draw benefit from oral therapy (Rabben *et al.* 1999), e.g., 1.5−2.5 mg/kg 5−6 times a day of ketamine, and long-term oral treatment may result in hepatotoxicity and severe psychic complications. NMDA blockade with dextrorphan/dextrometorphan (D-isomer of methorphan, also a sigma opioid and 5HT agonist) or the modestly stronger adamantane drugs (amantadine and memantine) relieved few patients to a major degree, without disabling side effects (see Canavero *et al.* 2002; Taira 1998); no experience has accrued with cycloserine. While no published data on felbamate (another antiglutamatergic agent) exist, its potential for lethal complications limits its clinical usage.

Poor or modest relief in most patients and the narrow therapeutic ratio of clinically available NMDA antagonists speaks against their use (Sang 2002). However, these drugs provided invaluable information on the neurochemistry of CP, particularly IV ketamine (Canavero and Bonicalzi 1998). Importantly, case reports of patients with cortical disease who failed to demonstrate analgesia to surgical stimuli in spite of multiple doses of ketamine suggested that *an intact and functioning cortex is a prerequisite for ketamine analgesia* (Drury and Clark 1970; Morgan *et al.* 1971; Janis and Wright 1972). NMDA receptors are especially important for intracortical processing. In an fMRI study, subanesthetic doses of ketamine especially reduced acute nociceptive-related brain activity in the insula and the thalamus (Rogers *et al.* 2002).

c. Sodium channel blockers. Initially employed to quench abnormal activity in neuromas and demyelinated peripheral fibers of PNP patients, the bulk of evidence points to the efficacy of sodium channel blockers in CP (Tremont-Lukats *et al.* 2005). Both lidocaine and its oral congener mexiletine act in an activity-dependent manner: as doses increase, repetitive firing is blocked before axon conduction, providing a degree of selectivity for paroxysmal activity. Although a peripheral action has been established at doses below those achieving conduction block, *a central action is also likely* (Boas *et al.* 1982); the observed preferential antihyperalgesic and antiallodynic effects of lidocaine suggest a selective central action on the mechanisms underlying such evoked pains. In particular, they may have a specific action on brush-evoked and mechanical allodynia, unrelated to general analgesic effects (Attal *et al.* 2000). In healthy humans, a single IV bolus of lidocaine results in sustained and constant concentrations in the cerebrospinal fluid, with a faster plasma decay (Usubiaga *et al.* 1967; Tsai *et al.* 1998). Although the lidocaine test may predict analgesia from mexiletine in several patients, this is not generally indicated.

IV *lidocaine* has been administered at doses of 1 mg/kg (over 10 minutes) to 5 mg/kg (over 30–120 minutes) diluted in saline, sometimes via a pump. Pressure and EKG monitoring are mandatory. Dysarthria and somnolence call for immediate suspension and lidocaine is contraindicated with Adams–Stokes syndrome or severe atrioventricular heart block. The most frequent minor side effect is dizziness during infusion. *Mexiletine* is started at 200 mg and increased every few days to a maximum of 1000 mg, analgesia or intolerable side effects; it must be administered on a full stomach to reduce nausea. Other side effects include dizziness, tremor, "jitters" and headache. A yearly EKG is indicated. Patients with a history of heart disease, arrhythmias, atrioventricular heart blocks and other EKG anomalies must be evaluated by a cardiologist before starting PO mexiletine. *Lamotrigine* must be increased slowly starting from 25–50 mg to reach a maximum dose of 600–800 mg, analgesia or intolerable side effects. While generally well tolerated, lamotrigine very rarely triggers Stevens–Johnson syndrome, which can be fatal. *Carbamazepine* is often poorly tolerated at effective dosage, with several CNS effects (e.g., ataxia). It must be started at 100 mg bid and increased to a maximum of 1200 mg, analgesia or intolerable side effects (an analog, oxcarbazepine, may be better tolerated); moreover, white cell counts must be monitored frequently in the first few months to check for possible hematologic toxicity. *Valproate* (also a weak T calcium blocker and unspecific pro-GABA drug) has allayed pain in few patients. Clearly, safer drugs are needed.

Similarly to GABA agonists, only some sodium blockers relieve CP and mexiletine may be the most potent (Canavero and Bonicalzi 2005; see also Bowsher 1994), although a formal trial is needed. Topiramate (also an antiglutamatergic, GABAergic agent; but see discussion in Canavero *et al.* 2002), phenytoin (also a L Ca^{2+} and NMDA blocker and GABAergic agent) and carbamazepine (also a weak L Ca^{2+} blocker, proserotoninergic, antiAMPA (-20%) and antiadenosine-1 agent) are the least effective, except for paroxysmal MS/SCI pains (Wiffen *et al.* 2000). Phenytoin has a longer time dependence for frequency-dependent blockade and for recovery from it than carbamazepine; neither affect amplitude or duration of individual action potentials, but both reduce the ability of neurons to fire high-frequency trains of action potentials in a use-dependent manner. Lamotrigine (which is also a powerful antiglutamatergic and modest GABAergic agent) has been found effective, but it lost effect in all our initially published patients (Canavero and Bonicalzi 1996) after 2–3 years (unpublished observations). Sodium block also leads to reduced glutamate release and the differential potency of mexiletine and lamotrigine versus carbamazepine may relate to this factor (Canavero and Bonicalzi 1996). *Riluzole*, a sodium channel blocker and NMDA antagonist has proved scarcely effective for PNP (Sang 2002), and we do not expect major analgesia in CP either. *Zonisamide*, a sodium–T calcium channel blocker with some GABA, serotonergic and dopaminergic effects, may prove helpful (see also Finnerup *et al.* 2002 for further discussion on mechanisms of action of anticonvulsants). In contrast, agents that target specific sodium channel subtypes in peripheral tissues (e.g., SNS1/PN3) will most certainly have no impact on CP, although some believe that the Nav1.3 subtype is upregulated in first, second and third-order neurons of the pain pathway after contusive SCI, leading to enhanced excitability (Waxman and Hains 2006).

From a pathophysiological standpoint, reviewed data point to hyperactivity as a mechanism of CP (Canavero and Bonicalzi 1998; Max and Hagen 2000).

d. Antidepressants. Amitriptyline, a tricyclic, is useful for BCP, but not (or only insignificantly) for CCP, syringomyelia CP or MS CP (see also Beric 1999), where side effects have a larger impact. Even in BCP patients, only about half will benefit and often only partially; worse yet, many cannot tolerate its many and sometimes serious side effects. The NNT of amitriptyline and congeners in CP is 1.7 (McQuay *et al.* 1996; Sindrup and Jensen 1999). Continuous, lancinating and thermally (but less so mechanically) evoked pains may respond, with analgesic doses less – but not much less, at least in our experience – than antidepressant ones. Analgesia can appear days to 5 weeks after initiation, regardless of dose, and can increase slowly, even if plasma levels are stable: a trial of efficacy should never last less than 2 months, bar intolerable side effects. After suspension of therapy, analgesia is lost gradually, but slower than expected from plasma levels. Relief is seen in both depressed and nondepressed patients and depressed patients may have their mood improved, but not their CP. Side effects include, among others, orthostatic hypotension (alpha block), urinary retention, memory loss, cardiac conduction abnormalities (muscarinic block) and sedation (histamine block). Amitriptyline is usually started at 10 mg in the elderly and 25 mg in younger patients and increased by 5–10 mg every few days until benefit or toxicity or a maximum dose of 300 mg. Being sedating (but less than doxepin), it can be given before sleep, until divided doses become necessary. Tricyclics call for an EKG at onset and EKG and blood level measurements above 100 mg die. Artificial saliva is indicated to counter mouth dryness (an anticholinergic effect). Anticholinergic effects contraindicate tricyclics in SCI pains, as these can trigger constipation or bladder retention and pain exacerbations. Although some congeners may be better tolerated (e.g., nortriptyline and clomipramine), it is a general opinion that amitriptyline is the most effective of all antidepressants, with tertiary amines more effective than secondary amines and both more than SSRIs (Sindrup and Jensen 1999). In fact, serotonin-specific reuptake blockers (fluoxetine and congeners), but also atypical agents, such as trazodone and risperidone, although better tolerated, have not proved superior to tricyclics and actually relieved few patients to a meaningful extent, and so serotonin/norepinephrine (e.g., venlafaxine) and selective norepinephrine (e.g., reboxetine) blockers. Interestingly, Sicuteri (1971) had reported that 4 out of 18 cases of intractable migraine treated with parachlorophenylalanine and 2 out of 23 treated with reserpine (both drugs are serotonin antagonists) developed spontaneous pain, hyperalgesia and hyperpathia in the body, similar to CP. No experience has accrued with MAO inhibitors. Why amitriptyline should be the most effective agent remains controversial. The importance of norepinephrine and serotonin agonism singly has not stood up to scrutiny (Jasmin et al. 2003; Canavero and Bonicalzi 2004). Yet, the range of action of tricyclics is bewildering: besides NE and 5HT effects, they also are alpha-1 and histamine-1 antagonists, sodium blockers, NMDA antagonists, opioid agonists, anticholinergic, increase local levels of adenosine, potentiate neurogenesis, regulate synaptic plasticity and enhance endocrine function (see references in Jasmin et al. 2003).

e. Opioids, naloxone and cannabinoids. By the IV route, morphine (and congeners) relieved none or only few patients with CP and only at very high doses. Their place in the treatment of CP is very limited (Canavero and Bonicalzi 2003; see also Warms et al. 2002; Eisenberg et al. 2005); their long-term side effect profile, with serious endocrinological and immune function side effects, excludes them from life-long treatment of CP (Ballantyne and Mao 2003). The only exception would be those rare patients who draw major benefit from not too high PO doses of morphine (e.g., MS Contin) (Yamamoto et al. 1997: 2/39 BCP patients; Attal et al. 2002: 3/15 BCP/CCP patients) or other congeners (e.g., methadone and dextropropoxyphene, also NMDA antagonists) who are fully informed of long-term consequences. As we have seen, the first patient in history to be diagnosed with

CP was opioid unresponsive (Edinger 1891; see Chapter 1) and, among others, Davis and Martin (1947) found opioids ineffective for true CP of cord origin.

From a pathophysiological standpoint, opioid unresponsiveness may simply depend on low − rather than loss of − opioid receptor binding in human SI (Pfeiffer et al. 1982; Sadzot et al. 1990; Jones et al. 1991; Willoch et al. 2004): "medial pain system" brain areas (i.e., thalamus, ACC, PFC, insula, temporal cortex and others) have a high density of opioid receptors, and this would point to a critical role of the sensory cortex in CP mechanisms (Chapter 8). However, morphine may have some effect on non-thermal allodynia, a likely sensitization-driven event (Chapter 8). Interestingly, opioids inhibit GABA interneurons, and, in light of the high efficacy of GABA agonists, this would be further reason to limit their use. Opioid unresponsiveness of CP speaks against a functional impairment of the CNS opiate system. Naloxone has not proved analgesic in a RCT (see Tables 5.1−5.4), although the dose employed was lower than per initial claims of efficacy. One notes the impossibility for an agonist and its antagonist to have therapeutic effects on the same disease, bar invoking unknown mechanisms of action.

Cannabinoids have a mixed (short) track record up to now, but the impression is that they will not represent a substantial advance over currently available drugs (see also Warms et al. 2002).

f. Miscellaneous agents. The following agents had no impact in the treatment of CP: NSAIDs, misoprostol (except for MS-associated trigeminal neuralgia), calcitonin, IV adenosine (which triggers frequent headache) (Eisenach et al. 2003), cholinergics (despite M1 and M4 and nicotinic receptors' involvement in endogenous analgesia; Mullan 2002), atophanyl, phenotiazines (which have severe side effects, including tardive dyskinesia), antihistaminics, mephnesin, IV tetraethylammonium (Davis and Martin 1947). Topical pain (band-like area or patch) may be treated with an amitriptyline-ketamine or gabapentin cream, but there is no published experience for CP.

We do not expect to achieve relief of CP with anti-absence drugs, such as ethosuximide (a T Ca^{2+} blocker), while levetiracetam gave no benefit in one personal patient).

g. Combinations. These have never been addressed in a controlled manner. However, in our experience, a combination of high-dose mexiletine and gabapentin properly administered proved synergic and highly effective in more than 50% of the patients we treated, with manageable side effects; as these were almost all referral cases who did not respond to prior therapy (amitriptyline, carbamazepine), this can be considered a successful combination (Canavero and Bonicalzi 2005). In epilepsy, promising combinations have been found to include a sodium blocker and a GABA agonist, two GABA agonists or two glutamatergic drugs with different receptor profile (Deckers et al. 2000). Intriguingly, even for CP, a combination of a sodium blocker (mexiletine) and a GABA agonist (gabapentin) proved particularly worthy. Antidepressants and antiepileptics in combination have not yet been assessed in a controlled trial for CP. Contrary to animal data, we see no place for combinations of morphine with gabapentin or dextrometorphan.

2. Drug aggravation of CP

Some of the drugs reviewed worsened CP in a few patients: ketamine in 2 patients reported by Yamamoto *et al.* (1997), propofol in 3 and dextrometorphan (100 mg) in 2 of our patients (unpublished observations), but also IT baclofen (Loubser *et al.* 1996). These should not be dismissed, as they may point to focal neurochemical mechanisms in single patients.

We would also caution against the use of modafinil, a glutamatergic agonist and GABA antagonist used in the treatment of MS: this might worsen MS-associated CP.

6 NEUROMODULATION

"Perhaps we can now envision a day in which, with the use of stimulation techniques, we can take advantage of the brain's natural modes of organization and reinforce them in time of need, whether to control pain,...epileptic...discharge, or...tremor."

(**Ervin and colleagues, 1966**)

When oral or parenteral drugs fail, the problem is what to do. In view of the continuing efforts aimed at neural reconstruction in the human brain and thus "physiologically" revert pain, and progress in neuromodulation and drug therapy, today there is only little room left for ablative procedures. Despite temporary initial benefit with several of these, destructive surgery at any level of the CNS has only a low long-term (>5 years) success rate, with a high incidence of recurrence and only few lucky patients totally relieved in the long term (Tasker 2001). Moreover, all techniques carry a serious risk of permanent, disabling complications, including new or worsening of pre-existent CP, as ablation only adds further damage.

The only true option is neuromodulation. This can be mainly achieved through electrical stimulation of the damaged nervous system or intrathecal pharmacologic infusion through implanted pumps.

ELECTRICAL

The analgesic effect of electrical stimulation has been known since Roman (and perhaps even earlier) times, when the shock from an electric fish was used to relieve gout pain and other pains, a custom that was not lost in the following centuries. The eighteenth century witnessed a resurgence of this technique, despite strong opposition. With Galvani and particularly Alessandro Volta in the nineteenth century, electrotherapy was poised to make progress. One of the true pioneers in the field was the Frenchman Duchenne de Boulogne, who published a classic book in 1855, in which he reported his experience in treating a wide variety of conditions, and predominantly pain, with custom-made machines; Hermel too treated neuralgias with "electro-puncture" (historical review in Sedan and Lazorthes 1978). Riddoch (1938) noted that CP could sometimes be diminished by concomitant stimulation through faradization in the abnormal or adjacent normal body parts. Today, more sophisticated means are employed.

1. Extra- and subdural motor (MCS) and sensory cortex stimulation (PCS) (Table 6.1)

CP is the original disorder that led Tsubokawa and colleagues to try MI (BA4) stimulation in 1988. Currently, the procedure is performed under local or general anesthesia. A stimulating paddle is positioned on the dura overlying the motor or sensory cortex trough two burr holes or alternatively a small craniotomy or craniectomy under fMR and/or neuronavigational conditions and, if effective parameters are found after a test period, hooked up to a subclavear pacemaker. A subdural approach may be elected in cases of pain involving the foot and distal leg. Permanent disabling morbidity (including epilepsy and intracerebral hemorrhage) and mortality have not been reported. Stimulation parameters have been the most diverse, analgesia having been obtained with both high and low frequencies (even > 100 Hz), low and high voltage, continuous and intermittent stimulation. The choice of stimulation parameters is also dependent on the presence of the so-called post-effect. Many, but not all, patients have their pain relieved or improved almost immediately during intraoperative stimulation for periods ranging from several minutes to hours or several days without further stimulation. This effect has a tendency to abate over time and by the second month may stabilize at several minutes to a few hours. Analgesia also can fade over time. Repositioning of the electrode or intensive reprogramming may restore benefit in some cases, although often at a lower level. Tolerance and fatigue are proposed mechanisms of such effects. Best results are seen when the stimulating poles overlie parts of cortex corresponding to painful body parts, although some data suggest that precise, "millimetric," somatotopic localization of the electrode may not be required (see full-breadth review and operative indications in Canavero and Bonicalzi 2002, 2003, 2004, 2006).

Analgesia can be expected when patients display mild (but not severe) sensory loss – particularly normal or only mildly elevated thermal sensory thresholds within the painful zone – and intact or almost intact corticospinal motor function, but several exceptions exist making these relative criteria only (Canavero and Bonicalzi 2002, 2006). Most importantly, pharmacological tests can predict analgesia in the single patient. Barbiturate- and/or ketamine-responsive patients can expect pain relief. We found a good correlation between analgesia with CS and response to transcranial magnetic stimulation (TMS) and between these two and propofol test (Canavero et al. 2003); apparently, responsiveness to GABA marks patients that are particularly favorable for stimulation. TMS also appears to predict response to CS, but, just like CS, its analgesic effect is not as strong (Canavero et al. 2003, 2005), and even when conducted daily for five consecutive days at higher frequency than usual (20 Hz), the duration of effect tends to be short (less than 2 weeks), with patients unpredictably obtaining excellent or no benefit (Khedr et al. 2005: 12 CPSP patients).

Even transcranial direct current stimulation does not appear to improve substantially on these results, being particularly effective for paroxysmal pain rather than the more resistant continuous pain (SCI CP: Fregni et al. 2006, 11 active therapy patients).

TABLE 6.1. Motor cortex stimulation (MCS) (arranged by reporting groups)

Author(s)	Type of pain (no. of patients)	Results (follow-up)	Notes
Tsubokawa's group			
Tsubokawa et al. *Pain* 1990; *Suppl* 5:S491 (abs.952)	CP (25 pts)	Effective in 75% of cases (>7 mos)	**First report of MCS for CP (1988)** MCS vs. thalamic stimulation. MCS is more effective than thalamic stimulation. Improvement of motor function in some pts
Tsubokawa et al. (1991)	Thalamic pain (7 pts)	Excellent (5: no drugs needed) or good (2: some drugs needed) pain relief	MCS improved movements of the painful limbs. Pain subsided within a few minutes. 5–10 min ON, 4–5 h relief 5–6 times daily, then 2–3 times daily
Tsubokawa et al. *Acta Neurochir Suppl* (Wien) 1991; 52:137–9	CPSP (12 pts; thalamic lesion: 6 pts; putaminal lesion: 3 pts; pontine hemorrhage: 1 pt; other lesions: 2 pts)	Complete pain relief in 5/12 pts (1 yr), considerable pain reduction in 3/12 pts (1 yr). Long-term benefit in 8/12 pts (>1 yr)	Intermittent stimulation effective in 5/12 pts. No seizures; pain relief at stimulus intensities below movements threshold. Paresis improvement. Pain improvement in barbiturate-sensitive, morphine-resistant pts. Disappearance of the analgesic effect in 3 pts, with reappearance after revision of electrode placement
Tsubokawa et al. (1993) (*Also see Tsubokawa et al. Pain* 1993; 58 (*Suppl.*):150)	CPSP (11 pts; thalamic stroke: 8 pts; putaminal hemorrhage + small lesion in the posterior limb of the internal capsule): 3 pts)	Pain relief: **Immediate:** Excellent (>80%): 6/11 (54%) Good (60–79%): 2/11 (18%) Fair (40–59%): 1/11 (9%) Poor (<40%): 2/11 (18%) **Long-lasting:** Excellent (>80%): 5/11 (45%) Good (60–79%): 0/8 Fair (40–59%): 0/8 Poor (<40%): 3/8 (37%) (2 yrs)	Barbiturate-sensitive pts: 5 (+3?)/11; morphine-resistant pts: 10 (+1?)/11. Stimulation of area 4 ipsilateral to the inciting lesion. One week test period. Fair and poor responders not implanted. Satisfactory immediate pain relief in 8/11 pts (73%). Gradual effect reduction over several mos in 3/8 pts. Long-term response in barbiturate-sensitive and morphine-resistant pts (also for Vc DBS). No pain-relieving effect by high-frequency postcentral stimulation (11/11 pts): in 2, worsening of pain, similar to their spontaneous ones. In 3 pts, areas rostral to MI stimulated without relief. Nonpainful paresthesias unrelieved

(continued)

185

TABLE 6.1 (continued)

Author(s)	Type of pain (no. of patients)	Results (follow-up)	Notes
Katayama et al. *Stereotact Funct Neurosurg* 1994; 62:295–9 (*Tsubokawa's group*)	CPSP (6 pts; lateral medullary infarct)	MCS in 3 pts. Pain relief: 2/3 > 60%; 1/3 > 40% (4 mos)	Pain relief >40% in 1 pt previously unsuccessfully treated by Vc DBS. No satisfactory pain control by thalamic stimulation in any pts
Yamamoto et al. (1997) (*Tsubokawa's group*)	CPSP (39 pts; thalamic stroke: 25 cases; suprathalamic stroke: 14 pts)	28 MCS. Excellent/good (50–100%) pain relief: Thalamic pts: 10/19 (53%) Suprathal. pts: 3/9 (33%) (difference not significant) T+ or K+ & M+: 2/4 (50%) T+ or K+ & M−: 10/14 (71%) T− & K− & M+: 0/2 (0%) T− & K− & M−: 1/8 (13%) Overall: 13/28 (46%) (12 mos)	Suprathalamic stroke = infarct or hemorrhage of the posterior limb of internal capsule, or parietal lobe, sparing the thalamus. No pts with midbrain or medullary lesions. MCS test period: 1 wk. 8/39: morphine responsive (M+) 22/39: thiamylal responsive (T+) 11/23: ketamine responsive (K+) Thiamylal + ketamine sensitivity + morphine resistance may predict a positive effect of MCS
Katayama et al. (1998) (*Also includes:* Katayama et al. *Stereotact Funct Neurosurg* 1997; 69:73–9) Tsubokawa et al. *In: Abst. 3rd Int Congress INS, Orlando, 1996, p. 123*) Some of the pts already reported in Tsubokawa, *J Neurosurg* 1993, above (*Tsubokawa's group*)	CPSP (31 pts. Thalamic stroke: 20 pts; putaminal hemorrhage: 8 pts; lateral medullary infarction: 3 pts)	Early satisfactory (>60%) pain relief: 23/31 pts (74%). Long-term efficacy (≥2 yrs): 15/31 pts (48%)	Damage of the posterior limb of the internal capsule in pts with putaminal hemorrhage. Previous ineffective SCS. Pain relief >60%: 13/18 pts (73%) with no or mild motor weakness (70% of pts with inducible muscle contraction); 2/13 pts (15%) with moderate or severe motor weakness (difference statistically significant). Satisfactory pain control in 14/20 pts (70%) with inducible muscle contraction, but in only 1/11 pts (9%) without inducible motor contractions ($p < 0.01$). No relationship between pain control and presence of hypesthesia, dysesthesia, hyperpathia, allodynia or disappearance of SSEP N20 wave plus stimulation-induced paresthesias, or motor performance improvement. 3 pts with MCS or DBS became pain-free without stimulation for years (all 3 getting initial excellent relief at

Reference	Patients	Pain relief	Comments
Yamamoto et al. (2000)	Small thalamic stroke, then action tremor, then Vim DBS, then cardioversion, then CPSP	50% relief over 2 years	Thiamylal/ketamine responsive, morphine resistant (progressively longer stimulation intervals during intermittent stimulation)
Katayama et al. (2001) (Tsubokawa's group)	CPSP (45 pts)	Satisfactory pain control: SCS: 7% of pts; DBS: 25% of pts; MCS: 48% of pts	(See text) Sometimes SCS and DBS produced long-lasting pain-free intervals (stimulator switched off). DBS and MCS in 4 pts: better result: MCS 1/4 pts; DBS 2/4
Fukaya et al. (2003) Also includes: Katayama et al. Acta Neurochir Suppl. 2003; 87:121-3 (Tsubokawa's group)	CPSP (31 pts)	Unsuccessful MCS in 2 CPSP pts reporting abnormal pain sensation after stimulation of the motor cortex (see text)	Experimental study on conscious somatosensory response during surgery for electrode placement
Toronto group:			
Parrent and Tasker (1992) Tasker et al. 1994 Tasker 2001	CPSP (1 pt, large suprathalamic infarct) CPSP (2 pts)	Substantial pain relief with *ipsilateral to pain* MCS with gradual abatement over 6 yrs; relief with subdural stimulation over a few months. 1 relief, 1 failure	Contralateral MCS due to a lack of sufficient MI on the affected side. Stimulation-induced ipsilateral paresthesias
Hosobuchi (1993) Also includes: Stereotact Funct Neurosurg 1992; 59:76-83 Abstr. IASP Congress 1993	CPSP (5 pts; post-removal of parietal cortical AVM: 1 pt; brainstem infarction: 1 pt; thalamic lesion: 3 pts)	Pain relief: Initial: 5/5 excellent. At 2-3 mos: 4/5 excellent (>50%); fair. At 9-30 mos: 3/5 excellent (thalamic, parietal, brainstem)	Efficacy dramatically reduced in 2 thalamic pain pts, to 0% in 1 pt and 30% in 1 pt 2-6 mos after implantation
Karolinska group:			
Meyerson et al. Acta Neurochir Suppl (Wien) 1993; 58:150-3	CPSP (3 pts; thalamic hemorrhage: 2 pts; brainstem infarction: 1 pt)	Pain relief: CPSP: none: 3/3	In spite of multipolar electrode grid in 1 and relocation of paddle in another

(continued)

TABLE 6.1 (continued)

Author(s)	Type of pain (no. of patients)	Results (follow-up)	Notes
Paris group:			
Nguyen et al. *Acta Neurochir Suppl (Wien)* 1997; 68:54–60	CP (12 pts; parietal lobe infarct: 1 pt; basal ganglia hematoma: 3 pts; thalamic pain: 5 pts (4 stroke, 1 abscess); deep post-traumatic brain lesion: 1 pt; SCI: 2 pts)	Pain relief: (a) parietal lobe infarct 80–100%: 1/1 pt (14 mos) (b) basal ganglia hematoma <40%: 1/3 pts (30 mos) 40–60%: 2/3 pts (25 + 32 mos) (c) thalamic pain <40%: 2/5 pts (18 + 22 mos) 40–60%: 1/5 pt (28 mos); 60–80%: 2/5 pts (22 + 30 mos)* (d) post-traumatic lesion <40%: 1/1 pt (29 mos) (e) SCI <40% in a paraplegic pt (18 mos); 100% (visceral pain + substantial reduction of diffuse pain) in a tetraplegic pt (22 mos)	Disappearance of allodynia in 2, but reduction only of spontaneous pain in 1 pt in the thalamic pain group. Globally, continuous pain improved in 4/10, evoked pain in 6/8 and paroxysms in 6/7. Reduction of the initial pain relief (to less than 40% in 2) in 3 cases. Previous ineffective Vc DBS (basal ganglia, deep lesion). Best results in the parietal lobe infarct, the thalamic abscess, and in one thalamic infarct pt (almost normal life, drugs markedly reduced). *In sum:* 58% of pts getting >40% relief
Nguyen et al. *Mov Disord* 1998; 13:84–8	Facial pain + arm tremor after removal of an acoustic neurinoma (1 pt)	Complete pain relief (32 mos)	Complete tremor relief
Nguyen et al. (1999) *(Includes all pts from previous paper)* Virtually the same patients reported in Nguyen et al. In: *Proc 4th Int Congress of INS, Luzern,* 1998, *and both following papers:*	CP (parietal stroke: 2 pts; deep brain hematoma: 5 pts; thalamic stroke: 4 pts; thalamic abscess: 1 pt; brainstem lesion: 1 pt; head trauma: 2 pts; SCI: 3 pts)	Satisfactory/good (40–100%) pain relief: parietal stroke: 2/2 pts; deep brain hematoma: 4/5 pts; thalamic stroke: 4/4 pts; thalamic abscess: 1/1 pts; brainstem lesion: 1/1 pts; head trauma: 2/2 pts; SCI: 2/3 pts (3–50 mos) *(Mean follow-up 27.3 mos)*	Pain relief in 13 pts described as CP by authors: 5 good (70–100%), 5 satisfactory (40–69%), 3 poor (<40%). SCI CP: 1: 70–10 f, 2: <40% relief. Progressive loss of eff 32 pts (19%), due to electrode malpositionir 5 pts. After electrode repositioning, good ief. RCT in 5 pts; 5/5 positive response
Nguyen et al. *Arch Med Res* 2000; 31:263–5 Nguyen et al. *Neurochirurgie* 2000; 46:483–91	CP (16 pts; CPSP: 11 pts; thal. abscess: 1 pt; head trauma: 1 pt; SCI: 3 pts)	Pain relief: BCP: Good (70–100%): 5/13 brain; 1/3 SCI	Progressive loss of effect in some pts reversed in most by correct repositioning of paddle.

Reference / period	Patients	Results	Outcome / Parameters
Drouot et al. (2002) *Same pts as reported above* **1993–2000**	CP (13 pts; parietal stroke: 2 pts; thal. stroke: 8 pts; thal. abscess: 1 pt; SCI: 2 pts)	Satisfactory (40–69%): 5/13 brain. Poor (<40%): 3/13. Substantial pain relief: BCP: 10/13 pts (77%). SCI: 1/3 pts (33%) *(3–50 mos; mean follow-up 27.3 mos)*. Good pain relief (>40%): 9 (69%). Unsatisfactory pain relief (<40%): 4	*In sum:* 66% had 30–100% relief, but less with at least 50% relief. MCS effective in pts with normal or quite normal non-nociceptive thermal threshold within the painful area or in pts with improved sensory thresholds during MCS. QST testing bilaterally; in non-responders, MCS induced significant changes on the side of stimulation. Parameters: 3 h ON, 3 h OFF, 60 μs, 40 Hz, 1–3 mV
Lyon group:			
[includes: Nuti et al. (2005) Peyron et al. *Pain* 1995; 62:275–86 Garcia-Larrea et al. *Stereotact Funct Neurosurg* 1997; 68:141–8 Garcia-Larrea et al. (1999) Mertens et al. *Stereotact Funct Neurosurg* 1999; 73:122 Sindou et al. *9th World Congress on Pain, Book of abstracts, IASP Press,* 1999 Montes et al. *Neurophysiol Clin* 2002; 32:313–25] **1992–2003**	CP: 27 pts. Ischemic lesions: 11 pts (3 thalamic (Vc), 4 medulla, 2 cortical parietal, 1 parietal/insula/ACC, 1 parietal/insula). Hemorragic lesions: 11 pts (1 thalamic (Vc), 1 thalamus/midbrain, 5 capsulothalamic, 1 capsulolenticular/insula, 3 cortical parietal). Frontoparietal trauma: 1 pt. SCI (discal hernia-associated myelopathy): 3 pts. Spinal conus AVM: 1 pt.	Follow-up: 2–104 mos (mean 49 mos). Pain relief: BCP: excellent (>70%): 3; good (40–69%): 8; poor (10–39%): 8; negligible (0–9%): 4. CCP: excellent: 0; good: 3; poor: 1; negligible: 0. Decreased analgesic intake: 52% of pts (complete withdrawal 36%). Unchanged: 45% of pts. Unavailable data: 3%. Decrease/withdrawal of analgesic in 10/11 poor responders (contradictory results as noted by the authors). Favour re-intervention: 70% of pts	Prospective evaluation of MCS. Long-term outcome evaluated by means of: 1) % pain relief, 2) VAS, 3) postoperative VAS decrease, 4) reduction in drugs intake, 5) yes/no response to being operated on again. MCS efficacy not predictable by motor status, pain characteristics, lesion type, QST, SSEP/LEPs, pain duration, BCP vs. CCP, presence of evoked pain. No subjective sensations during active stimulation. Partial epileptic seizures in 3 pts in the early postoperative stage or during trials for increasing intensity. 1 speech disorder and 1 motor deficit resolved spontaneously. Long-term pain relief predictable from early pain relief. 1–2 paddles. Parameters: 0.5–5 V, 30–80 Hz, 60–330 μs. MCS may have adverse cognitive effects. The risk may increase with age (>50 yrs)

(continued)

TABLE 6.1 (continued)

Author(s)	Type of pain (no. of patients)	Results (follow-up)	Notes
Turin Advanced Neuromodulation Group (TANG)			
Canavero and Bonicalzi (1995)	CP (2 pts; CPSP: 1 pt; syringomyelia: 1 pt)	Pain relief: 30–50% in syringomyelia pt (2 yrs); no relief in CPSP	Syringomyelia pt: parietal somatosensory stimulation. Spreading of pain to contralateral side and vanishing of analgesia at 2 mos. Modest propofol response; CPSP pt: propofol unresponsive
Canavero et al. (1999)	CPSP (1 pt; thalamocapsular stroke)	Effective short-term pain relief (allodynia disappearance and 50% reduction of burning pain) (5 wks)	Propofol-responsive pt. Painful supernumerary phantom arm during MCS and lasting 6 mos after stimulator switch-off. Pain relapse after 5 wks
Canavero and Bonicalzi (2002, 2003) Includes: Canavero et al.: In: Proc 4th Int Congress of INS, Luzern, 1998 Canavero et al. Neurol Res 2003; 25:118–22	CP (CPSP 5 pts; SC pain: 2 pts) + 1 (algodystonia) **1993–2003**	Effective (30–100%) pain relief with MCS/PCS in 2/7 pts. Long-term efficacy (4 yrs) in 1 pt (MS CP). Ineffective MCS in 4/7	Effective SI stimulation in 1, then resubmitted to MCS with same benefit plus 50% opioid reduction (however, patient unsatisfied and explanted). Overall efficacy: 3/7 CP pts, all propofol-responsive. Ineffective MCS in 4/7 CP pts, all propofol-unresponsive, but 1 who could not be assessed due to intermittent nature of pain. Algodystonia: temporary benefit
Saitoh's group:			
Saitoh et al. Neurosurg Focus 11(3), article 1, 2001 Includes Saitoh et al. J Neurosurg 2000; 92:150–5	CPSP (thal. stroke: 6 pts; putaminal hem: 1 pt; pontine hem: 1 pt) SCI (1 pt) **1996–2001**	Pain relief: Immediate + long-term (mos) CPSP (8 pts): Excellent 1 [+1] (3); Good: 1[+1] (48) (putam.); Fair: 2 [+2] (4, 25); Poor: 4 [not implanted with IPG] SCI: Excellent: 1 + 1 (1)	*Pain relief categorization:* Excellent (80–100% relief) Good (60–79% relief) Fair (40–59% relief) Poor (<40% relief) Poor responders not implanted. Pharmacological test with phentolamine, lidocaine, ketamine, thiopental, morphine, placebo. Reduction over the time of MCS pain relieving effect in 3/10 implanted pts. *Some pain reduction by SI stimulation.* Ineffective prefrontal stimulation. Subdural placement in some pts (5),

Tani et al. J Neurosurg 2004; 101:687–9			interhemispheric in 3. Dual IPGs driving 2 paddles in 2 pts. First report of bilateral cortical stimulation for SCI pain. 4 mos interval between implants. Thiamylal, lidocaine, ketamine, phentolamine, morphine, and placebo unresponsive pt. Pain control with 3–4 periods (30 min each) of stimulation a day, followed by 5–6 h benefit without stimulation. Left pain relapse after right system removal (infection, 6 mos after surgery)
Saitoh et al. (2003) Includes all previous pts	CP (11 pts; CPSP: 9 pts; brainstem injury: 1 pt; SCI: 1 pt)	Overall pain relief: Excellent: 6/19 pts; Good: 3/19 pts; Fair: 5/19; None: 5/19	Modified MCS protocol: subdural MCS within the central sulcus. Implants in interhemispheric fissure: 5 pts (lower limb pain); within central sulcus: 5 pts (area 4 and area 3b stimul.) + surface of the precentral gyrus. Area 4 within central sulcus seems to be the optimal stimulation point. Ketamine-sensitive pts seem to be good candidates for MCS
Saitoh et al. (2004) Likely included in series above	CPSP (1 pt)	Immediate successful pain relief (VAS decrease from 8 to 1)	PET study (see text)

Oxford group:

Nandi et al. (2002) Includes all pts reported in Carroll et al. Pain 2000; 84:431–7 Smith et al. Neurosurg Focus 2001; 11(3):article 2	CPSP (cortic. stroke 1 pt; thal. stroke: 3 pts; brainstem stroke: 2 pts). Gunshot brainstem injury (1 pt)	Appreciable pain relief: 1 pt, cortical (4 yrs); 2 pts (weeks to months)*; No pain relief: 4/7 pts (thalamic, brainstem); *Brainstem injury: 50–60% (31 mos): 1 pt	The only pt where it was tried: propofol-sensitive. Pain disappearance for 5 mos after stimulator switched off in the responder. Enduring benefit in 1 pt only

Other groups:

Cioni et al. Proc XLV SINCH Congress, 1996	CP (4 pts; thalamic pain)	Pain relief (50–60%): 1/4 pts, but unsatisfactory relief at 1 yr	Extradural multipolar (16–20) grid in all plus electrophysiologic mapping; several combinations assessed over 12 h

(continued)

TABLE 6.1 (continued)

Author(s)	Type of pain (no. of patients)	Results (follow-up)	Notes
Dario et al. Long-term results of chronic MCS for CP. A185 In Abstr. 9th World Congress on Pain, IASP Press, 1999 Also includes Dario et al. Riv Neurobiol 1997; 43:625–9	CPSP (thal. stroke: 2 pts; brainstem stroke: 1 pt)	70% pain relief in 1 thal. pt. (3 yrs) Gradual abatement of pain relief over 2 yrs. 60–90% relief, then 50–70%, then 20–30% at 3–41 mos (ave: 27 mos)	All pts propofol-responsive. 2–2.5 V, 50–75 Hz, 120–210 μs, continuous mode.
Franzini et al. (2003) Also includes Franzini et al. In: Abstr. XLVIII Congresso SINCH, Copanello, 1999 Franzini et al. J Neurosurg 2000; 93:873–5	CPSP (3 pts, A, B, C)	Satisfactory (30–50%) pain relief: Pts. A (>4 yrs) and B (>2 yrs). Short-term pain relief (6 mos): pt C	2 responders propofol-sensitive. Pain abolition after a second stroke in pt B. Unsatisfactory pain relief (30%) by further stimulation in pt C. Complete abolition of thalamic hand
Herregodts et al. (1995)	Thalamic pain (2 pts)	Immediate pain relief: >50% in both pts. Long-lasting: 1/2 (full relapse in one at 4 mos)	
Migita et al. (1995)	CPSP (2 pts; putaminal hemorrhage: pt A; post-20 mos stereotactic thalamotomy: pt B)	Pain relief: 70–80% in pt A (1 yr) No relief in pt B	Pt A: morphine and barbiturate unresponsive. 30% pain relief with TMS Pt B: previous 6 mos effective Vc DBS. Barbiturate responsive, morphine and TMS unresponsive
Fuji et al. (1997)	CPSP (thal. infarction: 2 pts; thal. hemorrhage: 5 pts)	Satisfactory pain relief: 6/7 pts (1 mo) Unsatisfactory pain relief: 5/7 pts (3 mos)	Lesions included internal capsule, Vc and pulvinar (MRI confirmed, 5 pts). Early electrode removal in 1 pt after unsatisfactory test stimulation
Barraquer-Bordas et al. (1999)	CPSP (1 pt: capsuloinsular hemorrhage)	MCS trial ineffective (motor response elicited)	Hemisoma burning pain, + evoked pains. DBS reduced CP for 5 mos and evoked pains, until glioma displaced electrode with relapse and death
Kuroda et al. (2000)	CPSP (evacuated putaminal hematoma) (1 pt)	MCS ineffective. Later SI/SII CS effective for 4 yrs	
Mogilner and Rezai (2001)	SCI (1 pt)	Relief (not broken down) (mean follow-up 6 mos)	
Rodriguez and Contreras (2002)	SCI CP (1 pt)	Evoked pain dramatically improved.	SCI pain following cervical ependymoma removal. Third party analysis of results. Tremor improvement.

Study	Diagnosis (patients)	Result	Comments
Frighetto et al. (2004)	CPSP (1 pt)	Steady burning pain moderately relieved (2 mos)	No reduction of analgesic intake after MCS. 7.1 V, 5 Hz, 450 μs, ON 2 h, OFF 3 h, 0−/2+
Henderson et al. (2004)	CPSP (1 pt)	Relief (no details given); Relief, then loss, then new relief (?) after intensive reprogramming	Previous ineffective thalamotomy
Brown and Pilitsis (2005)	CPSP, Wallenberg (1 pt) CPSP, thalamic (1 pt)	0%; VAS 10 to 8; McGill Quest. Index from 65 to 32 (both sensory and affective scores)	Follow-up max. in whole series (PNP and CP): 10 mos. Contrary to Nguyen, they conclude that precise, somatotopic localization of the electrode may not be required, because the optimal interelectrode distance determined during cortical mapping and afterwards with subjective patient evaluation of pain control was fully 3 cm. Intraoperative neuronavigation and cortical mapping for stimulation site targeting. Strength and discriminative sensation improvement from MCS in 3 pts with facial weakness and sensory loss. Dysarthria improvement in 1 pt More than 50% reduction in pain medication dose
Savas and Kanpolat (2005)	CP (1 pt)	No relief	They state that some experienced authors have expressed to them dissatisfaction with MCS. MCS performed at many more centers than those which publish; most of the failures go unreported and only series with good results are published
Slawek et al. (2005)	CPSP, brainstem (1 pt)	20% reduction on VAS; withdrawal of narcotic and decrease of non-narcotic medications, ability to introduce rehabilitation and improvement of sleep	Follow-up: 4 mos. No side effects

(continued)

TABLE 6.1 (continued)

Author(s)	Type of pain (no. of patients)	Results (follow-up)	Notes
Gharabaghi et al. (2005) *Also includes Tirakotai et al. Minim Invasive Neurosurg 2004; 47:273–7*	CPSP (hemorrhage) (3 pts) CP; insular (1 pt)	70–100% relief (follow-up: 6–18 mos) 90% relief (follow-up: 24 mos)	Frameless neuronavigation. Single burr hole and vacuum headrest. Awake patient. No complications. Third party evaluation. Description of an integrated protocol for precise electrode placement (functional image guidance: volumetric rendering of a 3-D MR data set with superimposed fMR imaging data plus intraoperative electrical stimulation)
Pirotte et al. (2005) *Also includes Pirotte et al. Neurosurg Focus 2001; 11(3)*	CPSP; subcortical (3 pts); capsular (2 pts); brainstem (1 pt); MS pain (1 pt); cervical syrinx (1 pt); SC ependymoma (1 pt) **1998–2003**	Pain relief (%) 100%/50%/worsening 83%/ failure (both plegic) 87.5% 100% 70% Failure	50–75% drug dosage reduction among responders. Third party evaluation. Plegia **not** an unfavorable prognostic factor. Study evaluating the usefulness of the combination of fMRI and intraoperative cortical brain mapping (iCM) as functional targeting methods for MCS
Rasche et al. (2006) *Includes: Tronnier VM. Schmerz 2005; 15: 278–9*	CPSP (thalamic): 7 pts **1994–2005**	3 responders (−31%, −41%, −62%) 2/7 pts placebo responder. Duration of positive effect: 2, 4, 1.5 years (4.5–6.0 V, 50–85 Hz, 210–250 μs). Relief of dysesthesia, allodynia and hyperpathia in 2 CPSP pts (pts were able to touch the painful area without having painful sensations).	Test trial including a double blind test. Results evaluated by means of VAS. Mean follow-up 3.6 years (range 1–10 years). Single burr hole, neuronavigation. No sensation evoked by stimulation. All responders on continuous stimulation. After implantation, intermittent stimulation. Lasting pain reduction with minor changes of the stimulation parameters. Immediate or almost immediate (30–60 min) pain reduction after turning the MCS on. MCS effect lasting from 30 min up to several hours after cessation of the stimulation

CS is the only electrical neuromodulatory technique which allows for blinded, placebo-controlled assessments: CS does not generally induce any motor activation, even at high voltage, or any sensory phenomena in a majority of patients. A pure placebo effect has been excluded (Canavero and Bonicalzi 2002; Rasche *et al.* 2006). In a few cases, though, sensory effects can be evoked with both MCS and PCS, but are unrelated to eventual analgesia. Although no analgesia was seen in the initial series of Tsubokawa of CS with SI stimulation, PCS has been confirmed to be analgesic in CP (see Table 6.1).

More than half of BCP patients gain 40% or more relief at 4 years. A suggestion of greater response of evoked versus spontaneous pains (see Table 6.1) is not confirmed in most series and MCS does not relieve nonpainful paresthesias.

Worsening of the original pain via ipsi- or contralateral stimulation of MI/SI has been reported in a few patients, and one of our CP patients developed a painful supernumerary phantom arm after MCS (see Canavero and Bonicalzi 2002).

Tsubokawa's group also reported a few patients with excellent analgesia and increasing periods of post-effect who, after having the stimulating apparatus switched off in 2 years, never had their pain return, interpreted as a sign of neuroplastic phenomena induced by MCS in SI (1 case also in Peyron *et al.* 1995). Analgesia via ipsilateral stimulation is on record. Nguyen and colleagues (see Table 6.1) saw no major modification of somatotopic arrangement in their patients, but one obtained bilateral benefit from unilateral stimulation. Rainov and colleagues (see Table 6.1) found that, by changing the polarity of the electrodes, it was possible to induce tingling sensations and muscle activation not only contralaterally to the stimulated MI but also in the ipsilateral part of the face.

Mechanism of action. Tsubokawa's original hypothesis (based on animal experiments) that MI, but not SI, stimulation restores the inhibitory surround of hyperactive SI pain-coded cells by anti-/orthodromic activation of non-nociceptive neurons has been disproved by successful cases of PCS and he later rejected it. Nonetheless, Drouot and colleagues (2002) concluded that MCS reinforces the control of non-nociceptive sensory inputs on hyperactive nociceptive SI cells, at least when these sensory afferents are partially preserved (implying that lemniscal fibers inhibit STT fibers), with improvement of sensory discrimination. In poor responders, MCS did not modify the sensory thresholds measured within the painful area, but induced significant changes on the opposite side, i.e., ipsilateral to stimulation. Lack of effect was ascribed to more severe disturbances of the sensory systems. However, the literature reports patients with impaired lemniscal transmission who were relieved by MCS (see Table 6.1) implying that a normal lemniscal system ("gate control") is not required to obtain good results. We have seen CP patients relieved by propofol, who also had restoration of normal sensation (see Canavero and Bonicalzi 2004). Parenthetically, MI is actually one of the areas activated after acute noxious stimulation in humans (Coghill *et al.* 1999).

Some authors believe that MCS does not act at cortical levels below the electrode, but through descending axons. For these, pyramidal neurons or their efferents (perhaps relaying to SI or thalamus) are important, as these can be activated even at intensities below the muscle contraction threshold; previously, Fields and Adams

(1974) stimulated pyramidal fibers in the internal capsule to relieve human pain, as they believed that CP is due to loss of intracortical inhibition, with relative preservation of excitation. However, in humans, there are few descending fibers from SI to the dorsal horn, and these do not end in laminas I–III (Schoenen and Grant 2004). Similarly, there are no or few descending fibers from MI to the superficial dorsal horn in man (Schoenen and Grant 2004). It is difficult to believe that CS in humans acts by descending direct inhibition to the spinal cord (see also Meyerson and Linderoth 2001). Other authors believe a cortical effect is foremost in this regard.

Neurometabolic studies of this problem have been published. Garcia-Larrea and colleagues (1997) studied 7 CPSP and 3 PNP (brachial plexus avulsion, BPA, pain) patients submitted to contralateral MCS (in 3 medially, i.e., subdurally). $H_2(15)O$ PET was done before, during – 5 and 20 minutes – and 30 minutes after a 20 minute session of stimulation. Results were not differentiated between CP and BPA. There was no significant difference in regional cerebral blood flow (rCBF) between the two controls or the two stimulation conditions. The only locus of significant CBF increase during MCS was observed in the motor thalamus. Sizable, but insignificant, CBF increases during MCS were seen in the left insula, BA24–32 and upper mesencephalon (plus a rCBF decrease in BA18–19 bilaterally). No significant change was seen in MI (SI could not be resolved with their machine). All changes were reversible upon stopping MCS, although BA24 and mesencephalic changes persisted or even increased slightly after stoppage of MCS. They compared 3 patients with 80–100% relief and 4 with less than 40% relief. Mean thalamic CBF was enhanced in both groups with a similar time course, albeit rCBF increase was greater in those with 80%-plus relief. In contrast, mean CBF in BA24-32 appeared to increase during MCS only in patients with good relief and to decrease in poor responders, even in individual analyses. The same group (Laurent *et al.* 1999; Garcia-Larrea *et al.* 1999) evaluated 10 patients with CP and BPA (likely including the above-mentioned patients, although time from implantation to PET does not correspond). MCS was stopped 24 hours before PET. Four consecutive scans were first recorded (A). Then PET was recorded at 5, 15, 25 and 35 minutes after switching on MCS (B). MCS was subsequently stopped and PET recorded at 15, 30, 45, 60 and 75 minutes after MCS had been turned off (C). MCS (B versus A) was associated with increased rCBF in rostral ACC contralateral to the electrode. During MCS stoppage (C versus A) there was strong activation up to 75 minutes after MCS discontinuation of rostral ACC, orbitofrontal cortex, basal ganglia and brainstem. MCS (B+C versus A) was associated with decreased blood flow (suggesting constriction) on the dura immediately below the electrode. Images of CBF changes in the brainstem did not cover the localization of the PAG. They did not find MCS activation of SI, a likely consequence of the spatiotemporal resolution limits of their PET machine. The low-threshold analysis (Z-score $\geq$ 3.5) of the two-step procedure yielded some regions of significant CBF increase: the whole thalamus (ipsilateral to MCS), the ACC (mostly contralaterally to MCS, plus midline), orbitofrontal areas, a region comprising the insula and descending towards the inferomedial temporal lobe – including amygdala (exclusively contralateral to MCS), subthalamic-upper brainstem region (ipsilateral to MCS). The second (high-threshold) step of the analysis (Z-score $\geq$4) restricted spatially the above results and limited the anatomical region of significant CBF increase to thalamic VL ipsilateral to MCS, with extensions to VA and subthalamic region. Vc was outside the region of increased CBF in both high- and low-threshold analyses. The sequence included condition A (CBF assessed basally, 15 minutes before MCS with stimulator turned off for 18 hours), conditions B and C (2 consecutive scans performed respectively after 5 and 20 minutes of continuous MCS) and condition D (scan after 30 minutes after MCS discontinuation). Pain ratings during PET were 4.8 $\pm$ 2.6 during condition A, 4.3 $\pm$ 2.9 and 3.69 $\pm$ 2.8 in conditions B and C and 3.69 $\pm$ 2.8 in condition D. In spite of a trend to pain decrease from A to D, differences were not significant. As far as rCBF changes are concerned, in all cases there was an abrupt CBF increase during the first scan under MCS (5 minutes after onset) which remained stable during PET 20 minutes after MCS onset. These effects were reversible 30 minutes after MCS interruption in all sites, except in ACC where rCBF had not yet reverted to pre-stimulation values 30 minutes after MCS discontinuation: here two spots of increased rCBF appeared in right and left ACC/orbitofrontal boundaries and stayed almost so after switching off the stimulator. No significant change related to MCS was observed in SI or MI. CBF decreased in BA18–19 areas and were totally reversible upon discontinuation of MCS. In CP and BPA patients with >80% versus <20% relief, while lateral thalamic CBF appeared to increase in all patients (albeit to a greater extent – 15% versus 5% – in those relieved), BA32 CBF increased in responders (+5% at 20 minutes), but decreased in nonresponders (−10% at 20 minutes); upon close scrutiny, this does not seem a strong finding as in their two reported CP cases this was not the case. These studies suffer from limited statistical power due to small number of patients and shortcomings of ROI measurements (analysis was based on ellipsoidal ROIs placed over the lateral thalamus and BA32, with other regions not studied due to their irregular shape) and the authors themselves considered their results exploratory and deserving confirmation. Also, VAS values reported here correspond to those obtained during the week preceding PET, and thus may have not fully reflected current pain intensity. They (Garcia-Larrea et al. 1999) also recorded CO_2 laser-evoked potentials (LEPs) and flexion nociceptive reflex (RIII) in these same patients. LEPs (amplitude and latency of each component) and RIII (surface) were studied with MCS turned off, on and at least 30 minutes after MCS interruption. LEPs were obtained after stimulation of both the painful and the intact side, while RIII was obtained after stimulation of the painful side only. In one patient, after stimulation of the non-affected side, LEP amplitudes of the vertex component decreased significantly during active stimulation. In the group as a whole, after stimulation of the non-affected side, LEP amplitudes tended to decrease under MCS, although not statistically significantly. RIII was not modified in the three conditions. Electrophysiological responses did not correlate with VAS. There was a lack of any significant acute change in SEPs during MCS in any of the recorded patients with central lesions. None of the 4 patients whose nociceptive reflexes remained unmodified by MCS was satisfied with the attained analgesia. Although the 7 patients with CP had sizable epidural SEPs during intraoperative monitoring, only 4 retained scalp-recorded SEPs of enough amplitude to permit assessment of MCS effects. Parietal somatosensory responses up to 50 ms post-stimulus did not exhibit any significant change in amplitude, latency or topography in relation to MCS. Thus, significant modulation of spinal nociceptive reflexes was seen during MCS in 3/7 patients, while it was unchanged in 4. Modification thereof corresponded in every case to attenuation of the responses during MCS. Two of 3 patients with MCS-related reflex attenuation experienced good to very good relief, while the third reported >60% abatement of allodynia during MCS, but only 30% of spontaneous pain. These data too do not add substantially to our understanding of how CS works.

Saitoh and colleagues (2004) submitted a right-sided CPSP patient to MCS, with excellent analgesia (VAS 8 to VAS 1) after 30 minutes of stimulation. $H_2(15)O$ PET pre- and post-stimulation revealed significant rCBF increases in left frontal areas (BA9 and 11, BA32) and the left thalamus and decreases in temporo-occipital areas (right BA22 and left BA19). The efficacy of MCS was mainly related to increased synaptic activity in the thalamus, whereas all other changes were related to emotional processes.

We (Canavero and Bonicalzi 1995; Canavero et al. 1999) and Tsubokawa's group (Tsubokawa et al. 1991) found that cortical stimulation changes both local cortical (SI/MI) and thalamic rCBF with pre- and post-stimulation SPECT. F-MR studies showed MCS to have inhibiting effects on SI/MI cortex as well as contralaterally, supporting a cortical mechanism of analgesia (see references in Canavero and Bonicalzi 2002). Moreover, subdural MI stimulation appears to activate axons in the cortex, which excite both corticospinal neurons and local inhibitory neurons. The effects are greater with cathodal stimulation (Hanajima et al. 2002).

We may conclude that CS may act locally by modulating ("unscrambling") the MI/SI dipole and the long thalamocortical reverberating loop, with subsequent fall-out effects on other brain regions. Physiologically, inhibition of nociceptive neurons and neurons with non-sensory discriminative response characteristics may be involved in cognitive modulation and in the interaction of pain and touch (see references in Schnitzler and Ploner 2000). This modulation may engage inhibitory interneurons to quench local hyperactivity and/or synchrony, or even ongoing inhibition (see Chapter 7). From a cellular point of view, it is important to note that different classes of GABAergic neurons are not distributed homogeneously among the different cortical layers (reviewed in Defelipe and Farinas 1992) and no less than 14 subclasses according to histologic and electrophysiologic (9 subclasses) criteria exist in SI (Gupta et al. 2000). The majority displays depression at low frequencies, but prominent facilitation at higher frequencies (50 Hz) and some show a burst response at the onset of depolarization. Specific interneurons form specific types of synapses on pyramidal cells and probably on other interneurons; while the temporal dynamics of transmission of glutamatergic synapses is highly heterogeneous, GABAergic interneurons form synapses with virtually identical temporal dynamics onto different targets of the same class (GABA group). It is clear that the exact mechanism of engagement of inhibition will require much more detailed work.

The tight coupling of sensation and motricity may also explain CS effects. Suppression of natural pain-related behaviors clearly engages a potent volitional motor control process, yet movements are known to increase the threshold for detection and decrease the perceived intensity of somatosensory stimuli, including those at a painful level (active movements having greater and more consistent effect than passive movements). Humans perceive forces they exert as weaker than identical forces acted upon them: in fact, a corollary discharge of the effort attenuates the subject's sensory feedback (Shergill *et al.* 2003) and pain interferes with mental representations of movement (Schwoebel *et al.* 2002). Tonic painful input leads to inhibition of MI and SMA during motor performance on the painful side (and contralateral one – though less) (Binder *et al.* 2002). TMS studies show that under normal conditions sensory afferents limit the activity of inhibitory neurons in MI, and that after pure thalamic sensory stroke, MI intracortical inhibition is increased (Liepert *et al.* 2005). In one possible scenario, the CP generator tonically inhibits MI, but, if this is too intense, CS may not be able to engage inhibition itself.

Finally, a relatively high stimulation frequency can induce a tonic depolarization and cortical inactivation effect, which is known to inhibit thalamic relays.

2. Deep brain stimulation (DBS) (Table 6.2)

In 1960, Mazars and colleagues first reported attempts to stimulate the somato-sensory pathways, particularly the neospinothalamic tract at its termination in Vc, for the treatment of chronic neurogenic pain. Their theoretical framework was the theory of Head and Holmes, which held that CP might be the consequence of an imbalance between protopathic and epicritic sensory functioning: stimulation of the thalamic sensory relay nuclei would presumably increase the epicritic component and hence inhibit the protopathic inflow (an anticipation of the later gate control theory). Acute thalamic stimulation was later found to suppress the aversive behavior in patients with facial postherpetic neuralgia (White and Sweet 1969). However, the real interest in DBS for the treatment of chronic pain in humans arose in the 1970s. Reynolds' (1969) discovery that electrical stimulation of the rat midbrain could produce profound analgesia without the concurrent administration of drugs and the gate control theory (Melzack and Wall 1965), according to which stimulation of large-diameter fibers is capable of inhibiting nociceptive information, paved the way to most electrical stimulatory procedures. Despite initial optimistic reports, it soon became clear that DBS was not as successful as was initially hoped. The clinical data did not fit with animal findings, and large discrepancies were noted between the results of different neurosurgical groups.

The targets for DBS include thalamic Vc nuclei and/or the posterior limb of the internal capsule, the caudal medial thalamic areas around the third ventricle, includ'ing CM-Pf and the junction of the third ventricle and the sylvian aqueduct (rostral ventral PAG-caudal ventral PVG). CP is generally treated by contralateral Vc stimulation, which is effective only unilaterally. The internal capsule (posterior limb) may be used if thalamic tissue is unavailable (e.g., after an infarct or encephalomalacia). A few groups also simultaneously stimulate the PVG area and Vc.

Mechanism of action

a. PAG-PVG: Numerous observations made in patients, such as an increase of the endorphin content in ventricular fluid after PAG-PVG stimulation, cross tolerance between SPA- and narcotic-induced analgesia, and naloxone reversal of PAG-PVG stimulation-induced suppression of chronic pain, support the notion that pain relief by PAG-PVG stimulation is mediated by endorphin-containing neuronal

TABLE 6.2. Deep brain stimulation (DBS) arranged by reporting groups

Author(s)	Type of pain	Target	Results/notes
Mazars (1976)	Thalamic lesion (3 pts)		Failure
Mazars et al. (1979)	Brainstem lesion (6 pts)		Relief in 5
Includes all previous papers by this	SCI (4 pts)	Vc (bilat. in SCI) or IC PAG/PVG	Relief in 4
pioneer group on the topic	BCP/CCP		Poor results
			First group to stimulate the thalamus starting 1960
Richardson and Akil (1977)	Paraplegic pain (5 pts, then 19)	PAG-PVG	Significant pain relief in 2 (18 mos). 1 pt previously submitted to failed rhizotomy/ cordotomy.
Richardson et al. (1980)			Further series: good relief at 1 yr in 6 pts
Lazorthes (1979)	Thalamic CP (28 pts)	Vc	Successful pain relief in 5
	SCI (8 pts)		Successful pain relief in 2
Schwarcz (1980)	CP (thalamic pain: 2 pts; partial SCI pain: 3 pts; postcordotomy CP: 1 pt)	Medial posteroinferior thalamic areas	Pain relief (deep background pain and hyper-pathia): >75% (but never 100%) relief: 2 50–75% relief: 2 Failure: 2 pts Hyperpathia abolished, deep background pain only reduced. No reversal by naloxone. Follow-up: 6–42 mos
Mundinger and Salomão (1980)	BCP (incl. CPSP) (5 pts)	IC/ML (4 pts) Pulvinar (1 pt)	>70%: 1; 50–70%: 1; 50%: 3 (1 pulvinar) (max. follow-up: less than 2 yrs). No relief at longer term.
Mundinger and Neumuller (1982)	SCI (5 pts)	IC/LM (3 pts) Pulvinar (1 pt) PAG/PVG (1 pt)	0%, 50% and 50–70% >70% 50% (except one, follow-up shorter than 2 yrs)
Ray and Burton (1980)	CPSP (thalamic) (1 pt) CCP (iatrogenic) (2 pts)	CM-Pf	>50% relief in all, drugs not stopped, effect abates in time
Plotkin (1982)	Thalamic pain (1 pt) SCI pain (1 pt) SCI pain (2 pts)	Vc Vc PVG	0% (?) 0% (?) 0% (?) successes (follow-up: 6–42 mos)

Dieckmann and Witzmann (1982)	CP, thalamic (5 pts)	PVG/Vc	5 *slight* late reliefs (6 mos–4.5 yrs)
Andy (1983)	CPSP (2 pts)	Right CM-Pf and left CM stimulation	Good or excellent results (follow-up: up to 18 mos)
Broggi et al. (1984)	CPSP; thalamic (2 pts)	Vc	40–60% pain relief (12–18 mos)
Turnbull (1984) *Also includes Shulman et al. (1982) and other previous papers by this author*	CP (including SCI)	Vc	Of limited efficacy, particularly ineffective in SCI pain. One pt with brainstem stroke relieved over a few years
Namba et al. (1984)	CP (thalamic and putaminal stroke: 9 pts; extrathalamic subcortical: 1 pt; MS CP: 1 pt)	IC (8) IC + Vc (1) IC + Vc + ML (1)	At discharge: 100% (3), 50–95% (3), fair (drugs needed, 2), 0% (3; 1 with thalamotomy, pulvinotomy, mesencephalotomy). Best stimulating point for analgesia not in the center of posterior limb but in most posteromedial part (area triangularis)
Frank et al. (1984)	SCI pain (1 pt)	Vc	Poor result
Tsubokawa et al. (1985) Katayama et al. (2001) *Includes all CP patients submitted to DBS by Tsubokawa's group*	CP above brainstem (8 pts) Myelopathic CP	Vc PAG PAG Vc	Short-term relief: 80% in 2/8 pts; 60–80% in 3/8 pts; <60% in 3/8 pts. Long-term relief: 33% No relief No relief 60–80% relief in 2
Hosobuchi (1986) *Includes all previous published pts*	BCP (cortex, thalamus, brainstem) (13 pts) Paraplegia CP (8 pts) Postcordotomy CP (9 pts) **1970–1984**	Vc, lemniscal, PAG	8 early successes, 5 failures; 6 late successes, 2 failures 3 early successes, 5 failures; 2 late successes, 1 failure 8 early and late successes (75–100% relief); 1 early bleeding PAG DBS: ineffective; lemniscal: 36% success Follow-up: 2–14 yrs
Heiss et al. (1986)	Thalamic CPSP	Vc (likely, not specified)	Pain relief (follow-up: unavailable)

(continued)

TABLE 6.2 (continued)

Author(s)	Type of pain	Target	Results/notes
Levy et al. (1987) Includes Fields and Adams (1974), Adams (1977–1978)	CP (25 pts)	Vc or IC	Test stimulations: 14 VPL, 11 VPM, 6 IC. Pain relief sufficient for internalization in VPL: 9/14 pts (64%); in VPM: 9/11 pts (82%); in IC: 1/6 pts. Initial success rate: 56%; long-term pain relief: 24%.
	SCI CP	Vc or PAG/PVG	14 electrodes implanted (7 Vc, 7 PAG-PVG) in 11 SCI pts. Pain relief sufficient for internalization in 2/11 pts (18%).
	CP, thalamic (3 pts)	PAG/PVG (both in 3)	No persistent (> 6 wks) pain relief.
	Paraplegia pain (7 pts)	PAG/PVG	Unsatisfactory pain relief, no internalization
	Postcordotomy CP (5 pts)		7 electrodes implanted; 2 internalizations; no persistent pain relief (0%). 6 Vc and 2 PAG-PVG electrodes implanted; 2 Vc and 1 PAG-PVG electrodes internalized. 3/5 pts (60%) with initial successful stimulation, 2/5 (40%) long-term pain relief. Follow-up: 24–168 mos; paresthesias independent of analgesia, not vice versa. **CP relief approaches 30% (rate close to that expected from placebo)**
Siegfried (1991) Includes all previously published personal cases	Thalamic CP (19 pts)	Vc	Long-term: 5 very good, 7 good, 3 fair, 4 poor. Better results in parathalamic lesions than true thalamic lesions
	Partial SCI pain (17 cases) 1973–1989	PVG	Pain relief in 3
		Vc	5 very good, 8 good, 3 fair, 1 poor DBS for MS CP: effect lost in time
Crisologo et al. (1991)	Case 1: thalamic stroke with left pain; 6 mos later, left stroke with right pain	Vc	Insignificant relief
Tasker et al. (1991, 1992) Includes all published cases from Toronto Western Hospital	CP (12 pts)	Vc/IC	Relief in 5 (3 with evoked pain: 2 relieved), failure in 7 (6 with evoked pain: stimulation painful in 3)

Reference	Patients	Target	Results
		PVG	PVG either ineffective or inferior to thalamic stimulation with the exception of 1 CCP pt whose severe allodynia and hyperpathia disappeared acutely after 5–10 min of PVG stimulation
	CCP (13 pts) (complete lesion or incomplete lesion unresponsive to SCS)	Vc (mostly bilat.)	Steady pain relief >50%: 20% of pts; 25–50%: 16% of pts; Intermittent pain relief: 0%; Evoked pain relief 25–50%: 16% of pts; Global: relief in 3
Gybels et al. (1993)	Thalamic pain (5 pts), SCI pain (5 pts), Postcordotomy CP (1 pt)	Vc	3/5 pts initial pain relief, 1/5 long-term benefit; Short-term pain relief in 3/5; long-term pain relief in 2/5 pts; Failure
Hariz and Bergenheim (1995)	CP, thalamic (6 pts)	Centrum medianum	4/6 reliefs; follow-up: 16 mos; CP, thalamic. Failure
Young et al. (1995) Includes all pts appearing in previous publications	BCP (14 pts), CCP (12 pts) 1978–1993	Unilat. PAG + Koelliker-Fuse nucleus (1 pt); PVG + Koelliker-Fuse nucleus (2 pts); PAG-PVG; Vc +/– PAG/PVG	Excellent pain relief in 2 pts suffering from SCI CP (follow-up 2 yrs and 8 mos, respectively). In 1 pt cessation of stimulation after 2 yrs was not followed by a full-fledged return of pain. Additive effect from PVG-Koelliker-Fuse n. simultaneous stimulation (but KF > PVG). Excellent or good pain relief from PAG-PVG DBS only in 35% of pts (median follow-up > 7 yrs) (From previous series.) Excellent pain relief (Vc): 1; partial relief (Vc + PAG-PGV): 9; ineffective: 6. (Of SCI pts, 4 had ≥50% relief at 2–60 mos) Apparently unsatisfactory long-term results from PVG stimulation in CCP. Analgesia onset: within minutes; long after-effect in some pts

(continued)

TABLE 6.2 *(continued)*

Author(s)	Type of pain	Target	Results/notes
Kumar et al. (1997) *Includes all pts from 1990 paper*	CPSP (thalamic) (5 pts)	Vc (1) IC (4)	Short- and long-term (3.4 yrs) successful (50–75%) pain relief in 1; early failures (0–50% pain relief) in 4
	SCI pain (3 pts)	Vc	Early successful pain relief (51–100%), 1; early failures (0–50% pain relief), 2; late failures (2 yrs), 3 Analgesia within 10 min (bipolar stim.); duration of pain pre-DBS not prognostic
Barraquer-Bordas et al. (1999)	CPSP (1 pt)	Vc DBS	Partial relief (analgesic reduction) of spontaneous and evoked pain. MCS ineffective. Painful relapse after tumoral displacement of electrode
Blond et al. (2000)	CP (brainstem or suprathalamic origin) (6 pts) SCI (3 pts) (Eur. Coop. Study) 1985–1997	Vc DBS	Unsatisfactory results. Paroxysmal pain refractory Pain relief > 50%: 1/3 pts
Phillips and Bhakta (2000)	CPSP (1 pt)	PVG	Improvement
Krauss et al. (2001)	CPSP (thalamic stroke) (1 pt)	CM-Pf + Vc	Failure
Nandi and Aziz (2004)	CPSP (14 pts) (+1 pt) (cortical: 5;	Vc + PVG (16 pts)	In 1 patient, trial PVG DBS provided 0% relief.
Owen et al. (2006)	thalamic: 8; pontine: 1; IC: 1) Other CPs (5 pts) 1995–2005	PVG (1 pt) Vc (1 pt)	12 patients seen for an average of 16 mos (3–36 mos). One patient had less than 3 mos follow-up. 11 of 14 were satisfactorily relieved and opted for IPG. 13 of 19 consecutive CP patients had satisfactory control with PVG and/ or Vc DBS. Trial relief maintained over an average 16 mos in all but 2 pts. Vc stimulation alone reasonably suppressed the pain in 4 pts (MS, tractotomy, post-SAH stroke, Chiari); however, in the first 2, paresthesias were intolerable. In the other 2 PVG DBS alone was

		superior. Combined Vc-PVG DBS was never synergic and worsened the pain in 2 pts. Their Fig. 2 with results on 14 pts (2 pts not shown having less than 3 mos follow-up): 3 pts not implanted (2 having less than 10% relief but 1 40%: why not implanted?). In 7 relief at follow-up was slightly better than test relief, but in 4 it was less, in 1 case half of it; never 100% relief or somewhat less. Final series of CPSP pts only (2006): 15 pts, evaluated with VAS, MGPQ, PRI-R. Pts with Vc strokes only implanted in PVG-PAG; avrg. follow-up: 27 mos, but results plotted at 2 yrs; *mean relief (VAS) for cortical strokes: 42% – for all others: 54%*; opposite results with PRI-R (!). Wide range of improvements: from slight worsening to 91.3% improvement. 7 pts stopped all analgesics. Post-effect: for over 24 hours **Severe burning hyperesthesia most responsive.** **Most pts preferred PVG DBS to Vc DBS (results thus refer mostly to PVG DBS)** Once burning abates, pts note the background crushing, aching sensation more strongly (past authors may have exchanged this phenomenon for tolerance and relapse)
Romanelli and Heit (2004)	CPSP (1 pt) Vc DBS	100% relief over >55 mos with several changes of parameters

systems (see references in Gybels and Kupers 1995; Meyerson and Linderoth 2001). However, this hypothesis has been firmly challenged by Young and Chambi (1987). Using a double-blind, placebo-controlled study design, they found no evidence that PAG-PVG-induced SPA in humans is mediated by an opioid mechanism. In a study, low- (1–20 Hz) and high-frequency (50 Hz) stimulation of the PAG produced neither relief nor reproduced pain in 8 thalamic CPSP, 1 tumor thalamic CP, 1 SCI pain and 1 tabes dorsalis patients, despite a modest-to-significant increase of CSF endorphin levels (Amano *et al.* 1982): this increase was interpreted as a psychological response.

The Oxford group (Nandi *et al.* 2003; Nandi and Aziz 2004) found that pain suppression is frequency-dependent. During 5–35 Hz PVG stimulation, the amplitude of thalamic field potentials (FPs) was significantly reduced and this was associated with pain relief; at higher frequencies (50–100 Hz), there was no reduction in the FPs and pain was made worse. Switching on the stimulation was followed immediately by a change in the thalamic potentials; however, the FPs did not revert to baseline immediately on cessation of stimulation, but only after a lag of 5–15 minutes depending on the duration of stimulation. The FPs consisted of a very low frequency potential, of 0.2–0.4 Hz, in Vc: their amplitude seemed to correlate with pain intensity, being much stronger off or with 50 Hz stimulation when there was no pain suppression, than with 5–35 Hz stimulation with accompanying pain relief. This suggested a fairly direct neuronal circuit between PVG and Vc mediated by reticulospinal neurons. All patients were also stimulated in Vc, alone or simultaneously with PVG. The PVG FPs were independent of both the pain scores and the state of stimulation of Vc. In non-responders, there was no flattening in the slow wave thalamic FPs across different frequencies of PVG stimulation.

b. Vc: The mechanism by which Vc DBS works is not likely to result from the activation of an endogenous opioid system (or other descending fiber tracts), because its analgesic effect is not reversed by naloxone. Although investigators found that, after thalamic stimulation, beta-endorphin levels were more than twice the resting level, no differences in beta-endorphin levels could be demonstrated between patients reporting complete pain relief and those reporting only partial relief (Tsubokawa *et al.* 1984); a much higher increase in beta-endorphin levels was found after PAG stimulation. In humans, administration of an antidopaminergic agent antagonized the analgesic effect of Vc, but not PAG, DBS (Hosobuchi 1990). However, Velasco and colleagues (1998) found that acute CM-PF stimulation at 60 Hz elicited pain in epileptic patients and this reaction was blocked by an opioid agonist. Tsubokawa and Moriyasu (1975) found that Vc DBS in 2 of 4 pain (non CP) patients at 50–100 Hz inhibited Center Median nociceptive responsive thalamic neurons, while stopping the pain.

A direct action on spinal STT neurons has been excluded, even via relay in the brainstem (Vilela Filho and Tasker 1994); also in light of results of drug dissection of CP, it is not clear if NE, 5HT or other fibers/nuclei are involved, and to what degree (see discussion in Gybels and Kupers 1995; Meyerson and Linderoth 2001). Andy (1983) suggested that altering the excitability state and/or the thalamic discharge patterns by artificially induced electrical stimulation underlie the pain-relieving effects of DBS, i.e., "jamming a low threshold discharging pain system (Emmers)." However, an exclusive depolarization block is an unlikely explanation. A differential effect on both gray (inhibition) and white matter (excitation) should also be considered (Bejjani *et al.* 2002). Electrical stimulation of the neuropil in general affects axons rather than cell bodies, thick before thin myelinated axons and preferentially fibers parallel to the stimulating current more than those transversally (Nowak and Bullier 1998; Ranck 1975). Neural elements up to 2–5 mm from the stimulating cathode may be excited (Ranck 1975). Presently, a GABA release is considered a likely mechanism (e.g., Obeso *et al.* 2000), although inhibition may adapt with continuous stimulation (Ashby and Rothwell 2000). A possibility would be orthodromic stimulation of inhibitory afferents to a target structure or recruitment of local inhibitory interneurons (Ashby and Rothwell 2000). Vc stimulation too can suppress medial thalamic hyperactivity (Tasker *et al.* 1983). Since the thalamocortical loop probably works more like a nonlinear dynamic system that is not solely based on a firing-rate code, DBS may actually work by rebalancing a skewed oscillatory pattern (Canavero 1994).

Neurometabolic studies have been published on this problem. These studies reported stimulator-induced signal increases to be higher than task activations (maximum 2%). Heiss and colleagues (1986) studied one CPSP case with PET. At rest (pain condition), the lowest metabolic rate was in the infarcted thalamus; some areas showed decreased glucose consumption in the otherwise normal ipsilateral cortex. A second PET during DBS (off-pain condition) revealed markedly decreased glucose metabolism in most brain regions. Rezai and colleagues (1999) scanned (fMRI) two patients who had steady-burning CP due to traumatic SCI (a third had PNP). PVG DBS – in contrast to Vc DBS – did not activate SI, but the cingulate cortex (compare to Vim DBS for tremor). Low-frequency stimulation of PVG led to activation of the medial thalamus (compare with Nandi *et al.* 2003). Activations near the electrode were written up to a possible, local nonspecific CBF increase rather than neural pathway activation. At paresthesia-evoking intensities, Vc DBS resulted in the activation of SI in all 3 pain patients. In most cases, areas of cortical activation corresponded to the homuncular somatotopy of paresthesias (3 V, 75–100 Hz, 150–200 μs). With no paresthesias, SI was not activated. In addition to SI, there was activation of thalamus, SII and insula. In a similar study, Duncan and colleagues (1998) submitted 5 patients with neuropathic pain (perhaps inclusive of CP) to Vc DBS. All had obtained relief for more than 3 years to reduce a placebo confounding role. Three patients were relieved, while two had no immediate relief. They reported that <100 Hz Vc DBS increased rCBF in and near the thalamus and some cortical areas, the effect being more prominent with continued stimulation. Their data did not support activation of tactile thalamocortical pathways being the sole mechanism underlying successful Vc DBS. Their most prominent cortical rCBF increase was in ipsilateral anterior insula, both with relief *and not*, although somewhat stronger with relief. Patients perceived both paresthesiae and cold and warmth during stimulation. The close proximity of microstimulation sites evoking tactile and thermal sensations indicates that bipolar stimulating electrodes could easily stimulate neurons within both the insular and SI pathways. They also observed a *nonsignificant* trend toward activation in ACC with Vc stimulation. Davis and colleagues (2000) studied two patients with CCP (plus 3 other neuropathic pain cases) submitted to Vc/ML stimulation. The first was a paraplegic suffering from unilateral leg pain: he obtained 100% relief after 30 minutes of stimulation. This analgesia disappeared immediately upon cessation of DBS. Follow-up was 9 months. On PET day, he was on amitriptyline, baclofen, diazepam and oxycodone. The second suffered from spinal AVM-related CP to left leg. Follow-up was 16 months. Analgesics were retained for 12 hours before PET. There was 0% relief at follow-up, but some relief immediately postoperatively (thalamotomic effect?). Paresthesias were strongest at the beginning of stimulation and subsided as stimulation continued. There was *no* clear relationship between the degree of stimulation-evoked pain relief and the magnitude of rCBF change in either region of the ACC (BA32–24). Activation of posterior ACC was detected after 30 minutes of DBS, but not at the onset of stimulation, in contrast to the ACC, which was activated throughout the period of DBS. Thus, posterior ACC was not related to direct activation from thalamus, but to other structures. Duncan and colleagues (1998) also noted that some of their DBS-induced activations were stronger after 30 minutes of DBS than at DBS onset; unlike this study, patients in Davis' study did not experience thermal sensations during DBS and *no insula activation* was seen. Lack of activation of SI-SII could be explained by low statistical power (only 2 responders), paresthesias in different body regions, thus activating different portions of SI-II, or diminishing paresthesias in the course of DBS. Other CBF changes may have involved other cortical and subcortical areas.

c. OTHER AREAS: Septum and caudate nucleus stimulation has never been reported in CP patients. Basal ganglia, known to process noxious information, and medial thalamic nuclei (Haber and Gdowski 2004) are closely interconnected, but stimulation at these levels is not expected to relieve CP.

Mayanagi and Sano (1998) state that "patients with chronic pain of thalamic or spinal origin failed to experience pain relief with hypothalamic DBS-like stimulation." Failure of stimulation to relieve CP may be similar to generally ineffective results of PAG-PVG DBS.

Stimulation of the Koelliker-Fuse nucleus, a pontine satellite of the locus coeruleus and the major source of catecholamine-containing fibers to the spinal cord, has been attempted in CP cases, but patients were too few for meaningful conclusions.

Other areas of possible interest, but not yet clinically explored, include the anterior pretectal nucleus.

Efficacy. Results of DBS for CP have not lived up to expectations, providing no long-term benefit, but in a few cases in most series.

Whereas patients referred for DBS are those in whom the success rate of many prior therapies has been zero or close to it, this notwithstanding, long-term results remain unsatisfactory.

According to Gybels and Kupers (1995), in their review up to 1993, results of DBS are as follows.

a. Vc DBS: **Thalamic pain**. Of 100 reported cases, mean success rate was 36%. The median success rate based on seven studies was 30% (range 0–63%).

SCI pain (mostly paraplegia pain). In 63 patients, mean success score was 35%. The median success rate based on eight studies was 25% (range 0–100%).

Postcordotomy pain. Of 26 patients, 19 (73%) responded well to DBS. Median success rate of four studies was 84.5% (range 40–100%).

b. PAG-PVG DBS: These are generally poor for thalamic and paraplegic pain, with some exceptions.

First, there can be a large placebo effect (Marchand *et al.* 2003). Secondly, CP includes several components (Tasker 2001) which may be differentially responsive to stimulation. Moreover, CP fluctuates, and a few successes may simply be due to a spontaneous downward fluctuation.

In the longest followed-up series of Vc-IC DBS (Levy *et al.* 1987), CP relief approached 30%, a rate close to the level expected of a placebo effect. They reported 0% relief for paraplegia pain. All patients with thalamic pain had a long-term success rate of 24%; the success rate of Vc DBS was about 43%, and if cases in whom Vc DBS produced paresthesias only are considered, the long-term success rate was about 55%. Long-term relief was obtained in 40% of postcordotomy pain. Gybels and Kupers (1995) stress the fact that true relief may be lower than suggested by the literature.

It is interesting to compare some series of DBS for CP with regard to long-term successes. Those with a short follow-up boast successes in the 70–80% range, while the longest followed-up series (Levy *et al.* 1987: mean, 80 months) reported long-term relief in about 30% of patients. The lesson is clear: pain relief abates with time (see also discussion in Nandi and Aziz 2004; Owen *et al.* 2006). So-called "tolerance" to DBS, despite initial claims, has not been reversed by disulfiram, L-tryptophan, amitriptyline, temporary holidays, while alterations in stimulus parameters have sometimes proved effective (Young and Rinaldi 1997): this is not due to tissue or endorphin changes (Tsubokawa *et al.* 1984), but electrophysiological adaptations. Young (1995) originally believed that most patients who experience declining effectiveness of DBS did so over the first year, but long-term follow-up over more than 15 years indicates a steady decline: total pain relief remained possible only in a few cases. According to Kumar and colleagues (1990), there is an initial two-year fall-off of pain control caused by idiopathic tolerance, with stable results thereafter, regardless of site of implant, suggestive of some biochemical modification of tissues around the electrode. Romanelli and Heit (2004) suggested that changing parameters at the first hint of relapse may block tolerance and restore relief; however, relief can be lost suddenly without warning.

According to the thoughtful review of Duncan and colleagues (1991), (1) the majority of the clinical reports are case histories rather than well-controlled studies, (2) the pain measures described usually involve imprecise questions about pain relief that do not allow a rigorous statistical evaluation, and (3) studies are rarely conducted in a double-blind fashion, and data from placebo-controlled experiments are seldom included. The potential for at least short-term placebo responses is substantial, considering the elaborate nature of the surgical procedure, the mysterious electronic technology involved and the close interpersonal relationship that develops between the pain patient and the attending clinician. No study provided a statistical analysis of the clinical pain changes. The absence of well-controlled studies and statistically significant results prohibits an objective appraisal of the clinical efficacy of DBS. In fact, there appears to be an astounding variability in reported results from several centers. It is improbable that this variability can be accounted for by differences in pain pathology because (1) in the larger studies, the major pain syndromes are all approximately equally well represented, and (2) even when the results obtained in a particular diagnostic category are compared, the same variability between the authors remains. The larger and older series generally reported much more favorable results than did the smaller and more recent series. The data of Marchand and colleagues (2003) suggest that for some patients DBS can be helpful in reducing clinical pain, but effect is *moderate*, as with SCS (see below). Importantly, patients reported the presence of paresthesias even in placebo conditions (the ability to induce paresthesia in the painful area is considered important for target localization!). Patients' expectations are an important factor in the DBS placebo effect. DBS – but not placebo DBS – was found to produce a significant reduction in thermal noxious (but not tactile) perception. The conclusion was that a *strong placebo effect may be involved in the efficacy of any form of DBS and placebo effects can last even for up to 5 years.* Interestingly, Wolksee and colleagues (1982) found no statistically meaningful difference between Vc and sham stimulation.

The PAG–PVG region responsible for analgesia is small (Gybels and Sweet 1989; Duncan *et al.* 1991), and also thalamic size varies considerably from patient to patient (Young 1989); thus, extreme precision is needed for deep stimulations, otherwise results will be jeopardized. Stereotaxic atlases are only a starting point and MRI and microrecordings are employed for fine positioning. Several factors have been proposed to influence therapeutic outcome and hence account for the observed variability between different authors. However, most of these explanations are based on empirical observations, and they have not been confirmed in controlled studies. Among these are stimulation parameters and electrode configuration (5–20 Hz versus 30–100 Hz; stimulation intensity below or above the level at which paresthesias are felt; brief periods of stimulation versus longer periods; dissociation between pairs of contacts producing analgesia versus paresthesias), exact target localization, patient selection (e.g., long-term success is largely reduced in a hysterical personality or a patient with secondary sickness gain), pain type (steady versus evoked). Since physiological studies of Vc stimulation indicate that strong inhibition of nociceptive neurons occurs at frequencies higher than those frequently used clinically, it may be that human stimulation parameters have not been systematically optimized (Duncan *et al.* 1991). The review of Gybels and Kupers (1995) found that not all authors reported early treatment failures (i.e., failure during test stimulation), and hence results overestimate the real therapeutic efficacy. Decrease in success rate occurred both in patients with PAG-PVG stimulation and in patients with Vc stimulation. Finally, many authors use as a criterion of success a pain relief of 50% or more, implying that several patients continue to be unrelieved of their pain: even moderate pain may be crippling and only a few patients obtain total relief over several years. Tasker's group (Vilela Filho 1996) reported 6 BCP (not brainstem) with evoked pain complaining of unpleasant paresthesias with Vc-ML-IC DBS. They all had unpleasant paresthesias with previous SCS, restricted thalamic lesions on CT and associated intermittent pain. Minor risk factors were cold allodynia-hyperpathia and no sensory loss.

Most importantly, DBS has complications which can be lethal. Bleeding is associated with a mean mortality of 0.3% and a permanent disabling morbidity rate of 1.4% (Favre *et al.* 2002). The risk of bleeding from DBS is related more to the patient (vascular fragility, various coagulopathies, unstable blood pressure) than to the type of stereoprocedure performed. Young and Rinaldi (1997) in 178 patients had 3.9% permanent complications and 0.6% indirect deaths. Higher mortality was reported in older series of DBS (<1.6%) (Bendok and Levy 1998).

3. Spinal cord stimulation (Table 6.3)
The gate control theory of pain (Melzack and Wall 1965) inspired Shealy to implant the first dorsal column stimulator in a cancer patient, the dorsal columns being rich in the large, low-threshold A-beta fibers, alleged to "close the gate" against nociception-subserving afferents – and also led to peripheral nerve stimulation. However, pain reduction without paresthesias can be obtained also from electrodes placed over the anterior cord surface (references in Gybels and Sweet 1989).

Mechanism of action. This is basically unknown. Certainly, SCS does not activate any gating mechanism, or it would also block acute pain. SCS may modulate local spinal networks, but also thalamocortical areas: the amplitude of evoked potentials in the human somatosensory cortex (Larson *et al.* 1974) and thalamic CeM nucleus (Nyqvist and Greenhoot 1973) is reduced by SCS; SCS also reduced the firing rate (including bursting) of thalamic Centrum Medianum neurons, with a post-stimulation effect of a few hours, at parameters achieving partial relief, in a patient with mixed nociceptive–neuropathic–central pain (Modesti and Waszak 1975). Tasker's group (Kiriakopoulos *et al.* 1997) reported on a SCI pain patient who described paresthesias and relief of her left leg pain at 2V, but not 1V: fMR showed increased activity in the right sensory cortex at 2V compared to 1V stimulation.

SCS may modulate several transmitters and peptides (5HT, glycine, adenosine), but the evidence favors GABA; in consideration of the efficacy of different GABA agonists, a role for both GABA A and B receptors can be envisioned, with an action on WDR cells (also see Meyerson and Linderoth 1999). If SCS acts by engaging GABA neurons, some may have died following excitoxic post-trauma injury (human studies show an increase of glutamate in such situations; see Canavero *et al.* 2003), and are no more available.

Efficacy. A prerequisite for successful pain relief by SCS has usually been a coinciding or blanketing of the painful area by the generalized paresthesias, but evoked paresthesias do not guarantee pain relief, and evoked sensations can also be outside the painful area.

Marchand and colleagues (1991) provided the first placebo-controlled study of SCS for chronic pain (other than CP). The conclusion was clear-cut: reduction in

TABLE 6.3. Spinal cord stimulation (dorsal column stimulation) (SCS)

Author(s)	Type of pain	Results/notes
Nashold and Friedman (1972)	SCI pain (leg pain; 6 pts)	Excellent: 1/6 pts (follow-up: 11 yrs) Partial: 4/6 pts (mild analgesic still required) Unsatisfactory: 1/6 pts
Nashold (1975)	CPSP (3 pts)	Initial pain reduction with stimulation of the trigeminal tract in the upper cervical cord
Urban and Nashold (1978)	CCP (3 pts)	Pain relief: 1; unsuccessful test stimulation (no paresthesias): 1; lost to follow-up but initial pain relief: 1
Sweet and Wepsic (1974, 1975)	Postcordotomy dysesthesia (7 pts) MS (3 pts) SCI pain (4 pts) Myelopathic pain (7 pts)	Good relief: 2 Good relief: 1 Failure Failure *Hyperpathia never relieved*
Hunt *et al.* (1975)	Radiation myelitis CP (1 pt)	0%
Long and Erickson (1975)	SCI CP (1 pt) Postcordotomy CP (2 pts)	Failure Failure
Lindblom and Meyerson (1975)	SCI pain (2 pts)	1 early success
Sedan and Lazorthes (1978)	Cord CP (postcordotomy pain: 14 pts; SCI: 16 pts)	Postcordotomy pain: review of Sweet, Shelden, Nashold and Long reports (14 pts). SCS results: excellent: 3/14 pts; bad: 1/14 pts; failure: 10/14 pts. SCI pain: review of Sweet and Long reports (16 pts). SCS results: excellent: 1/16 pts; fair: 2/16 pts; failure: 13/16 pts (**at least 1 pt with above-lesion SCS**). *No screening test in any pt*. BCP in anybody's experience: SCS totally ineffective
Rosen (1979)	MS	Good relief in 20%, 0% in 60% of pts
Richardson *et al.* (1980)	Paraplegia pain (10 pts)	**SCS rostrad to lesion**. Pain relief >50% from test stimulation: 5 (3 with incomplete cord lesion). At 1 yr follow-up: 4/5 lost to follow-up (2 pts died, 1 lost after 3 mos); 1/5 pain relief (presumably from recovered lesion) Failure of test stimulation in 5 pts (3 with complete cord lesion)

Author(s)	Type of pain	Results/notes
Demirel et al. (1984)	CP (10 pts)	Positive trial test in 6/10 pts. No late results
Vogel et al. (1986)	CP (3 pts)	No response to trial stimulation in all
Wester (1987)	MS CP (3 pts), SCI CCP (3 pts), tumor CCP (1 pt)	Benefit at 15 mos (median; range: 4–60 mos): 0% MS CP, 33% SCI CCP, 0% tumor CCP. Comment: global effect restricted, dwindling effect in time, "**DCS not of any great help**"
Mittal et al. (1987)	CP (8 pts)	Positive trial test in 3 pts. Persistent pain relief (3 mos, 8 yrs): 2 pts
Beric et al. (1988)	CP	SCS may worsen CP with absent STT function and preserved DCs
Buchhass et al. (1989)	SCI pain (7 pts)	6/7 good/very good relief at 3–72 mos
Krainick and Thoeden (1989)	CCP (transverse spinal lesions: 2 pts, other spinal injuries: 2 pts; incomplete conus-cauda lesion: 4 pts; tetraspasticity after cervical disc operation: 2 pts)	Initial pain relief in all pts; no long-term follow-up. Overall (CP plus other pains) long-term (2–3 yrs) results: 50–75% pain reduction in 39% of pts. ≥60% had complications requiring removal of the stimulator
Michel et al. (1990)	CPSP (5 pts; parietal)	50% pain relief in 2
Cole et al. (1987, 1991)	CCP (4 pts)	0% (1 worsened)
Simpson et al. (1991)	Thalamic CP (9 pts)	3 significant, 3 modest, 2 no benefit, 1 worsened (one after initial modest benefit)
	Post-thalamotomy CP (1 pt)	Worsened
	Painful paraparesis, paraplegia and hemiparesis (10 pts)	6 complete/partial, 1 nonsubstantial, 2 failures (1 worsened) (Relief: significant [complete or partial pain relief, with significant effect on medication and life-style, praise of the apparatus by the patient], modest [no substantial benefit, no significant change in medication, activity, sleep pattern], failure) Long-term follow-up data not available for single disease. Median overall follow-up: 29 mos (2 wks–9 yrs)

(continued)

TABLE 6.3 *(continued)*

Author(s)	Type of pain	Results/notes
Simpson (1999)	1 new CP, thalamic	Worsened. Conclusion: SCS relief very unlikely in complete SCI and reasonably likely in partial SCI; unlikely in BCP
Spiegelmann and Friedman (1991)	Cord CP: SCI, MS (6 pts)	Positive stimulation test: 4 pts. Long-lasting 50–100% pain relief: 3 pts. Mean follow-up: 13 mos (3–30 mos). No further pain relief after a change in the distribution of paresthesias in 1 SCI pain pt (initial 1 yr benefit). TENS was not predictive (TENS failures could respond to SCS, as found by many other groups)
Ohta *et al.* (1992)	SCI pain (4 pts)	At 1 wk, 100% relief in all. However, at 3–5 mos, no relief in 3, while in the fourth 70–80% relief at 19 mos only when SCS turned on
Tasker *et al.* (1992) *Tasker's group*	SCI complete (11 pts)	Steady (burning or not) pain unrelieved in 80% of pts. 25–50% relief in 20% of pts. Intermittent or evoked pain unrelieved in 100% of pts. All cases drawing benefit had T10–L2 lesions.
	Incomplete (24 pts)	(22/24 implants): steady pain relief ≥50% in 27% of pts and 25–50% in 14% of pts. Intermittent pain unrelieved. 25–50% evoked pain relief in 25% of pts. Of cases relieved, two thirds had T10–L2 lesions. *Authors' conclusions:* SCS is more effective for relief of steady pain (36%) than of intermittent (0%) or evoked pain (16%) (statistically significant difference). SCS is ineffective even for steady pain in cases with complete lesions (20% relief) Follow-up: > 1 yr Failures usually associated with an inability to induce paresthesias in the area of pain, due to severe cord lesions inducing dorsal column atrophy (dieback), difficulty in accessing the epidural space

Author(s)	Type of pain	Results/notes
		(trauma or previous surgery), difficulty in producing paresthesias over the large area of patients' pain. **Failures not due to intrinsic resistance of CCP to SCS**.
Kim *et al.* (2001) (Tasker's group)	BCP 12 pts CCP 20 pts	Pain relief >50% for 1 yr only in 1 Positive stimulation trial: 7 pts; test worsened pain in 2 pts with evoked pain (just like Vc DBS in BCP pts with allodynia). Early failures (pain relief <50% within 1 yr of implantation): 2/7 pts (early success probably a placebo effect); late failures (past 1 yr): 3/7 pts Long-lasting (mean follow-up: 3.9 yrs, range 0.3-9 yrs) >50% pain relief: 2/7 pts. Drug reduction not specified nor enhanced ability to work
North *et al.* (1993)	SCI pain (11 pts) **1972–1990**	Permanent implants in 90% of cases. No detailed follow-up reported
Italian cooperative study (Broggi *et al.* 1994)	Paraplegia pain (23 pts)	Failure in all implanted pts within 1 yr of surgery, despite initial benefit in several in this highly select group
Cioni *et al.* (1995) *Includes all previously published cases of Meglio's group in Rome (PACE 1989; 12:709-12, J Neurosurg 1989; 70:519-24)*	SCI pain (25 pts)	Pain due to trauma or surgery at all spine levels. 75% relief at the end of the test period: 40.1% of pts. Patients with more than 50% pain relief at a mean follow-up of 37.2 mos: 18.2%. Better results in patients with painful spasms and constrictive pain in the transitional zone in pts with incomplete thoracic lesions. Below-level burning pain unrelieved. *Authors' conclusions:* the relative integrity of the dorsal column is an important prerequisite for analgesia. 0% benefit without paresthesias evoked in the painful area. **SCS not effective in treating true SCI CP**

(continued)

TABLE 6.3 *(continued)*

Author(s)	Type of pain	Results/notes
Lazorthes *et al.* (1995) *Includes all pts operated on and previously published by both Lazorthes and Siegfried*	SCI pain (101 pts)	SCI pain included traumatic paraplegia pain, iatrogenous lesions or following cord tumor surgery, herpetic myelitis and spondylotic damage. Successful pain relief: Short-term: 50–58% of pts; long-term: 30–34% of pts *Authors' conclusions:* cord CP and even more BCP respond poorly to SCS, with increasing degrees of denervation. Analgesia is much less significant for SCI CP or iatrogenic CP following surgery on the cord (e.g., for tumor). Failures due to degeneration of lemniscal fibers
Barolat *et al.* (1995, 1998)	SCI pain (11 pts)	Short-term successful pain relief: 45% of pts. 55% of pts never experienced any pain relief (half never felt paresthesias in the painful area) Long-term successful results only in 27% of pts, with good ($>50\%$) pain relief in 2/11 pts and moderate (25–50%) pain relief in 1/11 pts. *Authors' conclusions:* results of SCS on SCI pain have been disappointing in the vast majority of pts
Peyron *et al.* (1998)	CPSP (Wallenberg) (3 pts, with evoked pain)	Failure
Anderson and Burchiel (1999)	CPSP	*Authors' conclusions:* CPSP is not particularly responsive to SCS
Tseng (2000)	SCI pain (1 pt)	Relief at 19 mos
Eisenberg and Brecker (2002)	Cord CP (postspinal cord tumor removal) (1 pt)	Pain relief for 9 mos. Above. Lesion SCS
Sindou *et al.* (2003)	Cord CP (30 pts; MS: 9 pts; trauma: 7 pts; spinal tumor: 5pts; syrinx: 5 pts; spondylotic myelopathy: 4 pts)	Long-term results (mean follow-up: 18.8 mos, range 11.2–19.2 mos): pain relief $>50\%$ (and minimal drug use): 12/30 pts (40%) All pts had incomplete spinal cord damage (CP pts with complete spinal cord damage or midline pain excluded). SCS: paddle. Previous TENS course, but results not given. No differentiation between end-zone pain and diffuse CP. At least some retained sensibility in the painful areas and normal or near normal somatosensory evoked potentials in most responders

Author(s)	Type of pain	Results/notes
Quigley et al. (2003)	Spinal cord/root compression (4 pts) MS (4 pts) Paraplegia pain (3 pts) **1989-2000**	Relief ≥50% in 4 SC-root compression, 3 MS and 0 paraplegia pain (doctor's assessment), 2 of 3, 2 of 3 and 0 of 2 (patients' assessment). **General anesthesia, laminotomy in most patients,** >80% receiving a quadripolar plate. Almost 60% inserted at T9-12. Then C1-4, C5-7, T5-8. 62% radiofrequency, 38% IPG.TEST: 5 days, retrospective study via questionnaire. No routine antibiotics. Majority of ALL patients used the SCS every day for about 12 h, 21% only during exacerbations, 10% did not use it anymore. Average time from implantation to data collection: 4.2 years. 64 revision operations out of 102 pts, due to electrode complications, generator complications, connecting lead fracture. Global infection rate was 4.9% (2 of 5 pts needed explantation). Globally (CP plus all other pains), pts who had used SCS for 5 years or more had lower levels of substantial pain relief compared to those using it for less (65% vs. 81%). It is unclear if this is due to tolerance, an initial placebo response, hardware failure or some other phenomenon.
Rogano et al. (2003)	CCP (12 partial lesion pts)	VAS from 9.9 to 3.6 (no details given). Minimum follow-up: 6 mos (mean 19.1 ± 13.5 mos)
Kumar et al. (2006) *Includes all pts operated on and previously published by this group*	MS CP (19 pts) SCI pain (15 pts)	Initial pain relief: 17/19 pts Long-term success (50-100% relief): 15/17 pts Initial pain relief: 7/15 pts Long-term success (50-100% relief): 5/7 SCI pts Mean follow-up whole series (including CP): 97.6 mos Limb pain considered to be due to cord injury. Favorable response in cord lesion pts with incomplete paraplegia and with the majority of pain felt below the lesion level. No benefit with SCS in pts with complete paraplegia complaining of either pain at the level of injury or diffuse pain below the injury level
Kim et al. (2006)	CCP (cavernoma) (1 pt)	Failure

clinical pain is small (less than 30%), and patients submitted to SCS all reported that they felt some sensations, when in fact the stimulator was not activated. Even today, there is a lack of high-quality evidence, no double-blind randomized trial (admittedly rather difficult to set up in this context) and serious flaws in blinding, recruitment and assessment in nearly all studies (Cameron 2004; Carter 2004).

When pain is below the lesion, SCS can be effective only if the corresponding dorsal column(s) retain sufficient functional value. If the territory below the lesion is totally anesthetic, SCS will not work. As a matter of fact, if the dorsal columns are totally interrupted, electrodes – even if implanted above the lesion – cannot stimulate the degenerated contained lemniscal fibers. Imaging and measurement of SEPs may be useful to check integrity of the dorsal columns. Instead, SCS appears to be effective in some patients with incomplete lesions, painful spasms, at-level pain or postcordotomy pain. Poor results are seen with complete lesions and intermittent and burning pain. Most studies report a decline in efficacy of SCS over time. Generally, the best results have been obtained with multipolar electrodes, with laminotomy epidural placement (Carter 2004), when electrodes are localized above the pain segments, if stimulation paresthesias and pain segments are superimposed and when the pain is localized rather than diffuse.

In conclusion, despite occasional spectacular successes, SCS is not indicated for CP of brain origin and only a minority of well-selected CCP patients may obtain relief in the long term (years) (see also Warms *et al.* 2002).

4. Transcutaneous electrical nerve stimulation (TENS) (Table 6.4)

TENS was first introduced in the 1960s as a screening procedure for SCS. It is applied at high frequency (80–100 Hz) (also known as *conventional* TENS) aimed at activation of myelinated cutaneous sensory fibers or low-frequency stimulation (short trains of impulses at 1–4 Hz over the motor nerves, known as *acupuncture-like* TENS), aiming at activation of muscle efferents/cells and thereby evoking muscle afferent input to CNS. Stimulation must be directed over the most painful region, with dual-channel stimulators to cover a large body area with pain.

Mechanism of action. TENS can apparently reduce CP only if the dorsal column–medial lemniscal pathways are uninjured or only mildly injured (i.e., paresthesias are evoked), perhaps by segmental conduction block of spinal projection fibers. At appropriately high stimulation frequencies, after-hyperpolarizations seen in dorsal horn neurons could coalesce and maintain the cell in a hyperpolarized and, therefore, inhibited state (just as PNS would on neuromas) by tetanic hyperpolarization. However, in the clinical situation, the intensity of the stimulating current for pain relief is commonly below the threshold for activation of C- and A-δ fibers, and the relief may last days and occasionally weeks. Also, if central sensitization renders low-threshold afferent input painful, it would be hard to explain how augmentation of such input through TENS (or SCS) would suppress the pain, and, in fact, TENS may exacerbate CP during stimulation. Suprasegmental mechanisms are, however, possible (Sjolund 1993).

TABLE 6.4. Transcutaneous electrical nerve stimulation (TENS)

Author(s)	Type of pain	Results/notes
Banerjee *et al.* (1974)	SCI pain (5 pts)	100% relief at short term (30 min three times per day)
Long and Hagfors (1975)	Pain secondary to CNS injury	TENS relatively ineffective
Davis and Lentini (1975)	SCI CP (11 pts) plus other SCI neuropathic pains	2 successes, 2 partial successes, 18 failures; 4/4 failures for cervical lesions, 5 successes and 6 failures for thoracic lesions and 50% success for conus-cauda lesions
Hachen *et al.* (1978)	SCI pain (39 pts)	49% early success, 28% late (3 mos) successes
Heilporn *et al.* (1978)	SCI pain (3 pts)	Failures
Guilmart (thesis, detailed in Sedan and Lazorthes 1978)	Brain CP (2 pts) SCI CP (9 pts)	1 relief Failures (Conventional TENS)
Long *et al.* (1979)	CP of any origin	Patients with CP of any origin do not respond to TENS in significant numbers and responders do not seem to maintain the response over a long period of time. TENS usually worsen hyperesthesia
Eriksson *et al.* (1979, 1984)	BCP (7 pts), CCP (11 pts)	In 6 pts acupuncture-like TENS, conventional in others. BCP: pain relief (continued for 3 mos.) in 5 CCP: pain relief at 3 mos in 7 (in 6, at-level pain, not below-level CP) Successful pain relief probably in incomplete lesions
	Brainstem facial CP (5 pts)	Not broken down from group: probably some reliefs
Sindou and Keravel (1980)	Thalamic pain (5 pts) Cord CP (17 pts)	Failures Relief in 2 (late follow-up not specified)
Bates and Nathan (1980)	Thalamic CP (12 pts)	8 stimulated beyond 1 wk. Stimulation up to 8 h daily; frequency up to 70 Hz. 0/8 helped by TENS. Pts did not notice any interaction between the sensation and their pain, except that when the intensity of stimulation was increased, this suddenly added to their pain.

(continued)

TABLE 6.4 *(continued)*

Author(s)	Type of pain	Results/notes
	Cord CP (16 pts; postcordotomy: 2 pts; intrinsic spinal cord lesions: 8 pts; syringomyelia and syringobulbia: 6 pts)	10 stimulated beyond 1 wk. Detailed results not given
		Globally, of 235 patients with chronic pain and 160 passing test, 20–25% used TENS at 2 yrs or more of follow-up, sometimes only to help them over crises of pain
Leijon and Boivie (1989b)	CPSP (infratentorial lesions) (15 pts)	Pain relief from conventional or acupuncture-like TENS in 4 (3 after 2 yrs). 3 pts (2 brainstem infarction, 1 unknown lesion site) continued to report pain relief after 2 yrs. All 3 had normal or near normal touch-vibration thresholds. One pt with Wallenberg syndrome had facial pain on one side and extremity pain on the other. High-frequency TENS for facial pain used without effect on arm and leg pains. High- and low-frequency TENS had approximately equal effect in the other 2 pts. The study applied rigid schedules not taking into account the varying distribution of pain and the subsequent need to apply the electrodes over the region with the most intense pain.
Tasker (2001)	CP	TENS is seldom useful in pts with pain over a wide area of the body. It may be useful for pain in the trigeminal area
Kabirov *et al.* (2002)	CCP (syrinx) (14 pts)	30–100% relief in 12 (TENS 10 sessions, 60 min each)
Nuti *et al.* (2005)	CP: > 10 pts (including 3 Wallenberg's CPs)	No significant analgesia

Efficacy. Controlled trials are lacking, and so are long-term studies. While certainly less expensive than SCS, DBS or MCS, and with almost no adverse effects, TENS cannot cover wide body areas and requires prolonged use several times a day, basically hampering a patient's daily activities. While a trial may be warranted before other more invasive procedures are contemplated, few patients gain long-lasting pain relief, both with BCP and below-level CCP. TENS may relieve some SCI patients with muscular or at-level pain. For MS spontaneous CP, TENS is ineffective (Rosen and

TABLE 6.5. Gasserian ganglion stimulation

Author(s)	Type of pain	Results/notes
Taub et al. (1997) *Tasker's group*	CPSP (brain 3 pts; brainstem 3 pts; bulbar tractotomy: 1 pt)	Successful pain relief: 5/7 pts (100%: 1 pt; 75%: 1 pt; 50–74%: 2 pts; 50%: 1 pt). The 2 failures had an initial success which was lost within a month (placebo effect?). Among these 5 pts, a patient with thalamic infarct experienced relief for 21 mos and then found the stimulation was no longer effective. Another stroke case found that he no longer needed the stimulator because the pain had subsided. Median follow-up: 21 mos. CP better relieved than PNP in this unique series

Barsoum 1979; Young and Goodman 1979; Tasker 2001). Even cutaneous field stimulation (16 metal pin skin cathode with single 1 ms, 4 Hz pulses, 30 minutes bid at twice the sensory threshold) in TENS-resistant (low and high frequency) adds little (20% more relieved patients) in PNP – and maybe CP – at 3 months.

The recently introduced scrambler therapy has yet to be tried on CP (Marineo 2003).

5. Gasserian ganglion stimulation (Table 6.5)

This was introduced in 1978 by Steude (see in Meyerson and Linderoth 2001). Presumably, the efficacy depends on an intact afferent pathway in the periphery along which nerve impulses generated by stimulation can reach the trigeminal nuclei in the brainstem and continue transsynaptically up to the cortex. Its place in the treatment of CP is virtually nonexistent.

6. Vagal nerve stimulation

There are no reports as far as CP is concerned. Given its possible unspecific effects on catecholamines (Kirchner *et al.* 2001), this technique is likely not to have an impact in the treatment of CP.

7. Electroconvulsive therapy (Table 6.6)

Introduced in 1938 by Ugo Cerletti, this has also been employed for pain control (see complete bibliography in Canavero and Bonicalzi 2001).

Mechanism of action. Bilateral ECT sends electric impulses through the thalamus, the hypothalamus and the brainstem. While ECT affects many neurotransmitters and neuroendocrine substances (e.g., endorphins, acetylcholine, (nor)epinephrine, dopamine, serotonin and GABA), Salmon and colleagues (1988) found no significant correlations between endorphin levels and ECT in CP; they also noted no placebo effect. Such changes of neurotransmitters – but also changes in gene expression – repeated over the course of a series of ECT treatments could modulate neural function at numerous sites throughout the nervous system. The α4 subunit of GABA

TABLE 6.6. Electroconvulsive therapy (ECT)

Author(s)	Type of pain	Results/notes
Von Hagen (1957)	CPSP (thalamic) with evoked pains and depression (1 pt)	Great improvement for about 10 mos from 8 bilateral ECTs, then relapse (1955). Further pain control from 3 additional treatments. Previous ECT for depression
White and Sweet (1969)	CCP (postcordotomy) (? pts)	Relief only during the confusional state
Salmon *et al.* (1988)	CPSP (thalamic) (4 pts)	Failure with *unilateral* ECT. No depressed pts
McCance *et al.* (1996)	CPSP (3 pts)	2/3 CPSP of immediate onset. 3/3 pts with allodynia. 1/3 depressed pt. **(Few months CP remission in 1 pt after an epileptic fit)** A course of six bilateral ECT sessions over 2 weeks slightly improved CP only in 1 pt, while 2 worsened
Doi *et al.* (1999)	Brain CP (12 pts)	Abstract. *CP remission in 1 depressed pt after ECT.* Bilateral ECT (110 V for 5 min) for 6–12 sessions at 1–7 day intervals. Complete relief of both steady and evoked pain in all suprathalamic cases. Partial relief in thalamic cases. Pain recurrence relieved by a new ECT course in 9 pts
Harano *et al.* (1999)	CPSP (thalamic pain) (39 pts)	Abstract. Convulsions (plus nausea and vomiting) lasting 2–3 min induced by intracisternal (cerebellar) methylprednisolone sodium succinate 125 mg in 5 ml syringe mixed with CSF. Excellent results in 54.4%, good in 38.6% and poor in 4%. Lateral position; 22G 6 cm block needle inserted at crossing point of bilateral mastoid line and sagittal halfline under fluoroscopy. 57 injections in 39 pts
Fukui *et al.* (2002)	CPSP	Relief with bilat. ECT (paper not available for review)
Canavero and Bonicalzi (2003)	Cord CP (1 pt)	No pain relief after injection of 125 mg of methylprednisolone in the lateral ventricle. No frank fit

A receptors may be implicated in the clinical effects of ECT (see in Olsen and Avoli 1997).

ECT likely has direct, acute effects on the cerebral cortex. In the words of Von Hagen (1957): "Electroshock therapy may produce its effect . . . from a reduction in the influence of the cortex on . . . reverberating . . . (circuits)." We proposed that ECT interferes with a corticothalamic reverberation mechanism (Canavero 1994; Canavero and Bonicalzi 2001). Seizures may be a natural example of spontaneous ECT: case 3 of Bornstein (1949) reported that a phantom sensation slowly shrunk before an epileptic fit to recede totally at the moment of the fit. After recovering consciousness, the phantom reappeared only after a certain lapse of time, a possible sign of the warm-up period required by the reverberation to restart.

The minimal electrical intensity needed for a generalized seizure of a specified minimal duration appears to vary by approximately 40-fold in the population (Sackeim *et al.* 1993): this range may also apply to reverberation *strength*.

Efficacy. Some patients with CP have been meaningfully relieved by ECT for more than a short time. Given the high rate of relapse (perhaps particularly in previously drug-refractory cases), the need for multiple courses, possible permanent side effects (amnesia) and non-uniformity of response, ECT should be considered as a last resort in highly refractory cases.

8. Conclusions

The most important paper providing conclusive evidence about the role of electrical neurostimulation for CP is that of Katayama and colleagues (2001). These authors analyzed a series of 45 patients with CPSP, all tested with percutaneous SCS. Satisfactory analgesia was set at ≥60% reduction on a VAS scale. In the long term only 7% (3 patients) achieved satisfactory analgesia with SCS. Of the remaining 42, 12 underwent Vc DBS (in 7 also of IC and/or medial lemniscus): 25% (3 patients) obtained satisfactory relief in the long term, while 31 patients in whom SCS was ineffective underwent MCS (1 underwent both MCS and Vc DBS): 48% (15 patients) obtained long-term relief. In particular, 9% (3/35) thalamic-infrathalamic and 0 of 10 suprathalamic obtained long-term relief from SCS; 0 of 2 suprathalamic and 30% (3/10) thalamic-infrathalamic obtained long-term relief from DBS; 37.5% (3/8) suprathalamic and 52% (12/23) thalamic-infrathalamic obtained long-term relief from MCS. In sum, CS is superior to all other techniques.

Thus, in light of minimal invasiveness, no reported mortality and disabling permanent morbidity, and the possibility of running placebo tests, CS is the technique of first choice in BCP patients in whom oral drugs as previously suggested have proved ineffective. In CS failures, DBS with simultaneous implantation of Vc (or ML) and PVG should be attempted as a second step. For CCP cases with some retained sensibility in painful areas, SCS is the first choice; in failures or totally anesthetic patients, there is as yet not enough evidence to support CS over DBS. CS may be a first option for reasons discussed above. TENS may be an option if cost is at issue or patients refuse surgery.

These conclusions must be tempered by the expensive nature of such treatments, including changes of batteries, loss of efficacy in several to many patients depending on the technique and explantation for intercurrent problems. Whereas SCS and CS appear to be safe, DBS carries a small risk of mortality and disabling morbidity.

CHEMICAL (Table 6.7)

Spinal administration of several drugs has been spearheaded by the not-well-understood observation that drugs ineffective by the systemic route often are effective

TABLE 6.7. Chemical neuromodulation (spinal intrathecal [IT] or epidural [EPI] infusion)

Author(s)	Type of pain	Drug	Results/notes
Pollock et al. (1951)	SCI pain	IT tetracaine 1 ml (0.5%)	In a number (unspecified) of cases, spinal anesthesia below level: burning pain did not disappear. In 4 cases with CSF block, anesthesia above level: in 3 distal pain gradually disappeared, then slowly returned (in 1 case, absent for 24–56 min, full relapse at 3 h)
Davis et al. (1954)	SCI pain	IT local anesthetic	Completely relieved spontaneous, diffuse, burning, below-level pain
Waltz and Ehni (1966)	CP; thalamic (2 pts)	IT pantocaine (6 mg)	Immediate abolition of leg pain, **even before sensory block.** In one case, leg pain was abolished, while arm and face pains were reduced
Namba et al. (1984)	CPSP (1 pt)	IT morphine	Failure
Glynn et al. (1986)	CCP (15 pts)	EPI clonidine (150 µg) EPI morphine (5 mg) EPI buprenorphine (0.3 mg)	Non-RCT, single-blind, crossover, single-dose study. EPI clonidine vs. EPI morphine. Pain relief: EPI clonidine: 7 pts (morphine unresponsive); EPI morphine: 5 pts (3 clonidine responsive). 3 pts unresponsive both to morphine and clonidine, 2 of them buprenorphine responsive
Crisologo et al. (1991)	CPSP (3 pts)	IT lidocaine (0.5%, 2%, 2 mL)	In all, complete or almost complete sensory block Case 1: thalamic stroke with left hemisoma CP; 6 mos later, left stroke with right hemisoma pain. IT lidocaine: at 0.5%: 0% relief; at 2%: 100% relief in left leg for 5 h Case 2: right hemispheric cortical stroke with CP in left arm/leg. Lidocaine at 0.5%: 0% relief; at 2%: 100% relief for 1 h, then gradual relapse at 5 h

Reference	Subjects	Drug (dose)	Results
			Case 3: thalamic CPSP (longer duration and higher intensity than cases 1 and 2): 0% relief at both concentrations, despite complete sensory block
Loubser and Donovan (1991)	SCI (21 pts)	IT lidocaine; 50–100 mg (2 injections 1 h apart)	RCT. Spontaneous burning pain and intermittent sharp pain. IT lidocaine effects: (1) sensory level of anesthesia above the level of injury in pts with lumbar and thoracic injuries and to T4 in pts with cervical injuries; (2) significant reduction of pain intensity when compared with placebo (13 vs. 4); (3) analgesia lasting for a mean time of 123 min, exceeding the expected duration of action for interruption of nociceptive messages. IT lidocaine effects on pain: overall: 65% relief of pain (mean) in 12/16 pts. Pts with spinal canal obstruction, sensory block above SCI level: no change in 4 and 20% relief of pain in 1. Negative response in 4 pts (2 with incomplete anterior cord syndromes), despite sensory anesthesia rostral to the level of SCI (pain generator more rostrally?) When spinal anesthesia proximal to SCI level was adequate, 9 of 11 had a positive response vs. 4 of 10 who did not obtain anesthesia above SCI level, because of spinal canal obstruction or high lesion level
Herman et al. (1992)	CCP (MS: 4 pts; spinal cord compression: 1 pt; transverse myelitis: 2 pts) SCI (2 pts)	IT baclofen (50 μg)	Cord CP: RCT (crossover with placebo = vehicle) assessing the efficacy of acute IT baclofen on chronic, dysesthetic and spasm-related pain. IT baclofen significantly suppressed dysesthetic pain and, after the suppression of neuropathic pain, spasm-related pain Non-RCT

(continued)

225

TABLE 6.7 (continued)

Author(s)	Type of pain	Drug	Results/notes
Glynn et al. (1992)	CCP (6 pts)	EPI clonidine (150 µg) + IT clonidine (1 pt)	Pain relief ≥50%: 3 (all with spasm). IT clonidine: excellent pain relief in 1 pt. Better relief with higher clonidine concentrations in the CSF
Triggs and Beric (1992)	CCP, ASAS (1 pt)	IT morphine	Failure
Loubser and Clearman (1993)	SCI CP (1 pt)	IT lidocaine (50 mg)	Dysesthetic and cramping pain in both arms and legs following a C6 incomplete injury. IT lidocaine produced a sensory block to light touch to the T8 level, with disappearance of both spasticity and pain
Reig (1993)	BCP (thalamic CP: 3 pts; CNS injury: 1 pt) CCP (paraplegia pain: 1 pt; postcordotomy pain: 1 pt)	IT morphine (initial dose, 1 mg, final dose 3.4 mg/day)	At 3 yrs of follow-up: never > 75% relief. None returned to work. 50–75% pain relief: some; unsatisfactory pain relief: some (numbers not clear). Congress abstract
Fenollosa et al. (1993)	SCI pain (12 pts)	IT morphine (0.3–1 mg/day, continuous infusion)	Non-RCT. Pain and spasticity improvement (>50% relief): 8/12 pts. Minimal tolerance in 6/8 pts (after 3 yrs final dose range: 1.6–6.0 mg/day)
Taira et al. (1994, 1995)	CPSP (8 pts) SCI pain (6 pts)	IT baclofen (50–100 µg)	Substantial pain relief starting 1–2 h after a single injection and persisting for 10–24 h in 9/14 pts (3 SCI). Allodynia and hyperalgesia, if present, also relieved. Placebo when tried ineffective. Incomplete data on CP components. Study prompted by a CPSP suppressing effect from 25 µg of IT baclofen in 1 pt with spasticity (not relieved by baclofen) and pain

Study	Pain type (patients)	Treatment	Results
Hassenbusch et al. (1995)	SCI CP (1 pt)	IT morphine (0.2 mg/h) (IT sufentanil)	NRS reduction from 9/10 to 5/10 1 mo after the pump implant. At 2 yrs follow-up, NRS = 6/10 in spite of IT sufentanil trial and oral propoxyphene addition. At last follow-up, pain relief judged fair (25%) by the pt and a failure by the authors. Positive preimplantation test
Loubser and Akman (1996)	SCI pain (12 pts: 7 at-level pain and 2 below-level CP; musculoskeletal in 6 pts also present)	IT baclofen infusion (implanted pump)	Non-RCT. Effects on neurogenic pain at both 6- and 12-mos interval: no significant change in pain severity in 7/9 patients; pain increase in 2/9 pts. Significant decrease of musculoskeletal pain (5/6 pts). *Authors' conclusions:* IT baclofen does not decrease SCI CP. Results of other studies were possibly positive due to higher doses achieved by bolus injections and continuous infusion resulting in comparably lower CSF doses; moreover, pain relief was assessed over only 24 h
Middleton et al. (1996)	Cord CP (1 pt)	IT baclofen and IT clonidine	Anterior cord syndrome case with incomplete C5 tetraplegia. Symptoms not improved by the administration of IT baclofen through an existing programmable infusion pump. Immediate pain relief after clonidine was added to baclofen in the pump reservoir and combined IT administration started
Winkelmuller and Winkelmuller (1996)	Thalamic pain (1 pt) Paraplegia pain (6 pts)	IT opioids (implanted pump)	Mean follow-up: 3.4 yrs (range 6 mos to 5.7 yrs). Continuing IT opioids infusion 6 mos after the pump implantation: 1/1 thalamic pain and 3/6 paraplegia pain pts. Initial mean morphine dosage: 2.6 mg/day; at the first follow-up: 3.6 mg/day; at the last follow-up: 5.2 mg/day No separate analysis results of BCP/CCP.

(continued)

TABLE 6.7 (continued)

Author(s)	Type of pain	Drug	Results/notes
Meglio (1998)	SCI CP (8 pts)	2 pts: IT baclofen (50 μg) 5 pts: IT morphine 1 pt: both Test: 0.5 mg IT morphine	Baclofen failure. Relief in 3, then 2 (due to side effects in 1) with >50% relief at 1 yr Average morphine dosage: 3 mg/day At- and below-level pains not distinguished
Angel et al. (1998)	Cord CP (syrinx) (1 pt)	IT morphine	Initial IT morphine dosage: 0.5 mg/day; 2 yrs later, the pt needed 3 mg/day of IT morphine to maintain the best possible analgesia (VAS reduction from 10 to 2)
Nitescu et al. (1998)	Cord CP (ischemic myelopathies: 5 pts; MS: 2 pts; post-traumatic myelopathies: 3 pts)	IT opioids (morphine or buprenorphine) and IT bupivacaine	Non-RCT. Drug dosage: morphine 0.5 mg/ml, buprenorphine 0.015 mg/ml, bupivacaine 4.75–5.0 mg/ml. Daily volumes tailored to give the pts satisfactory to excellent (60–100%) pain relief, with acceptable side effects Results: MS-related pain: effective; ischemic and post-traumatic myelopathy: ineffective in 5/8 (63%) pts (due to "centralization" at higher levels of pain). Several refused to continue treatment
Anderson and Burchiel (1999)	CPSP (1 pt) CCP (2 pts, 1 syrinx)	IT morphine	Outcome of CP patients (out of 30 sundry pts) not specified, but all 3 had >50% relief at test injection
Belfrage et al. (1999)	CP (CPSP?) (2 pts)	IT adenosine	Reduction of spontaneous and evoked pain. Results not broken down according to pain type (CP vs. other pains)
Becker et al. (2000)	MS incomplete T5 CP (1 pt)	IT baclofen (110 μg/day, continuous administration) (450 μg at each refill)	Complete pain relief for 20 mos. Pain reappearance soon after baclofen discontinuation (pump explanted on patient's request after progression of MS)

Reference	Patients	Treatment	Failure
Gatscher et al. (2002)		IT morphine (up to 3 mg/die)	
Siddall et al. (2000)	SCI CP (15 pts) (below level: 13; at-level: 4 pts; both types: 3 pts. Figures not in agreement!)	IT morphine (0.75 mg (mean) (IT, bolus 0.2–1.5 mg) and/or IT clonidine (50 μg (mean) (IT, bolus 50–100 μg or 300–500 μg over 6 h). Combination: half of each dose. Minimum 4 injections, 1 day apart	6-day double-blind crossover, placebo-controlled RCT. Overall pain relief (4 h after drug administration): IT morphine alone = IT clonidine = placebo. IT morphine (median minimal effective dose = 0.75 mg) + IT clonidine (median dose 50 μg as bolus injection or 300–500 μg over 6 h) produced significantly more pain relief than placebo 4 h after administration. Pain relief ≥50% (mixture): at-level pain: 50% of pts; below-level pain: 35% of pts (in this group of patients, IT placebo was pain relieving in about 30% of cases). Conclusions: at-level pain appears to be more responsive. The concentration of morphine in the cervical CSF and the degree of pain relief correlated significantly, so drugs should be administered above-level NNT: 7.5 (combination)
Siddall et al. (1994)	SCI CP (1 pt)	IT morphine (10 mg/day) & IT clonidine (17 μcg/day)	Pain unresponsive to IT morphine alone. Marked decrease in pain from IT morphine + IT clonidine combined administration
Ridgeway et al. (2000)	SCI CP (2 pts)	IT ziconotide (and opioids coadministration) up to 144 μg/day	No relief at end of trial. 47% CP decrease at 14.4 μg/day. No further decrease at 28.8 μg/day. Dramatic pain increase over time, requiring an increase in concurrent opioid administration. Trial stopped and IT baclofen restarted after appearance of confusion and sedation
Penn and Paice (2000)	MS CP (1 pt) plus other 2 chronic pain pts	IT ziconotide up to 5.3 μg/h	Ineffective. Very serious side effects. Infusion stopped. Coma. Residual memory impairment

(continued)

TABLE 6.7 (continued)

Author(s)	Type of pain	Drug	Results/notes
Margot-Duclot et al. (2002)	SCI pain (low lesions) (14 pts) (plus 19 cauda lesions pts)	IT baclofen (50–150 μg)	Placebo-controlled study. 8 had > 60% relief; 5 implanted with pump. Effect lost in a few. Cauda pts: 12 had > 60% relief and 10 implanted. **Paroxysmal component more responsive than steady pain**
Canavero and Bonicalzi (1998, 2003)	BCP and CCP	IT midazolam (2.5–6 mg/day)	Analgesia from IT midazolam correlates with positive propofol test. Pump implanted in a few pts. Satisfactory analgesia, although tolerance may occur. Follow-up is entering a few years. No side effects observed to date
Rogano et al. (2003) Plus congress abstracts	CCP (18 pts), most spinal traumas	IT morphine (1–6 mg)	VAS from 9.2 to 3.6, both in complete and incomplete lesions. Minimum follow-up: 6 mos (mean 19.1 ± 13.5 mos). No details are given and data are inserted shortly in discussion. No differentiation between at- and below-level pains. Follow-up short. Nausea and vomiting frequent
Nuti et al. (2005)	CCP (1 pt)	IT morphine	Failure

when given spinally (references in Siddall 2002). Unfortunately, although several drugs have been administered intrathecally (IT) in attempting to treat CP, there is only a small number of papers reporting the effect of continuous IT administration of drugs on CP and the vast majority of them deal with CP after SCI. These studies are not randomized, nor controlled, and often patients with CP are no more than 1 or 2 cases among several other pain conditions or just single case reports. In most papers, only the outcome of the mixed group of pain patients is reported and the outcome of patients with CP remains unknown. Well-designed studies with homogeneous groups of patients with long-term follow-up are needed before drawing definite conclusions on any of the reviewed drugs. Moreover, a positive preimplantation test does not guarantee long-term relief.

A review of the literature and of personal experience suggests the following conclusions:

1) IT lidocaine significantly reduces pain in a proportion of SCI patients, if access to the cord cephalad to injury level is preserved; however, relief may not be obtained despite a sensory block above the level of injury. Although good relief can be obtained, the effect is only temporary and even multiple local anesthetic blocks do not result in long-term relief of SCI pain.

2) IT midazolam (a GABA A agonist) has significantly relieved several patients with both BCP and CCP in our experience, without side effects of any kind, although tolerance can be seen.

3) IT baclofen relieved few patients of their CP in the long run, as relief is often lost (tolerance) due to long-term receptor changes (down-regulation at, for example, cord laminas I–II or higher levels) or other factors. It may even make pain worse in some patients. Although generally well tolerated, the general impression is that it has no major effects on CP (see also Slonimski *et al.* 2004).

4) Clonidine (epidural or IT, but only poorly PO) is efficacious in some patients with both BCP and CCP, but this effect may be no greater than placebo. Its noradrenergic effects (α2 agonist) may modulate pain centrally; however, there is no firm evidence that the analgesia due to activation of spinal adrenoceptors is long lasting. In humans, long-term IT clonidine infusion rarely produces pain relief beyond 3 months (Ackermann *et al.* 2003).

5) Epidural or IT morphine at a dose of 0.5–1 mg/day is initially effective against SCI CP in some patients (particularly with incomplete injuries): at-level, but much less below-level, pain appears to be responsive. The general impression is that opioid efficacy in pure CP is poor, with rare patients drawing long-term benefit (similar to what is observed with oral drugs).

6) The IT calcium channel blocker ziconotide had proved of little value (Bonicalzi and Canavero 2004).

Analgesia with all these drugs is due to targeting of spinal above-level or supraspinal sites. Drug combinations may be more effective. Tolerance to a combination of morphine and clonidine develops more slowly than with morphine alone, but side effects are not reduced even with reduced doses of clonidine (hypotension, sedation). While intermittent bolus and continuous infusion may not differ in efficacy, infusion with a totally implanted pump is preferred to lower the infection rate, even if initially more expensive. The pharmacodynamics of IT-injected drugs differs considerably on type of administration: a bolus dose produces much higher concentrations of CSF baclofen compared to continuous infusion, particularly at cervical and higher levels and a positive response to a bolus may not be duplicated during continuous infusion. Also, spasticity and analgesia may require different receptor subsets (Herman *et al.* 1992). An important caveat is that an excess of free GABA may cause postsynaptic receptor changes, leading over time to desensitization.

We recommend that, if spinal infusion is selected, a combination of IT midazolam/clonidine (on the basis of possible greater efficacy of GABA A modulation deduced by oral studies) or (in failed cases, due to GABA A downregulation) baclofen/clonidine be the first option, particularly in patients with extensive (hemisoma) CP, in whom CS may not ensure complete coverage of painful areas. However, cases are on record where CS controlled the pain beyond expected somatotopic limits.

PREVENTION

There are no known ways to preempt the development of CP, nor are there markers for identifying pain-prone patients. Prophylactic amitriptyline does not appear to exert any meaningful effect (Chapter 5). Neuroprotective agents have yet to deliver the promise they raised in the stroke-trauma setting (Canavero *et al.* 2003).

Zimmermann (1979) questioned whether implantation of an electrical stimulator immediately after a CNS lesion could prevent changes, like supersensitivity, leading to CP. While this is of course totally unfeasible, brain reorganization could be modulated by TMS and this may become a possibility in the future, once we identify CP susceptibility markers. Preemptive manipulations, such as those employed in amputees, e.g., with memantine (Flor 2003), to block SI reorganization and reduce phantom pain, may also be explored for CP.

ALTERNATIVE APPROACHES

No systematic data are available for CP on any one technique.

Peripheral/regional and epidural neurolytic blocks (phenol, alcohol, anesthetics) are basically useless in the long-term management of CP and some may be harmful: results are short-lived or disappointing. However, abolition of oncoming normal afferent stimuli can sometimes secure temporary relief; repeated or prolonged blocks can dampen at least temporarily a patient's suffering, sometimes for longer periods of time than the duration of the block (Tasker *et al.* 1991). Since permanent surgical neural interruption at the site of successful block usually fails to relieve the pain, anesthetics likely act as pain modulators (Condouris 1976).

Psychologic support may be useful in selected patients as a corollary measure. Pain is a highly intrusive event that is extremely effective at capturing attention. Cognitive factors can alter the perceived intensity of pain and, accordingly, can modulate SI activity in functional imaging studies (references in Schnitzler and Ploner 2000).

Cognitive strategies to deal with the situation may be used – sometimes with hypnosis – as coping may change not just the perception of pain, but also autonomic responses during noxious stimulation (Thompson 1981; Weisenberg *et al.* 1996). In this regard, the relative increase of activity in the lateral orbitofrontal cortex during pain may represent a source of cognitive modulation of emotional components that are produced by or interact with pain processing (references in Petrovic and Ingvar 2002). Coping aims at making pain comprehensible, planning activities, taking drugs, communicating and distracting oneself. One possible cognitive coping mechanism involves suppression of activity in ACC, OFC and PAG: cingulate cortex, for one, is known to regulate brainstem opioid network during opioid and placebo analgesia (Petrovic and Ingvar 2002). However, in our extensive experience and that of others (e.g., Warms *et al.* 2002), such strategies never provided substantial relief to CP patients: submitting anyone to psychotherapy is callous and unrewarding, except to help control depression, which may profoundly affect the perception of pain.

CP is life-long and a durable *rapport with doctors* is vital, particularly to rein in moments of despair: thus, a "placebo approach" is warranted in all cases. For instance, excellent interpersonal relationships, demonstration of caring by the therapist and enthusiasm, spending time with the patient, supplying accurate, rational information on the effects/results to be obtained, a predicted positive course, belief in treatment efficacy and charisma (the "surgical look") all affect placebo circuits. Patients with strong dependency needs and desire to please will respond positively, while those with more explicit conversion of negative affect and somatic preoccupation respond negatively (Nicholson *et al.* 2002). All this is reduced by informed consent, decreased physician paternalism/authority, and so on. When both context and expectations are completely eliminated (hidden therapy), pain relief is less than when therapy is in full view of the patient (Pollo *et al.* 2001). Anticipation of pain relief is closely tied to the *placebo* response and intimately tied with actual pain reduction. Since a high level of activity at prefrontal levels marks patients with high expectation of pain relief and high levels of actual pain relief, prediction of response to medication may become possible by looking at the "expectation component" in patients' brain scans. Also, the same sets of neurons activated both by experienced and imagined (empathy) pain (ACC and other areas, but not SI) are also set in motion by the anticipation of pain (Holden 2004 and references therein). However, it should be stressed that in CP patients a placebo response seems less common (unpublished observations) than other neuropathic pain states (Verdugo and Ochoa 1991), suggesting that placebo mechanisms may be disrupted in CP.

Riddoch (1938) already noted that CP could sometimes be diminished by concomitant stimulation (e.g., pinching, induced itching, fractures); also, pushing into the muscle tendons or bellies may relieve cramping pain up to a few hours (McHenry's website: www.painonline.org).

Distraction from pain through attractive and pleasant hobbies is indicated, as these compete for attention. We and others noted that orgasm can temporarily decrease CP, but also vice versa. A distracting task can reduce pain by reducing activity in somatosensory regions and the PAG. Cognitive distraction may attenuate the pain-evoked activity in the ACC, the insula and the thalamus, and in phantom pain this can be activated by simple hypnotic suggestion (see review and references in Petrovic and Ingvar 2002). Pain can be momentarily soothed by making comparisons and enduring the pain; consideration shown by others may also help.

Several *alternative approaches* have been attempted. However, trials of alternative medicine must be considered in the light of their quality (as for any other therapy): pot-pourris of several treatments such as EMG biofeedback, behavioral coping training, cognitive behavioral therapy and the like may be moderately effective for a short time (Edwards *et al.* 2000). On the other hand, several CP patients are poorly compliant with their drug regimens (justifying some apparent failures) and it may happen that, being under the "doctor's eye," the patient feels compelled to take drugs on a regular basis and thus obtain drug-related benefit.

There is uncontrolled evidence that eastern medical treatments can allay CP, particularly combined with western drugs (Yen and Chan 2003; Kong *et al.* 2004). Li (2000) treated 20 cases of "central pain after head injury" (1990–1998) by "invigorating blood circulation." Bi Tong Tang (a decoction of several herbs taken daily in divided doses for 14 days) was used for the pain. Acupuncture was used in some patients for 7 days, and infrared radiation (20 minutes die) for 7 days. Pain disappeared in 18 patients after 2 to 12 weeks of therapy, and in 2 was reduced. Follow-up was not specified. Perhaps, this is the natural history of brain injury-related CP.

No reports exist on biofeedback techniques (surface EMG, temperature/thermal, EEG-based) in the CP setting. A small controlled study found that people can learn to suppress acute pain when shown the activity of the rostral ACC in real time from fMRI represented on a computer screen as, for example, a flame of varying size in just three 13-minute sessions, the effect seeming to last beyond the sessions in the scanner (DeCharms *et al.* 2005). In this case, it would be important to define neurometabolic markers of CP for possible image-guided feedback therapy.

Autogenic and/or progressive muscle relaxation training, physical and massage therapy have only a minimal role to play in the vast majority of patients. However, they may help in treating secondary or associated musculoskeletal and other nociceptive components. Musculoskeletal pain arising from, for example, abnormal posture must be specifically addressed in all cases. On the other hand, physical activity may either increase or decrease CP in individual cases. Pain can be momentarily soothed by changing body position.

Acupuncture has never relieved our patients (as also experienced by Bowsher 1994), a sign that acupuncture only works if the CNS is intact. However, it may moderately help non-CP SCI pains (Warms *et al.* 2002).

Phantom pain has been reportedly reduced with mirror training: actually, only the clenching spasm and cramping pain, not the burning or lancinating pains, were reduced. Analogous treatment for CP has not been reported.

As regards CCP, it must be added that any factors that work to the detriment of general health will often worsen or contribute to the severity of pain, and any form of stimulation below injury level may worsen the pain (UTI, bladder stones, decubitus ulceration, paronychia, stress, psychological factors, etc.).

A FUTURE?

Neuroablative techniques as a whole have failed to relieve more than a few patients, often with intolerable side effects; sometimes, they have triggered new pains (Chapters 1 and 7).

Today, properly used oral drugs can allay the suffering of many patients and totally relieve a few. Neuromodulation as discussed may achieve similar results in the sizable proportion of patients who drew no relief whatsoever, or help boost relief in others. The "bottom line" is that only a minority of patients will not be helped by current strategies (Table 6.8). On the other hand, patients with good initial relief may later find that they can no longer tolerate even modest degrees of pain.

The literature is clear in this regard. For instance, in a SCI CP series (Falci *et al.* 2002), all patients were refractory to tricyclics, antiepileptics, baclofen, klonopin and

---

TABLE 6.8. Treatment of central pain: the TANG guidelines

A. ORAL DRUGS*

Step 1: mexiletine (up to 1000 mg) + gabapentin (up to 3600 mg); *timeline: 1 month*

Step 2: lamotrigine (up to 600–800 mg); *timeline: 3 months*

Step 3: amitriptyline (up to 150 mg) (*only brain central pain*); *timeline: maximum 3 months*

B. NEUROMODULATION

BRAIN CP

Step 1: (only if propofol AND/OR TMS responsive)

Extradural cortical stimulation (1-2 paddles)

OR (if hemisoma or diffuse pain)

IT midazolam/clonidine or IT baclofen/clonidine

Step 2: Bifocal DBS (Vc and PVG)

Step 3: Convulsive therapy

CORD CP

A. Some preservation of lemniscal conduction

Step 1: SCS

Step 2: IT midazolam/clonidine or IT baclofen/clonidine

Step 3: Extradural cortical stimulation (only if propofol and/or TMS responsive)

OR Bifocal DBS (Vc and PVG)

Step 4: Convulsive therapy

B. No preservation of lemniscal conduction

Step 1: IT midazolam/clonidine or IT baclofen/clonidine

Step 2: Extradural cortical stimulation or Bifocal DBS (Vc and PVG)

Step 3: Convulsive therapy

---

* If elected, TENS should be attempted at this time combined with drugs.

opioids (at most "taking the edge off the pain"), and in some to IT opioids, baclofen, clonidine, local anesthetic or SCS.

The promise of peptides (e.g., neurotensin; cholecistokinin modulation during opioid administration; growth factors antagonists) coming from animal studies has yet to materialize.

What options are available? It will be our contention that CP can be abolished, immediately and permanently, by a small focal lesion in the internal capsule (Chapters 7 and 8). We will try to prove that this is the only ablative technique with a place in the therapeutic armamentarium of CP – particularly at a time when neural reconstruction with stem cells or other engineered cell lines or implantation of cells secreting analgesic substances subarachnoidally in the nervous system is slowly becoming a reality (e.g., Kondziolka et al. 2002; Wirth et al. 2002; Szentirmai and Carter 2004; Fouad and Pearson 2004; Bang et al. 2005).

However, for those unwilling to undergo demolitive surgery of any kind, the benefit of combining different strategies (despite higher costs) may represent an interesting avenue. Recently, SCS analgesia has been found to be boosted by concurrent pump infusion of baclofen or adenosine in PNP patients over a few years (Lind et al. 2004). In CP, combining CS with IT drugs as discussed above could prove effective, and so could the combination of CS with DBS (although at a high cost). Given the pivotal role of GABA, the infusion of a GABA A agonist such as muscimol (a drug with a 15–20 minute posteffect seen in tremor patients; Levy et al. 2001) directly in the thalamus or cortex may become an option, and so may the transplantation of GABA (stem) cells. Mark and Tsutsumi (1974) have already reported on intrathalamic infusion of lidocaine in the treatment of chronic pain.

7 PATHOPHYSIOLOGY: HUMAN DATA

"To wrest from nature the secrets which have perplexed philosophers in all ages, to track to their sources the causes of disease, to correlate the vast stores of knowledge, that they may be quickly available for the . . . cure of disease – these are our ambitions." **(William Osler)**

"A theory that accounts for all the facts is bound to be wrong, because some of the facts are bound to be wrong." **(Francis Crick)**

A theory of CP must be able to explain:

1) its idiosyncratic character, i.e., why it arises only in some individuals and not in others with apparently identical lesions;
2) its immediate or delayed (even for years) onset;
3) why both a small lesion of the dorsal horn of the spinal cord or a huge infarct of the parietal cortex can equally trigger CP;
4) its continuous, spontaneous nature in the vast majority of patients, but also its evoked components (allodynia, hyperalgesia) – which, in some instances, can be the only or opening symptom, plus radiation and prolonged aftersensations;
5) its many different qualities, even simultaneously (including dysesthesias and pruritus);
6) referral to superficial and/or deep structures;
7) pain intensity fluctuations, from day to day or month to month, for no obvious reason and increases by both somatic stimuli and emotion;
8) constant somatotopical referral of pain to areas of sensory loss;
9) differential response of patients with apparently identical lesions, i.e., of the same size, site and nature, to some treatments but not others.

In the end, the winning theory is the one that leads to a cure. In this sense, all past and present theories fail.

We will make no reference to animal studies. In spite of veterinary evidence of "classical thalamic pain" following Vc lesions (e.g., Holland *et al.* 2000), a critical review clearly shows that current animal models of CP are wholly unsatisfactory – to say the least (see reviews by Willis 2002 and Pioli *et al.* 2003): not unexpectedly, no therapeutic breakthrough ever came from such studies.

Neuroanatomy and neurochemistry differ in humans and experimental animals. For instance, substance P has been considered a key substance in pain transmission on the basis of animal data, but the majority of clinical trials with human NK1 receptor antagonists for a variety of acute and chronic pain states (including migraine) gave negative results. Heat hyperalgesia, so commonly seen in animal models, is only present in a small proportion of patients suffering from CP. Even monkeys differ from humans, for instance in cognitive processing of pain. Autotomy, a "classic" sign of pain in animals, has been reported in several human patients without pain (e.g., McGowan *et al.* 1997; Tasker 2001). In the words of Gazzaniga (1998):

> Humans often turn to the study of animals to understand themselves . . . monkeys . . . It has been a common belief . . . that the brains of our closest relatives have an organization and function largely similar, if not identical, to our own. Split-brain research has shown that this assumption can be spurious. Although some structures and functions are remarkably alike, differences abound. The anterior commissure provides one dramatic example . . . When this commissure is left intact in otherwise split-brain monkeys, the animals retain the ability to transfer visual information from one hemisphere to the other. People, however, do not transfer visual information in any way. Hence, the same structure carries out different functions in different species – an illustration of the limits of extrapolating from one species to another. Even extrapolating between people can be dangerous.

Actually, animal data in the whole field of biomedicine show profound flaws (see review by Pound *et al.* 2004; Linazasoro 2004). Even capsaicin-evoked pain in human volunteers is not a model of neuropathic pain, as the latter is often delayed and generally permanent, whereas capsaicin-induced hyperalgesia develops within minutes and is transient.

Finally, CP differs from peripheral neuropathic pain (PNP) and, although they share clinical similarities, no attempt will be made to correlate the two.

The vast majority of theories proposed to explain CP until now are based on incomplete "current" anatomical knowledge, selective adaptation of anatomical data (often of animal provenance) to authors' needs, scarce appreciation of the full clinical spectrum of CP and its features, exclusion of contradictory findings or scarce familiarity with the full gamut of neurosurgical data (e.g., Melzack 1991; Cesaro *et al.* 1991; Jeanmonod *et al.* 1996; Craig 1998). Some are technology- more than idea-driven. Dismissal of exceptions – not just single cases, but whole groups of patients – is the norm in the field. It should not come as a surprise that different authors, based on similar evidence, reached opposite conclusions. As physicist Stephen Hawking (1988) put it, "you can disprove a theory by finding even a single observation that disagrees with the predictions of the theory . . . if ever a new observation is found to disagree, we have to abandon or modify the theory. At least that is what is supposed to happen." Finally, a few authors embarked on phreno-logical approaches that try to paste the CP sensation to a unique brain center, with scarce success.

Our thesis is straightforward: CP is the end result of a decorrelation of sensory information processing along the sensory thalamocortical loop. The only permanent cure, bar complete neural restoration, is a stereotactically guided lesion of the descending arm of this loop. This theory refutes "neuromatrix" approaches, which, in light of the wide network of interconnecting areas at the basis of acute pain, find surgical lesions useless (Melzack 1991). It also refutes the suggestion that the spontaneous, resting component of CP is the end result of different pathophysiologic mechanisms (see Garcin 1937): differential engagement of this single mechanism explains, for instance, different descriptions of the pain. This chapter reviews the evidence for such a theory.

Important sources of information regarding the genesis of CP are:

1) functional imaging studies;
2) neurophysiologic studies;
3) results of neuroablation for CP;
4) reports of sudden disappearance of CP;
5) pharmacological dissection data (see Chapters 5 and 6).

These will be reviewed in detail.

Throughout the text, no reference to psychological theories of CP will be made, not because of a dearth of such theories, but for the simple reason that CP is somatic pain that cannot in any way be understood in terms of a psychological (e.g., cognitive or psychodynamic) framework of any kind, but in reductionist terms. In addition, several studies indicate that CPSP is not part of a psychiatric disorder. A Danish group (Andersen et al. 1995) found no statistical evidence of an association between depression, social factors or major life events and CPSP. Mukherjii and colleagues (1999) found depression-dysthymia in 41% of CPSP versus 40% of non-CP stroke patients. Likewise, Stenager and associates (1991) found no differences between MS patients with and without pain with respect to depression (see also Osterberg et al. 1994). Thus, the presence of depression/dysthymia does not correlate with CP. Even suicidal ideation, which is frequent (up to a quarter of patients at some point of their history), is proportional to severity of pain and hostility, and not depression. On the other hand, like all pains (and medical conditions), the experience of CP may be influenced by so-called psychological factors.

FUNCTIONAL IMAGING STUDIES

With the advent of human neuroimaging over the last 20 years, there has been a trend to use this technique with its pretty pictures of colored blobs on brain slices almost as a modern-day phrenology. It is crucial that we remember that these pretty pictures can easily mislead us and that their interpretation needs to take into account the wealth of scientific evidence obtained with different methods from humans. There are many, sometimes quite small, populations of neurons with different responses to different types of stimulus or event in brain regions which may not all be revealed by functional neuroimaging, which rather reflects the average metabolic demands of a brain region. Further, brain imaging does not address the issue of the information that is represented by virtue of the different tuning of individual neurons (which are the computing elements of the brain), and so does not provide the evidence on which computational models of brain function must be based. It is thus very important to consider the results of human functional neuroimaging in the light of what is known from complementary studies using, for example, neurophysiology and the effects of brain damage (Kringelbach and Rolls 2004).

Not all neurometabolic studies provide the same degree of information. Some refer to the spontaneous component of CP; others assess the brain response to allodynic conditions. A few address receptor anomalies. It is important to keep these separate. For instance, the spontaneous, resting component of CP can only be assessed with single-photon emission computed tomography (SPECT) or positron emission tomography (PET) – but not functional magnetic resonance imaging (fMRI) as commonly used. Drugs with clear-cut pharmacodynamic profiles can dissect neurochemical mechanisms by modulating the resting state and provide crucial pathophysiologic information.

1. Studies assessing the spontaneous resting component and its modulation

1. Laterre and colleagues (1988) studied with fluorodeoxyglucose (FDG)-PET in the resting state (twice, with a 2 month interval) a woman who developed CPSP due to a small right infarct at the level of the posterior putamen and posterior limb of the internal capsule, with no visible extension into the thalamus on MRI. There was right hypoperfusion (17% asymmetry), particularly at the level of the posterior thalamic complex as well as in the putamen. No metabolic alterations were found in the cerebral cortex.

2. Lee and colleagues (1989) studied six CPSP patients with technetium-99m hexamethylpropyleneamineoxime (HMPAO) brain SPECT: 4 infarctions in the thalamus and internal capsule and 2 hemorrhages in internal capsule-putamen (4 left, 2 right). Three patients showed thalamic lesions and these had decreased rCBF in ipsilateral parietal (one bilaterally) and temporal cortex and one in frontal areas. Extrathalamic lesions showed no cortical anomaly.

3. Tsubokawa and colleagues (1991) studied at 4–10 days after implantation of a motor cortex stimulator 7 patients with CP with ^{131}I-amphetamine SPECT. The rCBF showed a marked increase (+150–200%) in the stimulated cortex and the ipsilateral thalamic and brainstem area, along with pain abatement. The skin temperature as assessed with thermography in the painful area increased to almost the same level as that in the contralateral non-painful area.

4. Hirato and colleagues (1993) submitted to PET studies with [18]FDG and a steady-state method with $C^{15}O_2$–$^{15}O_2$ nine CP patients. MRI and CT revealed definite thalamic (3), putaminal (3), thalamoputaminal (1) and cortical parietal (2) damage. Superficial pain was more marked in cases with definite thalamic damage. In patients with a thalamic lesion, there were many irregular burst discharges in the Vop-Vim area at stereotactic microrecording. The relative value of regional cerebral glucose metabolism (rCMRGlu) decreased in the lesioned thalamus, but increased in the cerebral cortex around the central sulcus on the lesioned side. However, the relative value of regional cerebral oxygen metabolism (rCMRO$_2$) did not increase (dissociated glucose/oxygen metabolism of the same area). In patients studied with both techniques, OGMUR (oxygen–glucose molar utilization ratios) in the premotor area and SI/MI decreased more in cases with a thalamic lesion than in those with a putaminal lesion. In a patient with a combined putaminothalamic lesion, neural activity was reduced in the Vim-Vc area, with peripheral receptive fields to electrical thalamic stimulation being predominantly in the face, hand and sometimes in the foot area. In this case, the regional oxygen extraction rate (rOEF) was markedly increased in the cerebral cortex around the central sulcus on the side of the lesion, despite the chronic stage of cerebrovascular disease. In two patients with cortical lesions, who showed mild superficial pain with or without deep pain, rCMRGlu was decreased in the lesioned cerebral cortex. Though no ischemic lesion could be demonstrated by CT, rCMRGlu was reduced in the lesioned Vc. In patients with a subcortical lesion, rCMRGlu commonly decreased in this area. Therefore, rCMRGlu in this area was decreased in all cases with CP including cortical cases. This study then showed that OGMUR in the cerebral cortex around the central sulcus was markedly decreased on the damaged side in cases with thalamic lesions. However, in patients with a putaminal lesion, it was only moderately decreased, particularly rostrally. In patients with subcortical lesions, the more severe the superficial pain, the higher was the relative value of glucose metabolism compared to that of oxygen (which was a reciprocal value of OGMUR) in the cerebral cortex around the central sulcus on the involved side. In the patient with combined lesions, rOEF was increased in the same area. Sensory thalamic hypo-activity (decreased rCMRGlu) was seen in all cases. In sum, in the thalamic lesion group with pain (superficial pain dominant), r-O_2 consumption was maintained in most brain structures, except in the lesioned thalamus, while in the cortical central sulcus this was normal, but the rO_2 extraction ratio was increased and so was the relative value of r-glucose utilization compared to r-O_2 consumption. In the patients with thalamic lesions and pain (deep pain dominant), both r-O_2 consumption and O_2 extraction ratio were reduced in all brain structures and so was glucose metabolism. They concluded that increased activity in SI/MI combined with a decreased activity in Vc appeared to be a marker of CP, with character of pain (superficial versus deep) depending on different processing at thalamocortical levels (see also Svensson *et al.* 1997, who show that acute skin pain increases thalamic CBF and decreases MI/SI CBF). The same group (Hirato *et al.* 1995) reported that in one putaminal hemorrhage case (included in the above analysis) PET renormalized after successful radiosurgical Vim thalamotomy.

5. De Salles and Bittar (1994) studied with FDG-PET a thalamic pain patient. CP appeared two weeks following a stereotactic biopsy for a midbrain lesion and worsened over one month. The patient complained of an annoying sensation of needles and at times a burning sensation on the right hemiface and hand with hyperesthesia to pinprick and light touch on the right face and hypoesthesia to pinprick on the right fingertips. MRI disclosed that the needle had passed precisely in Vc, plus the mesencephalon (where the medial lemnicus, which courses just caudal to Vc, could have been damaged). Two months after the biopsy, PET showed marked hypo/ametabolism of the left thalamic region, right cerebellar diaschisis

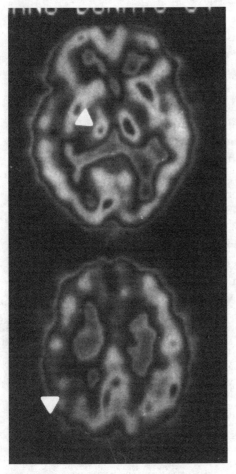

Figure 7.1: High-resolution SPECT (double-head camera) images of postcordotomy CP. Note both thalamic (upper scan, arrowhead) and parietal hypoperfusion (lower scan, arrowhead).

and left parietal cortex hypometabolism. Ten months later, allodynia with cold intolerance persisted in the right hand and face. At this time PET showed enduring thalamic hypometabolism, recovery of the parietal cortex anomaly (which, however, might be interpreted as a sign of hyperactivity) and of the cerebellar cortex.

6. We (Canavero *et al.* 1995; Pagni and Canavero 1995; Canavero and Bonicalzi 1995; Canavero *et al.* 1999) showed that patients with CPSP, CCP (intramedullary cyst, syringomyelia) and other CPs show basal parietal (SI) and/or frontal MI/ PM/PFC (in a few cases also temporal), plus thalamic hypoperfusion on HMPAO and ECD SPECT. These flow changes are promptly renormalized following successful treatment (propofol, evacuation, cortical stimulation) (Figure 7.1).

7. The Lyon group (Peyron *et al.* 1995) reported on 2 CP (both spontaneous and evoked) patients, one with a right mesencephalic infarct with left leg pain (spontaneous and evoked) and the other with a left parietal infarct sparing the thalamus, with right hemisoma pain, bar the face. In case 1, PET at rest showed no cortical abnormality, but right thalamic hypoperfusion (-9%). During MCS, CBF was increased in brainstem, orbitofrontal cortex (OFC), right thalamus and cingulate cortex (CC): 30 minutes after discontinuation, persisting CBF changes were seen in OFC and CC. In case 2, PET at rest showed widespread CBF decrease in left parietal cortex (-35%) and hypoactivity in left thalamus (-10%), this latter being normal on MRI. During MCS, CBF was increased in brainstem, OFC, left thalamus and CC, while the parietal cortex asymmetry was unmodified. Analgesic effects in both patients lasted at least 30 minutes after stopping MCS and this went along sustained CBF changes, particularly in the thalamus. CBF increases were of the order of 7–9%. An important sustained CBF increase was seen in patient 2's brainstem, while in patient 1 it was delayed, of lesser intensity and shorter duration (patient 2, but not patient 1, also showed modulation of nociceptive flexion reflexes RIII). No change was seen in SI. Thalamic CBF changes were almost superimposable in both patients, but pain relief was satisfactory only in one patient, in whom there was also brainstem activation. CBF changes in OFC and anterior CC (ACC) were stronger and more sustained in the patient with less pain relieving effect of MCS than the other.

8. Ness and colleagues (1998) studied a patient with paraplegia who, for many years, experienced rapidly fluctuating, severe, highly aversive (VAS 10), unilateral pain below the level of the lesion. The searing attacks lasted up to 10 seconds. SPECT was done in pain and non-pain conditions (threshold of significance: 10%). When experiencing pain, there was increased CBF to ACC (cingulate), increased thalamic CBF bilaterally and increased SI contralaterally, plus decreased CBF in caudates bilaterally. The patient responded to gabapentin, which reduced the anomalies (and also induced mirror pain).

9. Doi and colleagues (1999) showed renormalization of thalamic SPECT hypoperfusion after successful convulsive therapy in 5 suprathalamic CP patients.

10. Fukui and colleagues (2002) reported thalamic hypoperfusion with HMPAO SPECT in CPSP: ECT relieved the pain and renormalized thalamic hypoperfusion.

11. Cahana and colleagues (2004) studied a patient with encephalitis and CP, who showed left thalamic (Vc region) hypoperfusion. The patient complained of "hot" left-sided paresthesias and burning pain, particularly in the chin and left palm, plus evoked pains. SSEPs were normal. Lidocaine infusions relieved the pain and the anomaly.

2. Studies assessing the evoked components

1. Cesaro and colleagues (1991) studied 4 CPSP patients with ^{123}I-N-isopropyliodoamphetamine brain SPECT, with and without allodynic stimulation. In the two patients with hyperpathia (with the lesions involving the parietal subcortical white matter and the thalamocapsular area), there was hyperactivity (+20–26%) in the central thalamic region opposite the painful side. Amitriptyline relieved both the SPECT anomaly and the pain, and thermoalgesic deficits renormalized. The two patients without SPECT anomalies had subcortical or subcortical plus thalamic lesions.

2. We (Canavero *et al.* 1993, 1995) showed in CP patients that basal SPECT hypoperfusion of SI increases under allodynic conditions and that this anomaly spreads anteriorly to MI and other frontal areas.

3. The Lyon group (Peyron *et al.* 1998) studied 9 patients with acute unilateral CPSP after a lateral medullary infarct (Wallenberg's syndrome) with PET (resolution: 7 mm). They did *not* study spontaneous pain (present in 4 at a VAS value of 3–5), nor discussed baseline anomalies; brainstem and cerebellum were not studied. All patients showed cold allodynia (assessed with frozen water in a moving flat plastic container). During cold allodynia, statistically significant increases of rCBF were seen contralaterally to stimuli in the lateral half of the thalamus, SI, anterior insula and inferior frontal gyrus. R-CBF was increased *bilaterally* in SII and inferior (opercular) parietal areas (BA39–40) and significantly decreased contralaterally in BA10, ipsilaterally in BA24–32 and sub-significantly in ipsilateral BA23–31. *No rCBF change was observed in BA24 (ACC)*. A significant decrease was also seen bilaterally in BA18–19. During electrically (high-frequency) elicited pain to the normal side, rCBF increased significantly bilaterally in BA39–40 and SII, contralaterally in BA6 (anterior insula), ipsilaterally in BA44–45–47. rCBF decreased ipsilaterally to stimulation in BA10. Again, *no rCBF change was seen in BA24*. rCBF was significantly decreased bilaterally in BA18–19. Cold stimuli to the normal side induced significant increases in contralateral SII and BA39–40, without extending into SI, and ipsilaterally in BA46. No significant modification was detected in the thalamus and ipsilateral parietal cortex. rCBF was significantly decreased bilaterally in BA18–19 and ipsilaterally to stimulation in the caudate head. There was a sub-significant decrease in contralateral BA24–32 and ipsilateral BA10.

The same group (Peyron *et al.* 1999) studied with PET 8 patients with CP (1 CCP, 3 brainstem CP, 1 thalamic CP, 3 corticosubcortical CP). They compared rest, cold moving allodynia and thermal heat pain. They also studied 4 additional patients with fMRI. Cold allodynia was associated with rCBF increases in contralateral insula-SII and SI and bilaterally in posterior parietal cortex and ACC (plus ipsilateral cerebellum). Thermal pain induced increased CBF bilaterally in insulae-SII, posterior parietal, ACC and right prefrontal cortex (plus bilateral cerebellum), but *not SI*. MR analysis showed *individual variations* in the allodynic response, except for the contralateral insular-SII activity. Compared to thermal pain, allodynic pain induced a greater activity in contralateral SI (ascribed to moving stimulus). Allodynic pain compared to control stimulation of non-painful side showed higher activity in contralateral SI and ACC.

They (Peyron *et al.* 2000) also reported on a CPSP patient, who complained of spontaneous paroxysmal pain, mechanical and thermal allodynia and pinprick hyperpathia. She had severe thermal hypesthesia of the left hand and foot. SSEPs were diminished, but not absent. This case developed CP and allodynia in her left side after a bifocal embolic infarct following vascular surgery involving both the right parietal cortex (SI and SII) and the right rostral ACC (BA 24 and 32), plus a small anterior and inferior part of the inferior parietal lobule (BA40), plus BA6, 8, 9 and 10. Judging from the images, SI could have still been partially active, with reorganization posteriorly. SII was considered anterior to BA40 in the upper bank of the sylvian fissure. This patient was studied with both PET and fMRI, under basal conditions (PET only), control and allodynic stimulation. No rCBF increase was found in any part of the residual cingulate cortices, neither in the basal state (which included spontaneous pain and extensive hypoperfusion around the infarct), nor during left cold allodynic pain (see their previous study). No abnormality was observed in the left cingulate cortex. PET at rest (VAS 1) showed a wide hypoperfusion including the infarct and widely extended within the frontal and parietal cortices. Left parietal cortex, in the depth of SI, showed a significant increase of rCBF in the control condition, which remained below the statistical threshold for the allodynic condition. In the allodynic condition only, the rCBF was significantly increased in the right anterior insula-SII, immediately forward to (at the boundaries of the insular-SII infarct) the right parietal lesion; there were also prominent responses in the hemisphere *ipsilateral* to allodynic (but not control) stimulation: insula-SII and lateral thalamus and (sub-significantly) SI. Sub-significant rCBF increases were observed in the head of the right caudate during the control condition and in the right lateral thalamus during allodynia. *No rCBF increases, even at a sub-significant threshold, were observed in ACC on both sides.* No intracerebral significant rCBF decrease was observed. Results remained unchanged even on non-normalized PET images.

Finally, these authors (Peyron *et al.* 2004) studied the brain responses of 27 patients with peripheral (5), spinal (3), brainstem (4), thalamic (5), lenticular (5), or cortical (5) lesions with fMRI, as innocuous mechanical stimuli were addressed to either the allodynic territory or the homologous contralateral region. When applied to the normal side, brush and cold rubbing stimuli activated the contralateral primary (SI) and secondary (SII) somatosensory cortices and insular regions. The same stimuli became severely painful when applied to the allodynic side and activated contralateral SI/SII and insular cortices with, however, lesser activation of the SII and insula. Increased activation volumes were found in contralateral SI and primary motor cortex (MI). Whereas ipsilateral responses appeared very small and restricted after control stimuli, they represented the most salient effect of allodynia and were observed mainly in the ipsilateral parietal operculum (SII), SI, and insula. Allodynic stimuli also recruited additional responses in motor/premotor areas (MI, supplementary motor area), in regions involved in spatial attention (posterior parietal cortices), and in regions linking attention and motor control (mid-ACC).

4. Lorenz and colleagues (1998) studied a single patient who suffered Wallenberg's syndrome with selectively abolished pain and temperature sensitivity in the right leg. One year later, CP had developed in the leg, with touch and cold allodynia. P40m dipoles calculated from magnetoencephalographic (MEG) fields after electrical stimulation of both tibial nerves were localized in SI; however, stimulation of the affected side caused deep pain sensations and elicited a large N80m component best explained by an additionally co-active dipole in the cingulate cortex. Cingulate activation was in the medial part *slightly more posterior than BA24.* Electrophysiologically, the affected limb was characterized by larger components P40 and N80 of the tibial nerve SEP compared with the unaffected left limb. In particular, the enhanced N80 amplitude augmented in parallel with the enhancement of CPSP severity in the patient.

The same group (Kohlhoff *et al.* 1999) studied with MEG 4 patients with Wallenberg's syndrome and CP. They found that the component around 80 ms after tibialis stimulation showed side asymmetries in the patients which exceeded the normal interindividual variability and were also reflected in the equivalent current dipole parameters. The degree of asymmetry seemed to be related to the *severity of allodynia.* They concluded for CP possibly reflecting functional disorganization in SI.

5. Jensen and colleagues (1999) studied 10 CPSP women with $H_2^{15}O$ PET under resting conditions and following stimulation of the painful body part and the corresponding non-painful body part with phasic heat stimuli. They observed hypoperfusion of the affected thalamic region versus non-affected thalamus under resting conditions.

6. Olausson and colleagues (2001) studied a hemispherectomized patient with touch-evoked pricking and burning pain, plus a robust allodynia to brush stroking (enhanced at a cold ambient temperature) in her paretic hand. Psychophysical examination showed that, on her paretic side, she confused cool and warm temperatures. On fMRI, brush-evoked allodynia activated posterior ACC, SII and prefrontal cortex.

7. Morrow and Casey (2002) studied a CPSP man with $H_2^{15}O$ PET. He had sudden onset of constant persistent painful dysesthesias of left hemisoma. Sensory examination was normal, bar deep pressure allodynia on the left and elevated but symmetrical cutaneous heat pain thresholds. MR disclosed a lacunar infarction ($2 \times 4 \times 7.5$ mm) in Vc. At rest, rCBF was markedly reduced in the right Vc (as compared to left Vc) and insula. Heat stimulation (49–55°) of either side showed exaggerated rCBF increases relative to rest on the right (Vc and insula). They then studied another 4 CP (CPSP, CCP) male patients (age: 40–68), all with clinically detectable impairment of heat and/or mechanical pain sensibility on the side of CP. Each patient had abnormal, contralateral to pain, thalamic (3, hemithalamic hypoactivity; 1, hemithalamic hyperactivity) and/or cortical asymmetry at rest and increased thalamic and/or cortical responsiveness to contralateral stimulation following contact heat stimuli.

8. Bowsher and colleagues (2004) studied four patients with small cortical infarcts: one with a parietal operculum (SII) lesion, another with SII lesions encroaching on the posterior insula, a third with damage to both banks of the sylvian fissure plus the dorsal insula and the last with damage to the upper bank of sylvian fissure. In all, SI was intact. Patients 1 and 2, but not 3 and 4, had (mild) spontaneous pain and also pinprick and thermal anesthesia. In affected areas, mechanical pain was not felt in all. FMR following thermal stimulation in patients 1 and 2 showed SII involved in reception of innocuous and noxious thermal, mechanical and pinprick pains, and SI in non-painful mechanical stimuli, although SI was activated in one patient by innocuous cooling.

9. Seghier and colleagues (2005) studied a CPSP patient who suffered deep and superficial burning cold-like constant and paroxysmal pain in the left hemisoma, worse in the pectoral region, hand and foot. The pain was triggered by cold objects and cool temperatures. He displayed a prominent mechanical allodynia. There were severe left hypesthesia for heat, warm and cold temperatures, selective cold allodynia and pinprick hyperpathia. On MRI, there was an infarct of Vc and adjacent internal capsule (IC) along the STT. Under FMR conditions, the hand was stimulated with a plastic object filled with water at 22°, 15° and 5° (only 5° painful). Touch activated bilateral SI, right SII and supplementary motor area (SMA). Increasing temperature activated the right middle insula and right mesial SI. Hyperpathia activated BA24/32, BA5/7 and the left anterior putamen. The activation in the putamen and BA5/7 was *ipsilateral* to the stimulated hand. ACC activation was not correlated with the simple cold quality of the pain-eliciting stimulus, as innocuous cold correlated with activity in, for example, right insula and right SI.

10. Villemure and colleagues (2006) reported on a patient with typical iatrogenic cervical myelopathic CCP. The odor of cat litter, newspaper or popcorn triggered electric shock/shooting paroxysms and also slowly increased spontaneous pain after repeated challenge. Upon moving away from odors, pain abated. FMR under odor challenge showed larger activations after the termination of the unpleasant odors than after the termination of pleasant ones in the contralateral thalamus, amygdala, insular cortex (bilaterally) and ACC, with similar trends in contralateral SI. Odors triggered pain only on days they were judged unpleasant.

11. Ducreux and colleagues (2006) submitted 6 patients with syringomyelia and suffering CP to fMRI. Cold allodynia (felt like a deep, freezing sensation, sometimes burning, with a tingling sensation) under static conditions activated the mid-posterior insula, ACC, SII, inferior parietal areas, frontal areas (BA8, 9, 45, 46), mostly ipsilaterally and contralateral SMA. In 2–3 patients, activation in the lenticular nucleus, hippocampus and cerebellar lobes was also observed. Brush allodynia (felt like burning in 4 and electric shocks in 2) activated ipsi- and contralateral SI-SII, inferior and superior parietal cortex, ipsi- and contralateral middle frontal gyri (including BA 45-46), contralateral thalamus, caudate and SMA. No activation was observed in BA24-32.

3. Studies assessing biochemical changes

1. Pattany and colleagues (2002) compared 7 SCI (plus 1 tumor) (1 C8, 6 T9–L3) pain patients with 9 SCI (plus 1 ischemia) (4 C4–8, 5 T7–L3) non-pain patients and 10 controls in a magnetic resonance spectroscopy (MRS) study. A total of 74% of pain patients had complete injuries (versus 67% without pain). Pain was described as sharp, burning, aching or electric. Pain was generally above VAS 5 (86%). Statistical analysis showed no significant differences in metabolite concentrations between the two thalami. However, N-acetyl aspartate (NAA, a neuronal marker) correlated negatively with average pain intensity and myo-inositol (a glial marker) correlated positively. NAA also showed a significant difference between SCI patients with pain and those without. Other trends toward significance remain of moot significance. Limits of the study are inhomogeneity of ages between patient groups, exclusion of females, scanning without drug wash-out and no differentiation between diffuse versus end-zone pains.

2. Fukui and colleagues (2002) submitted to ECT a thalamic CPSP patient. ^{1}H-MRS ($2 \times 2 \times 2$ cm voxel in the thalamus bilaterally) was performed before and after a single course of ECT. The NAA/Cr ratio was calculated. Before ECT, the L/R thalamic ratio was 62.3%: after ECT (and during analgesia), the NAA/Cr ratio of the left thalamus increased by 32%.

3. Willoch and colleagues (2004) reported on 5 right-handed CP patients (aged 54 to 77). In 3 cases, CP arose following an ischemic stroke also involving the thalamus, in 2 after a hemorrhagic stroke (pons; parietal angioma). Both spontaneous and evoked components were present in all and involved the hemibody, bar the face in one. CP never started immediately after the insult. They assessed diprenorphine (DPN) binding with PET. Arterial sampling necessary for quantitative modeling could not be performed in 3 patients. Results were compared with 12 healthy controls with a mean age of 39 years. Given low opioid receptor (OR) binding, *SI* was *excluded* from the analysis. This disclosed a hemispheric asymmetry with significant relative reductions in OR binding in prefrontal BA44, parietal BA40, SII and insula (BA14) and Vc contralateral to symptoms. The insular cluster was adjacent to SII and probabilistically extended into SII. While Vc showed maximal peak difference, there was reduced binding also in anteromedial thalamic nuclei. A bilateral relative reduction in OR binding was shown along the midline in the ACC (BA24 and 32), PCC (BA7 and 31) and the PVG. The ACC revealed maximal reduction posteriorly, but stretched to BA24 and 32. Non-significant reduced OR binding was observed in BA6/8 and BA21/22/38. There were only reductions compared to controls and no increases. Actually, infarcts in the thalamus and parietal cortex could have been at the basis of the observed reductions. All 3 patients with thalamic lesions demonstrated binding levels below the control group, but the two patients with cortical or pontine lesions revealed reductions in the lowest range of the patient group. The global mean value of DPN binding for 2 patients was within normal range as compared to the control group.

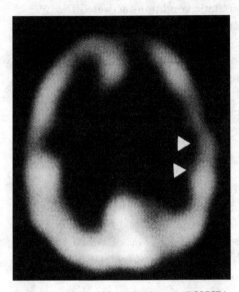

Figure 7.2: Iodine-123-labeled iomazenil SPECT in one BCP case. *Data processing*: one week after suspension of all drugs, and following thyroid block with oral potassium perchlorate, SPECT scanning started 70 minutes after intravenous injection of iodine-123-labeled iomazenil (MallinCkrodt), 111 MBq, with a rotating two-head SPECT device (Varicam, General Electric equipped with high-resolution, low-energy collimators). SPECT images (120 128 × 128 pixel matrices, 5 pixel thick slices, zoom 1, 30 angular 30-second-long steps; 160 keV 20% window recording at least 3500 kCnts) were reconstructed from projection data by a filtered backprojection technique with a Hanning filter (cutoff frequency 19 f/Nyquist, power factor 40). Cortical regions of interest were automatically marked by the dedicated GE reconstruction software on operator-chosen transaxial slices. Semiquantitative right-to-left ratios were immediately calculated by the package software with a ±10% significance limit. Arrowheads show the anomalous frontoparietal area.

4. Jones and colleagues (2004) performed a similar study in a group of CP patients (predominantly CPSP) compared to age-matched pain-free controls. They observed reductions in opioid receptor binding mainly in the dorsolateral (BA 10) and anterior cingulate (BA 24, with some extension into BA 23), plus insula and thalamus. There were also reductions in the lateral pain system within the inferior parietal cortex (BA 40). These changes in binding were outside CT/MRI areas of damage.

5. By means of iodine-123-labeled iomazenil SPECT, we assessed the regional distribution of benzodiazepine-GABA A receptors in the cortex in five patients with CP (three women and two men; aged 41–65; time from onset: at least three years; three patients with a neuroradiologically confirmed thalamic and/or capsular previous stroke, ischemic or hemorrhagic and two with pure spinal cord damage due to previous myelitis and no end-zone pain). Four patients showed reduced uptake at parietal and, in two cases, frontal cortical levels on the side opposite the painful syndrome (R/L 117, 116, 113, 114). In the fifth patient (a thalamocapsular hemorrhage), the ratio approached significance (R/L 0.91). Both brain and cord cases displayed similar binding anomalies, with reductions in CCP contralateral to worse pain, excluding direct brain damage of GABA receptors as a mechanism of such reduction (Figure 7.2).

interpretation: Neurometabolic studies suffer from serious drawbacks (Box 7.1). Thus, only general conclusions are possible regarding the genesis of CP:

1) The thalamus appears to be implicated.
2) Somatosensory areas (SI-SII) appear to be involved.
3) The ACC cannot be a prime actor: rCBF changes in ACC are also reported in PNP and other chronic pains (Hsieh *et al.* 1995), making it an unspecific finding, and a lesion of ACC does not prevent or is involved in the generation of CP. Allodynia does not necessarily activate ACC (as in studies of acute pain in healthy volunteers). Absence of change in ACC (plus SI-SII) has been reported for capsaicin allodynia as well (Baron *et al.* 1999).
4) Bilateral activation of brain areas in CP is possible simultaneously: normal inhibitory mechanisms cannot rein in incoming impulses, with spread of (de)activations (Box 7.2).
5) All CBF changes are functional and rapidly reversible, rejecting "entrenched neuroplasticity" theories (see Chapter 8).
6) Allodynia involves different changes from spontaneous pain: spread to frontal areas may signal engagement of avoidance networks, as unpleasantness degree increases.

Based on such evidence, several older and newer theories of CP collapse, as they ignore the role of cortex or ascribe the pain generator to a dedicated CNS area outside the thalamocortical sensory loop (see below).

Reduced transmitter binding may be due to direct neuronal damage, antero- or retrograde transneuronal degeneration, release of endogenous molecules and subsequent increased occupation of binding sites, internalization and/or receptor downregulation. In this regard, the study of Willoch and colleagues does not provide useful data. Decreased opioid binding (i.e., increased production of endorphins) is seen in many pain conditions. Aside from suboptimal receptor binding specificity of available markers and poor CP responsiveness to opioids, we never observed CP worsening during opioid challenge, and naloxone has been shown to be ineffective in the only controlled trial (see Chapter 5), refuting an opioid hypertonus as surmised by these authors. In this context, Morley and colleagues (1991) found reduced spinal (dorsal horn) enkephalin concentrations at segmental levels corresponding to the pain, at sites where primary sensory afferents terminate, in two cases of chronic pain. Proper control, i.e., non-CP patients with similar lesions, to study patients and homogeneous age (not a group of younger healthy subjects) was lacking. Finally, they erroneously compared their resting findings with imaging studies of CP during allodynic stimulation, two very different situations. A literature survey points to similar brain areas activated by evoked pain in both PNP and CP, making these findings unspecific. A simple corollary endorphin "fall-out" due to the primary lesions can explain their findings (along these lines, we might also expect possible

Box 7.1 Limits of neuroimaging studies

1. Very large discrepancy between actual decreases in spiking activity and rCBF decreases (by a factor 3 to 7): under pathologic conditions neuroimaging methods based on hemodynamic signals may only show small changes, although the underlying decrease in neuronal activity is much larger (Gold and Lauritzen 2002).
2. Complex mechanisms of cortical activation, even in cases of simple sensory stimulation: dissociations may occur between obvious neurological deficits and apparently normal activation patterns, i.e., *activation studies should be interpreted cautiously in patients with focal brain lesions* (Remy *et al.* 1999). Also, noxious stimuli produce arousal, orientation, escape or immobilization and help-seeking, which must be properly dissected.
3. False negatives due to arbitrary group analyses (averaging) that miss important individual rCBF changes due to intersubject variability (e.g., anatomical [cingulate gyry patterns, thalamic/pallidal size and location of tactile representation of various body regions – somatotopy – differ among subjects], attentional [requirement of attentional resources is longer after pain than other sensory stimuli], affective [e.g., anxiety], previous experience) or averaging over task duration. Various combinations of cortical and/or thalamic activations, uni- or bilateral, in individual subjects following the same stimulus and a high degree of variability in cortical activation patterns seem the norm, calling for repetitive single-subject analysis, particularly during heat- and cold-evoked pain. Intensity of a stimulus may be rated similarly among subjects, but overall sensory-cognitive experience of that stimulus may vary. Comparisons of different individuals have shown that fMR responses to the same stimulus within a particular area are variable in location and can also differ in extent over time depending on pain duration and intensity. *Hence the importance of single case studies.*
4. Different neural recruitment depending on methodology of noxious/non-noxious stimulation (contact versus noncontact, escapable versus nonescapable pain), type (cold pain, more unpleasant versus heat pain, less so, having only some regions in common; tonic cold pain and phasic heat pains having different sets of afferents and different sympathetic activation; pinprick engaging the lateral system, heat pain both lateral and medial pain systems), duration (tonic stimuli being more unpleasant than acute ones at any given level of pain intensity), location (skin, subcutis, muscle: frontal areas and SII more activated with skin than muscle pain), periosteum, vascular nociceptors and *side of the body*), quality and, most importantly, intensity (which bears on attention, arousal, orientation and intrusiveness) of stimulus (Bushnell *et al.* 1999). Responses are usually lateralized and most often contralateral to a noxious stimulus, but the side can be unpredictable. Different operational mechanisms recruited in processing a long-lasting pain state with persisting emotional distress versus acute pain with a low affective tone.
5. Low sensitivity of **fMR** to small, but important, differences in cortical activation, to cold pain and to deep structures.
6. Different spatial resolutions among studies (due to different techniques and different generations of machines) – fMR > PET > SPECT – which cannot yet resolve, for example, single thalamic nuclei or SII from insula, and may "wash out" small foci of activation during averaging over a wide neuronal population.
7. Different temporal resolution of chosen technique (PET/SPECT versus fMR versus MEG/EEG), with brief, transient changes or frequent fluctuations in neuronal activity, which may be a critical component of the brain process under investigation, going undetected: non-converted BOLD fMRI cannot capture the initial highly localized increase in O_2 consumption (proportional to initial changes in neuronal spike frequency) following a stimulus, with serious mapping consequences (Smith *et al.* 2002); dissociation between changes in synchronization of neuronal populations and (no significant) changes in mean neuronal firing rates ("mute imaging").

8. Different values of significance in rCBF changes (generally 3–5%).

9. Dependence of PET on a nitric oxide mechanism which is not evenly distributed (making absence of CBF change not equivalent to absence of activity) and unclear mechanisms of coupling of glucose and O_2 consumption to brain activity.

10. Inability of SPECT/PET to distinguish between increased inhibitory and excitatory activity.

11. Non-quantitative nature of fMR versus quantitative analysis (including of basal state) possible with SPECT/PET.

12. Poor slice selection and low signal-to-noise ratio.

13. Inability of fMR to scan the whole brain (unlike SPECT-PET) and the basal resting pattern of activation.

14. Widely different statistical factors among studies (number of patients, values of significance, correction for multiple comparisons versus no correction, wrong selection of control group, especially in CPSP study, controls being often younger), making comparison impossible; small differences in setting up superficially similar experimental tasks leading to markedly different neuroimaging results.

15. Nonhomogeneous degree of differentiation of sets of increasingly intense stimuli analyzed with subtraction analysis (e.g., subtraction between neutral and more intense, but non-painful, heat and neutral and painful heat yielding differences of greater magnitude than subtraction between intense, but still nonpainful, heat and painful heat), which calls for simultaneous correlation analysis.

16. Different data acquisition and analysis procedures between, for example, SPECT and PET.

17. Artefacts (e.g., bilateral increases in temporal muscle blood flow mistaken for brain activation; geometric distortion (MR techniques), interference with resolution from large veins (fMR), imperfect correspondence between fMR signal and locus of synaptic activity).

18. Unexplained participation of areas not believed to be involved in a task confounding interpretation (e.g., bilateral visual areas decreases).

19. Disregard of the high baseline activity in the awake resting brain; most functional imaging experiments show small fractional changes in CMR-O_2 from baseline values in response to stimulation, but not the larger increases in the overall cerebral metabolic rate of glucose consumption (i.e., uncoupling between utilization of glucose and oxygen). Importantly, such baseline activity might be high enough so as not to require incremental activity during performance, i.e., a particular region could still be actively contributing to brain function. Neuronal activity in the cortex is extremely efficient, with neurons requiring a minimum total amount of energy to process information. This would call for studying the magnitude of the total neuronal activity (baseline plus activation) using measurements of neuroenergetics (Shulman et al. 2004).

20. PET estimated CBF changes identified using the relative CBF analysis not necessarily reflecting functional change, particularly when the experimental conditions directly affect global CBF (absolute CBF analysis should be considered when conditions potentially evoke autonomic nervous system responses).

deranged NE/5HT neurotransmission). The same comments apply to the study of Jones and colleagues.

In our own study, reduced binding could have been due to decreased sensitivity of the postsynaptic membrane to GABA or a downregulation of receptors in response to enhanced release of GABA. A significant GABA A downregulation, in the course of long-standing CP, at fronto(MI/premotor/PFC)-parietal (SI) level (and not diffusely) is suggested by our data.

Box 7.2 Explaining deactivations

While hyperactivations imaged by current technologies can be more easily explained, deactivations have not yet been adequately explained. In particular, noxious input may initially activate, and after some time depress certain brain regions. Backonja and colleagues (1991) suggested that initial somatosensory activation in response to tonic pain (decreased alpha 1 power) progresses to somatosensory inhibition (alpha 1 augmentation) after the first minute of stimulation. Le Pera and colleagues (2000) showed that tonic muscle pain induces EEG increments of both delta and alpha 1 powers bilaterally over the parietal somatosensory areas (but not SII-insula or ACC), more so contralaterally to painful stimulation. Since enhanced slow waves are usually considered an expression of inhibition, these findings could be related to inhibitory processes occurring in SI. Apkarian and colleagues (1992) showed SI deactivation following contralateral stimulation with moderately painful hot water bath. A SPECT study found that thalamic perfusion increases just after onset of symptoms as a reaction to pain and then gradually decreases in more chronic phases (Fukumoto et al. 1999). High intensity stimuli produce SI deactivation. Thus, tonic pain may trigger an inhibitory response in these areas. The same line of reasoning applies to CP.

Possible mechanisms include the following. (1) Organized, baseline default mode of brain function, which is suspended during activating contexts (Raichle et al. 2001) or pathologic states. (2) Ongoing inhibition (Canavero et al. 1993): activity of GABA neurons demands energy (i.e., enhanced glucose metabolism; Ackermann et al. 1984), but the net inhibition may swamp their increased demand for energy. Also, few interneurons (whose firing rate tends to be higher than pyramidal neurons) can effectively inhibit many projection cells, particularly if GABA is over-released by these or GABA receptors are increased on target projection neurons. (3) Diminished input: this cannot be the explanation in the CP setting, since excitatory allodynic barrage is accompanied by further deactivation. Also, thalamic hypometabolism renormalizes, along with analgesia, after cordotomy (i.e., further input reduction) in cancer patients (Di Piero et al. 1991). (4) Passive shunting to nearby activated areas. (5) Decrease in thalamic firing between bursts (Lenz 1991), due to excessive inhibition in the thalamus trying to overcompensate excessive excitatory nociceptive input (this cannot be the case: see section on neurophysiology and Box 7.3). (6) Attentional focusing on an area and shutting down of another; even anticipation of a painful stimulus yields decreases in blood flow in areas of SI outside the representation of the anticipated stimulus (Drevets et al. 1995). (7) Diminution of ongoing neuronal processes as an outcome of increased neuronal activity elsewhere. (8) Diaschisis (Nguyen and Botez 1998), defined as a sudden inhibition of function produced by an acute or chronic focal disturbance in an anatomically intact portion of the brain remote from the original site of injury, but anatomically connected with it through fiber tracts. There are several forms: (a) the transhemispheric form acts through the corpus callosum and may be due to loss of facilitatory inputs; in the acute phases of stroke there may be reactive contralateral disinhibition or facilitation followed by depression; (b) the corticothalamic form, which follows pure cortical stroke, is accompanied by ipsilateral thalamic hypometabolism (e.g., Kuhl et al. 1980: 5 non-CP stroke patients); (c) the thalamocortical form, in which both small and large posterior thalamic infarcts can result in ipsilateral parietotemporal hypometabolism; unilateral thalamic stroke may induce bilateral (ipsilateral > contralateral) metabolic cortical depression, perhaps mediated by the corpus callosum; and (d) reverse diaschisis (i.e., increase in CRF) determined by contralateral structures (Weiller et al. 1992) (interestingly, isolated lesions of the internal capsule show no significant cortical hypometabolism). (9) Neuronal death. This has been excluded (Baron et al. 1986): cortical hypometabolism shows a trend toward renormalization over time. Most importantly in the CP setting, both pain and (de)activations can be promptly reversed.

Among these, inhibition is a prime candidate. For instance, different net effects of excitation and inhibition have been observed within SI, with nociceptive neurons even suppressed by noxious stimuli (see references in Bushnell et al. 1999; Schnitzler and Ploner 2000). Inhibitory effects within SI have also been demonstrated simultaneously with (Tommerdahl et al. 1996, 1999) and after excitation (Backonja et al. 1991), within (Tommerdahl et al. 1996, 1998) as well as outside the somatotopically appropriate regions of SI (Derbyshire et al. 1997). Inhibition within SI is known to enhance contrast both within-area and with contralateral SI for pain perception (Drevets et al. 1995). The net effect of exciting some neurons and inhibiting the spontaneous activity of others could have different effects on PET rCBF or on fMR measured venous blood oxygenation. Recently, a TMS study found that pure sensory thalamic stroke, which reduces or abolishes sensory input induces a hyperactivity of inhibitory cortical neurons and simultaneously induces intracortical excitability without affecting corticospinal excitability (Liepert et al. 2005).

Thalamic hypoperfusion has been reported not only in CP, but also in PNP and cancer pain (Di Piero et al. 1991; Hsieh et al. 1995), making it an unspecific finding. However, the underlying mechanism may be different between CP and other pains, as propofol only relieves CP, along with this anomaly (Canavero et al. 1995). Part of the normal tonic synaptic thalamic activity may be concerned with inhibition of pain perception/input and this may be defective in CP, the thalamus being hyperresponsive following innocuous or noxious stimuli (allodynia-hyperalgesia).

By focusing on the pharmacodynamic profile of propofol (Chapter 5), we may speculate on the origin of such deactivations. One possible mechanism would be disinhibition, that is, CP would be subtended by ongoing hyperinhibition at cortical and/or thalamic levels: our binding study may be explained by both reduction of GABA receptors and GABA hypertonus displacing the tracer. We know that, under normal conditions, there is tonic inhibition at both thalamic and SI levels and for some reason this would be increased in the CP setting. On the other hand, almost half of patients do not respond to propofol and we speculated that this might depend on too strong an excitatory tone in the cortex (Canavero et al. 1996). Since the end result in CP must be net corticothalamic facilitation (Chapter 8), this inhibition would be sufficient to produce deactivation, but not switching off descending input, which seems indefensible. In fact, ketamine can quench CP by antagonizing intracortical excitation and some studies actually point to cortical excitation and thalamic deactivation, so that one possible explanation would rest in study methodology (Hirato et al. above versus our data). Moreover, some patients with thalamic deactivation showed no anomaly at SPECT. Differential participation of separate cortical layers too may originate different findings on SPECT or PET. Feedback excitatory connections coming from a higher order cortical area densely project to layer I, where they may activate pyramidal neurons by synapsing on their apical dendrites. In parallel they might also activate GABAergic interneurons located in this layer and in turn may inhibit the same pyramidal cells, so that inhibition of an area may disinhibit another. This might explain hyper- and hypoactivations of different areas. In fact, GABA inhibition reaches both horizontally through long-range monosynaptic projections (surround inhibition) and vertically in the same column (vertical inhibition): pyramidal cells found in layers V–VI are under stronger inhibition than those in layers II–IV (Shepherd 2004). Inhibition, besides adapting receptive fields (RFs) of pyramidal cells to context, has also a synchronizing role; interlaminar inhibition, for one, has an important role: the synchronous activity of even a small number of inhibitory cells (unlike pyramidal cells) making many contacts onto postsynaptic cells could be sufficient to provide synchronization in a large population of pyramidal neurons. Specularly, the synchronous activation of a local group of many pyramidal neurons may provide an optimal stimulus for activation of inhibitory neurons, compensating for the sparse connectivity from individual pyramidal neurons onto interneurons. The extensive recurrent excitatory connections between pyramidal neurons allow positive feedback to dramatically amplify afferent signals, important in enhancing cortical sensory selectivity. However, these circuits are intrinsically unstable. This is kept in check by GABAergic interneurons, in a tightly regulated balance. Thus, it is not difficult to envision different degrees of activation and inhibition (even overinhibition leading to bursting: see Box 7.3), simultaneously or not, even in the same lamina. To this, we must add regional differences in GABA and glutamate release (Salin and Prince 1996; Castro-Alamancos and Connors 1997; Shepherd 2004). An imbalance in excitatory and inhibitory influences most likely will not consist of uniformly increased excitation and decreased inhibition. Spatial and temporal changes are the norm. Under physiological conditions, the shifting balance between these components serves the scope of promoting contrast enhancement to improve discrimination or curbing strong inputs (center-surround interactions), primarily in supragranular layers. The check is a shift over time that favors inhibition (i.e., prolonged firing induces a much stronger depression of pyramidal excitatory synapses than of interneuronal inhibitory ones, never vice versa), particularly at relatively high frequencies (Galaretta and Hestrin 1998; Nelson and Turrigiano 1998), or during prolonged sensory stimulation (such as during chronic pain). This high-frequency shift may be due to sensory adaptation of

> **BOX 7.2** Explaining deactivations *(continued)*
>
> excitatory neurons at lower frequencies than inhibitory neurons, increase of excitatory inputs to inhibitory neurons at higher frequencies and depression of excitatory inputs to pyramidal neurons in SI or feed-forward inhibition predominating at lower amplitude input (Moore *et al.* 1999). At shorter time scales, excitatory inputs to some classes of interneurons show transient facilitation, promoting stability by boosting recurrent inhibition.
>
> Thus, a general model for theoretical discussion emerges (Canavero *et al.* 1996; also based on Thomson and Deuchars 1994).The direct monosynaptic thalamocortical (TC) input and pyramidal neuron–interneuron inputs involves non-NMDA receptors, unlike local circuit pyramidal–pyramidal cell connections. These connections, which act at distal dendritic sites, can easily trigger a reverberant excitatory activity between interconnected pyramidal cells and recruit surrounding columns when they receive coincident TC afferent input. Random tonic activity will more readily recruit other pyramidal neurons, while burst firing will recruit interneurons. This simple circuit favors excitation and recruitment of surrounding columns when excitatory inputs to pyramidal neurons are weak or desynchronized, particularly when the input is repetitively activated. In contrast, it favors inhibition when inputs are asynchronous or strong, resulting in a strong inhibitory surround, limiting reverberant excitation amongst pyramidal neurons. In other words, when many columns are recruited for a long time, given the presence of powerful lateral inhibitory circuits, reciprocal inhibition between columns might exert an increasingly dominant role. The strongest excitatory connections between pyramidal neurons appear to involve connections between neurons within a column or very closely neighboring columns, which can recruit each other in a reverberant manner, i.e., vertically excitatory connections appear to predominate. In contrast, inhibitory circuits appear predominantly to involve lateral connections. Inhibitory inter-neurons with vertically oriented axons innervating cells within their own column might therefore receive excitation from surrounding columns. Conversely, an interneuron excited by pyramidal neurons in its own column would inhibit surrounding columns. This model must also take into account that NMDA receptor density and subtypes vary greatly between cortical areas and there may even be a decrease of NMDA activation with age (Castro-Alamancos and Connors 1997). Only further studies will determine the applicability of this model to CP.

NEUROPHYSIOLOGY

1. Human microrecording/stimulation studies

Findings in BCP

1. Obrador and colleagues (1957) failed to elicit pain by stimulating the thalamus in cases of CP.

2. Nashold and Wilson (1970) reported on 3 CP patients. One (V.H., female) was affected by severe paroxysms of right lancinating facial pain plus dull, aching pain ("thalamic pain"), both worse in the cheek (which became red), due to "vascular mesencephalic lesion" associated with subarachnoid hemorrhage. During the pain paroxysms, EEG recording demonstrated "in the left dorsal mesencephalic tegmentum epileptiform spike activity grouped in trains lasting for the duration of the pain," and less striking EEG spikes coincident with dull aching pain. Electrical stimulation of this area enhanced the paroxysms and a radiofrequency lesion eliminated both the abnormal EEG activity and the pain. Interestingly, despite gross anomalies in the anterior parietal lobe and left frontoparietal white matter (single spikes or multiple bursts at 6 s and beta rhythms mixed with spike activity, with bursts every 1–3 s, minimal beta activity and slow theta), stimulation at these sites elicited no subjective responses. A second patient (P.B., male) suffered burning CP to right face, arm and chest due to a traumatic parietal and stereotaxic midbrain lesion. Four lesions in the left dorsolateral mesencephalon, in the region in which stimulation reproduced the pain, relieved both the pain and the hyperalgesia, although an undefined discomfort in his hand lingered on. Two years later, he suddenly died from acute subdural hematoma. At autopsy, an atrophic lesion was found in the left parietal lobe. A third patient (S.M., female) suffered burning/freezing CP to the right hemisoma following thalamomesencephalic stroke. Two lesions were made in the left dorsolateral tegmentum where stimulation elicited the pain; pulvinar stimulation was silent. The patient still felt the "cold" sensation in the arm, but it was no more unpleasant.

3. Guecer and colleagues (1978) implanted electrodes stereotactically in (likely) Vc and nearby somatosensory nuclei and made thalamic EEG recordings (scalp EEG plus thalamograms) in 7 patients with thalamic CPSP. Excessive thalamic slowing was found in 4/7 (3 within range). One patient had marked rhythmical intermittent delta activity in the thalamus which was often triggered by arousing stimuli. Thalamic spindle activity was sometimes noted without concomitant spindle activity on the scalp and would occasionally occur in states of early drowsiness. All 3 patients with markedly abnormal scalp EEG recordings also showed excessive slowing in the thalamic leads. Marked thalamic and surface slowing of irregular (polymorphic) waveform was found to increase in the thalamic as well as the scalp leads when the patient became drowsy. In 2 of these 3 old patients, abnormal EEG scalp findings were likely due to advanced diffuse cerebrovascular disorder. Thalamic participation in the posterior alpha rhythm was absent or poorly developed in most patients: only 2 had good evidence of alpha rhythm, possibly depending on the electrode site (and on the degree of cortical alpha development). Marked thalamic delta activity likely marked a genuine pain-related abnormality (insertion trauma was ruled out by concomitant scalp EEG slowing and lack of subjective implantation complaints).

4. Namba and colleagues (1984) reported on 11 patients with BCP. Stimulation in mesencephalic lateral tegmental field elicited the most severe burning pain compared with Vc and internal capsule.

5. Barcia-Salorio and colleagues (1987) studied 2 patients with CPSP. The preoperative EEG of patient 1 showed basal activity and marked bilateral delta waves, worse on the affected stroke side in temporal regions. The second showed slow irritative activity on scalp EEG. Deep brain recordings of scalp EEG showed marked delta activity in the thalamus of patient 1 and a cortical focus in the second case. After radiosurgical Vc thalamotomy, these findings were unchanged, despite some pain improvement.

6. Ohye's group (Hirato *et al.* 1991), in a series of 11 patients with BCP (plus 5 Parkinson's disease controls), noted that "deep pain" was more marked in non-thalamic lesion (on CT) cases and "superficial pain" in cases with definite thalamic damage. Patients were submitted to microelectrode recording. In the *non-thalamic* lesion group with CP, the power amplitude voltage histogram showed a slight reduction with a mixture of various activities in and around the Vim nucleus and multiple peak configurations between 0 and 1000 Hz with a maximum at 200–300 Hz. Thalamic background neural activity in and around Vim was comparable to controls. Background neural activity in intralaminar nuclei (CL) was generally low. In *thalamic* CP, the power amplitude voltage histogram (i.e., background neural activity) showed marked decrease in and around the Vim nucleus (which shows clusters of STT fibers), suggesting damage in Vc. The background neural activity in CL was higher than in Vim, especially in its dorsal part, and was also higher than in the non-thalamic lesion group. In a case *without any CT lesion*, but a dominant superficial pain, the background neural activity in CL was relatively high. Thus, in non-thalamic CP (*deep pain* dominant) thalamic background neural activity was relatively high in Vim (where deep muscle sensation can be usually elicited), but *low in CL*, whereas in thalamic CP (*superficial pain* dominant), this was *higher in CL* than in Vim and markedly decreased in Vc. The initial small damage in Vc may have induced an abnormal state of activity in the surrounding areas in *surviving* Vc neurons and adjacent Vim neurons (and their projection areas). Ohye (1998) very often found that spontaneous activity in Vim and Vc of CP patients was considerably reduced, particularly with massive thalamic involvement. Many irregular burst discharges were encountered throughout the electrode descending in these nuclei, but he noted *no coincidence between pain sensation and moment of burst discharge.* The topographic representation in Vim and Vc was lost. He also found more responses related, for example, to face and arm and often convergent responses from different peripheral receptive fields (RFs). Moreover, a response to *ipsilateral* stimuli was found. Neurons of the face area (including eye movement neurons) seemed to occupy a wide area of Vim. Curiously, coagulation in this area did not change eye movements, but relieved deep pain.

7. Fukaya and colleagues (2003) reported on cortical stimulation findings in 31 CPSP patients (28 thalamo-putamino-capsular; 3 Wallenberg's syndrome). In 23 (84%), SI stimulation at 50 Hz elicited contralateral tingling versus 40% of non-pain patients; in 12 (39%), abnormal pain sensation or exacerbation of original CP were observed, versus 0% of non-pain patients. MI stimulation at 50 Hz had no motor effects, but evoked sensory tingling in 52% of the patients versus 20% of non-pain patients, and very unpleasant sensations (interpreted as a sign of extensive reorganization and unfavorable prognostic sign for MCS-induced analgesia) in 6% of the patients, versus none of non-CPSP cases. MI stimulation at 1–2 Hz evoked tingling in 25% of the patients. In these authors' experience, half of their CPSP cases submitted to Vc DBS reported more pain.

Findings in CCP
spinal recordings:
1. Loeser and colleagues (1968) recorded unit activity in the dorsal horn of a chronically denervated conus medullaris of a paraplegic suffering from burning rectal and thigh pain and hyperpathia following trauma: denervated cell groups (10 dorsal horn neurons *rostral to the site of injury*) had developed spontaneous high-frequency "epileptic" paroxysmal burst discharges.

2. Evidence of high-level spontaneous activity assumed to be abnormal focal hyperactivity within the superficial laminae of the injured cord has been recorded *up to 7 levels cephalad to injury site* prior to computer-assisted DREZ surgery for SCI and other pains (39% of cases had hyperactivity higher than 3 levels above injury site) (Edgar *et al.* 1993).

3. Falci and colleagues (2002) performed multilevel DREZ surgery on 41 CCP patients. Electrophysiological analyses of the DREZs were performed one level caudal to the injury site and *up to 5 DREZ levels cephalad*, exploiting an active electrode inserted free-hand 2 mm into the specific DREZ tilted 35–45° medially (the same as per coagulation). In 32 patients, additional DREZ recordings were carried out during transcutaneous C-fiber (inclusive of sympathetic fibers) stimulation in which a current perception threshold device was used (electrodes were in the distribution of a dermatome, with 5 Hz electrical stimuli activating the nerve fibers directly, but not the actual receptors in the skin due to too low current levels). The device was used for preoperative testing of dermatomal skin sensation in a C-fiber frequency band caudal to, at, and cephalad to injury level. A 5 Hz threshold above 0.35 mA was empirically assumed as significant. In general, the elevated thresholds were found in dermatomes at and cephalad to the neurological injury level in patients who were sensory complete (occasionally also in dermatomes immediately caudal to the sensory-complete neurological level); these same skin dermatomes with elevated and *presumed* abnormal thresholds received above-threshold stimulation intraoperatively. Intramedullary recordings were then made in the DREZs corresponding to the particular skin dermatome. Data were analyzed and filtered to obtain "spindles," *presumed* to signal abnormal neural activity when exceeding 3 s. These were corroborated by higher voltage and frequencies of the activities. The same recordings were obtained after lesioning. These data were in spatial correlation with those obtained with current perception threshold. In the first 9 patients, 7 showed areas of DREZ neuroelectrical hyperactivity: radiofrequency microcoagulations (90°C for 30 s) with 1 mm of separation were performed in order to silence all abnormal activity (otherwise, they were repeated). In the 2 cases without hyperactivity, lesioning extended at 2 DREZs cephalad to injury level and 1 below (90° for 30 s). Of the remaining 32 patients, 9, all with below-level pain, had no spontaneous DREZ hyperactivity; operative transcutaneous C-fiber stimulation of skin derma-tomes with elevated C-fiber sensory thresholds resulted in evoked neuroelectrical hyperactivity in specific DREZs, *presumed* pain generators, and used to guide lesioning: 8 were totally relieved, with 1 failure. In the rest, both techniques guided total silencing of hyperactivity (see results in Table 7.1, below). Lack of spontaneous neuroelectrical hyperactivity in 27% of the patients was ascribed to pain being cyclical and waxing and waning in intensity.

cerebral recordings: Lenz (1991 and references therein; Lenz *et al.* 1994) studied patients with CP following spinal cord transection. All patients experienced pain in the anesthetic part of the body; some also experienced dysesthesias in the part of the body adjacent to the area of sensory loss. They designated the area of thalamus representing the borderzone area and the anesthetic area as the borderzone/anesthetic area (BAA). Evidence of somatotopic reorganization was found. Neurons with RFs on the border of the area of sensory loss occupied more of the thalamic homunculus in Vc than in patients with controls (movement disorder patients), i.e., body parts bordering the anesthetic body part had *increased representation.* For instance, in one patient, the representation of the trunk occupied 1.2 mm of a trajectory through the part of the thalamus where the leg, anesthetic as a result of the spinal injury, is often represented. In another with clinically complete spinal transection at C6, the representation of the external ear, neck and occiput occupied 1.5 mm of a trajectory through the forearm representation, versus 0.1–0.3 mm of neck and trunk representation in controls. Stimulation of these neurons by whatever means (e.g., touching the skin near the border of the sensory loss) could produce an abnormal sensation in the anesthetic part of the body (mislocalization). A significant increase in the number of neurons in Vc (BAA) *without RFs* was also characteristic. Unlike controls, Vc microstimulation at sites with neuronal RFs on the border of the anesthetic area of the body characteristically revealed a dissociation between the RFs and projected fields (PFs) (*RF/PF mismatch*), with PF altered less than the somatotopic map of the inputs demonstrated by the RF; RFs were often located on the border of the anesthetic area, while PFs extended far into the anesthetic part of the body, suggesting to the authors that abnormal activity recorded in borderline regions might be reflected in sensations experienced in anesthetic areas, but also that the representation of sensory input (RFs) is much more plastic than the central representation of the part of the body (PFs). In other words, in Vc regions that would normally represent the anesthetic body part, neurons often had no RFs, although PFs were referred to the anesthetic body part, evidence that *a central representation of the anesthetic body part still exists years after total interruption of input from that part of the body*, an essential ingredient if pain is to be appreciated in that body part. Microstimulation at these Vc borderline regions often produced sensations in the anesthetic area. These regions of Vc representing parts of the body where the patient experienced pain (and possibly dysesthesias) showed *increased bursting activity.* Bursting activity was one- to three-fold greater for cells in the BAA without RF than for control cells (i.e., those representing body parts distant from the representation of the anesthetic part of the body). In control Vc, STT cells fired regularly at a rate of approximately 10 spikes/s and few spike trains exhibited high-frequency bursting. In contrast, cells recorded in BAAs showed a significantly higher likelihood of a bursting pattern. Here, bursts were preceded by a period of inhibition, with the initial interspike interval being less than 6 ms in duration, becoming longer throughout the burst (i.e., decreasing number of action potentials in the burst), a pattern typical of bursts associated with Ca^{2+} spikes (as seen in sleep) and involving a low-threshold rapidly inactivating Ca^{2+} current. Moreover, cells in the BAA region without RFs had longer preburst intervals (i.e., longer periods of silence before a burst) and lower primary event rates (i.e., action potentials outside bursts). In view of their inverse correlation, these cells were believed to have tonically decreased firing rates between bursts. The most intense bursting was found in cells that appeared to be located in the posterior aspect of the Vc core and in the posteroinferior area (Lenz *et al.* 1994), where nociceptive STT terminations are most dense (Lenz and Dougherty 1997). Thermal pain-responsive cells appear to be more frequent posteroinferiorly to Vc core, with warmth and cold coded cells contiguous, but separate (see references in Hua *et al.* 2000). The increase in spontaneous thalamic activity was more pronounced with more complete interruptions of somatosensory input from a particular body part. In further microstimulation studies (Lenz *et al.* 1998) of 12 neurogenic pain patients (CPSP $n = 4$, SCI CP $n = 4$; Lenz *et al.* 1994, and PNP [$n = 4$]; controls: 10 movement disorder cases) in parts of the thalamus representing the painful area (both the core and posteroinferior areas of Vc), there was an increase in the number of sites where pain was evoked by stimulation, with a corresponding decrease in the number of sites where non-painful thermal (warm and cold) sensations were evoked. Yet, the percentage of sites where pain or thermal sensations were evoked was not significantly different between parts of thalamus representing the painful and non-painful parts of the body (2%). Thus, *despite the central body image being relatively constant in the face of altered input, a reorganization occurs so that cold modalities are relabeled to signal pain in the thalamus of patients with CP*, possibly explaining cold hyperalgesia; spontaneous bursting activity at these sites may be more likely to produce the sensation of pain. In CP patients too, the number of sites where cold was evoked was significantly lower than in controls, whereas the number of sites where warmth was evoked was not different from controls (Lenz *et al.* 1994); moreover, there was a significant increase in the number of sites where pain was evoked, but no significant difference from controls in the number of pain sites plus thermal sites.

Findings in mixed series

1. Pain and burning can be elicited in CP/PNP (but not non-pain) patients by stimulating the STT in Vc (Hassler and Riechert 1959; Levin 1966), the mesencephalon (Nashold *et al.* 1974; Sano 1977; Tasker *et al.* 1983), thalamic radiations (Albe-Fessard 1973; Koszweski *et al.* 2003) and SI (Hamby 1961; Dierssen *et al.* 1969). In this latter case, the response is obtained *only* in an area related to a deafferented portion of the body (while the same stimulation in an area related to non-deafferented body parts gives only the usual paresthesias), mimicking the patient's spontaneous pain ("in the same body part as their own pain").

2. Epileptifom discharges related to pain paroxysms have been recorded in the lateral mesencephalic tegmentum inferior and posterior to the intralaminar nuclei in patients with PNP and CP, possibly at the site of termination of the spino-mesencephalic tract (Iacono and Nashold 1982).

3. Toth and collegues (1984) examined neurogenic pain (including 3 thalamic CP cases) and non-pain patients. They studied Vc, CM, pulvinar and mesencephalic reticular formation, with stereotactically positioned electrodes. Unlike non-pain patients, in patients with CP, the spontaneous activity in Vc and CM was strikingly dysrhythmic, contained many sharp steep waves and the amplitude was pronounced, sometimes more than in the cortical activity. The activity contained bursts composed of sudden spike-like waves. By stimulating Vc or CM with single stimuli, in the others, 4–6 Hz waxing–waning steep potential series could be recorded. During 100 Hz/500 ms train stimulation in Vc and CM, typical electroconvulsive paroxysmal activity occurred which was strictly localized within these structures. Only slight traces appeared in the frontoparietal cortical activity (unlike Guecer *et al.* 1978). These changes were most pronounced in phantom pain (4 patients), but could also be observed in CP. In CP, the spontaneous and evoked electrical activity in the specific and non-specific thalamic nuclei was characteristically paroxysmal and could be strongly enhanced from each other (Vc-medial thalamus autokindling).

4. Tasker's group in Toronto published an impressive series of papers on the topic. These authors (Hirayama *et al.* 1989) performed single-unit analysis of spontaneous neuronal activity in 3 patients with thalamic CP and 2 with complete cord transection at C3 and T4, respectively (plus 4 PNP cases and 4 non-pain controls: 3 MS cases and one patient with dystonia following a supratentorial thrombotic stroke which produced a painless Djereine–Roussy syndrome). They recorded three kinds of cells firing in bursts (types A–C) and one kind not firing in bursts. (1) In pain patients, 47% of the studied bursting cells were of type A, 42% of type B and 11% of type C. Some 43% of the cells were located in Vc, 32% in Vim, 19% in Vcpc, 4% in Vop and 2% in zona incerta. A total of 22% of bursting cells had cutaneous RFs. In other words, bursting cells typically fired at interspike intervals of 1–2 ms and interburst intervals of 50 ms. Microstimulation at sites where bursting cells were recorded usually induced no response. Bursting cells tended to be located in Vc and Vcpc (sites in pain patients believed to be in Vim could actually have been in Vc). (2) In non-pain patients, 59% of bursting cells were of type A, 23% of type B, 18% of type C. Fifty-three percent of the cells were located within Vim, 35% in centrolateralis intermedius, 6% in Vc and 6% in Vop. None had cutaneous RFs or responded to movements. Thus, *bursting cells were rarely encountered in Vc,* and those bursting cells encountered elsewhere tended to have lower mean firing rates and longer interspike and interburst intervals. *Stimulation in Vc never induced pain.* Although it was concluded that the Vc region of pain patients (CP and PNP) contained many more bursting cells than the comparable region in non-pain patients, with different characteristics than bursting cells in non-pain patients, "It is not possible to determine whether the bursting cells recorded in pain patients have anything to do with the pain the patient experiences."

They (Gorecki *et al.* 1989) reported thalamic exploration in 39 patients: 13 thalamic CP cases, 10 SCI pain cases, 4 postcordotomy pain cases and 11 PNP cases. Macrostimulation was carried out in the first 23 cases, with microelectrode recording and microstimulation performed in the last 16 cases. In these latter cases, abnormal neuronal firing was recorded in all, as spontaneous bursts of action potentials. The interburst interval was of the order of 50 ms; 76% of bursting units did not have RFs. Stimulation at 8% of the sites where bursting units were recorded induced burning or pain, being found both in close proximity to or remote from units subserving deafferented dermatomes. The time course of appearance of these units could not be determined. Non-pain patients also demonstrated bursting cells with intervals of the order of 200 ms, burst frequency of approximately 5 Hz, usually located more anterior and dorsally with respect to Vc. Unlike normal patients, in 17 cases, 16 of whom had a clear history of hyperpathia or allodynia, stimulation in Vc elicited painful sensations, often reproducing the patient's particular pain syndrome. In 12 cases, neuronal recordings at the stimulation site indicated that the neurons had low-threshold mechanoreceptive fields corresponding to the pain location and to the dermatomes affected by sensory changes, a response most frequently obtained in Vc. *The induction of pain was thus more frequent in patients with allodynia and/or hyperpathia.*

Altered thalamic somatotopy was observed. They divided the different thalamic maps into four categories: *normal, empty* (when there was a general lack of response to stimulation or lack of RFs over a large number of trajectories or when there were only lemniscal or spinothalamic tract responses in locations at which units with receptive fields would be expected), *displaced* (thalamic units possibly shifted by atrophy or sprouting at the sites of a lesion or by altered ventricular size) and with *abnormal receptive fields.* The majority of patients with thalamic CP (8/13) had an empty thalamus. At least one patient with a thalamic infarct, but no CP, demonstrated a typical empty thalamus. In two patients, the somatotopic organization was found to have a relatively normal sequence, but individual responses were located in sagittal planes more lateral than expected. In 5 cases (2 CCP and 1 thalamic CP, 2 PNP), somatotopic mapping demonstrated abnormal receptive fields. One patient with C5 clinically complete spinal cord transection had extensive RFs over the occiput and the back of the shoulders (a location where RFs have rarely been found), corresponding to the border of the deafferented region; in particular, the representation of the external ear, occiput and neck occupied 1.5 mm of a trajectory through the part of the thalamus where the hand, anesthetic as a result of the spinal injury, would normally be represented, versus a 0.1–0.2 mm trajectory length in movement disorder cases. In this patient, there were also statistically significant differences in neuronal firing patterns in the deafferented region of the thalamus, compared with the presumably normal region of the thalamus (patient included in Lenz's series discussed above). *Two patients had wide areas of bilateral as well as ipsilateral representation with bilateral pain induction on stimulation.* The remainder of the patients had *"normal" maps with a propensity for SCI patients to be in this category (6/10). These three types of altered thalamic somatotopy were present in patients both with and without pain states.*

They (Rinaldi *et al.* 1991) observed bursting in PNP and CP (2 cases), occurring in two patterns, short bursts of 2–6 spikes every 1–4 s or a long burst of 30–80 spikes, at an average rate of a burst every 1–4 s. This activity was found concentrated to the lateral aspect of MD, CL and only a small part of CM-Pf complex.

In an excellent study, this group (Parrent *et al.* 1992) reported on two patients with massive suprathalamic infarcts. Their first case, a 58-year-old woman, suffered a right hemispheric infarct following carotid endarterectomy. Shortly thereafter, she developed left hemibody CP. A cordotomy was ineffective. The pain was constant, burning, particularly significant in the shoulder. Aside from motor deficits, there was marked sensory loss on the left side, with preserved, though reduced, vibration sense in the left hand. There was no hyperpathia, bar a suggestion of cold allodynia in the left shoulder area. MRI showed parenchymal loss in the distribution of the right sylvian artery, with T1-hypointense areas in the right periventricular region. The right cerebral peduncle and thalamus were atrophic. Stereotactic exploration of the right thalamus with the patient awake and unsedated and exhaustive microrecording plus micro- and macrostimulation of Vc and medial thalamic nuclei revealed no motor or sensory responses of any kind and no receptive fields were recorded. PVG stimulation produced no subjective sensations or effect on the patient's pain and allodynia. Their second case, a 57-year-old man, suffered a right hemispheric infarct. Almost immediately following the stroke he developed CP. Constant sharp pain was experienced in the left shoulder and hand and in the lower back and left hip (worse in the latter two), with spontaneous exacerbations occurring every two minutes; steady burning pain affected the medial left thigh, knee and foot and cramping pain the left thigh and calf. Aside from motor and other deficits, there was a diminished to absent appreciation of light touch, pinprick and vibration in the entire left side of the body. There was allodynia to light touch and cold stimuli on the entire left side, and hyperpathia of left limbs and face. CT showed a massive infarct in the right sylvian artery distribution. Stereotactic exploration of the right thalamus with the patient awake and unsedated and microrecording plus micro- and macrostimulation obtained no motor or sensory responses. No stimulation-evoked responses were obtained in the right PVG region. Exploration of the left PVG obtained the typical stimulation responses of this region as well as acute relief of the patient's allodynia and hyperpathia. *They concluded for a major role of the thalamus ipsilateral to pain.*

Tasker and colleagues (1994) observed bursting cells in 64% and somatotopic reorganization in all of 29 CPSP (thalamic, suprathalamic and brainstem) patients. Recordings showed a lesion could leave deafferented structures "in neutral," but capable of electrical and (therefore presumably) intrinsic stimulation to possibly produce pain. Macrostimulation of the tegmental reticulothalamic pathways (and medial thalamic nuclei), normally unresponsive to stimulation, at threshold effective for ML/STT stimulation, induced a widespread nonsomatotopographically organized burning or pain sensation (mimicking the original pain) extending beyond the involved dermatomes, often similar to that from which the patient suffered (5 brainstem CPSP, 1 MS, 1 CCP). Stimulation tended to be painful in patients with evoked pain (14/16) but not without (1/4), even in the absence of contralateral functional SI (or massive hemispherectomy-like lesions); the reticular system was thus implicated in allodynia, ipsilateral structures in the mediation of constant pain (Tasker *et al.* 1983; Tasker 2001a).

Thalamic reorganization following denervation was tested by studying thalamic somatotopy (microrecording/stimulation) in 61 patients: 5 groups were compared according to body part in patients with pain in the deafferented body part and in controls (movement disorders). PNP and CP were considered together (Kiss *et al.* 1994). Trunk representation (RF) was significantly larger in patients with leg–foot deafferentation than in those without; however, microstimulation induced paresthesias in the face from a significantly larger thalamic area in facially denervated cases than controls (i.e., face RFs *increased*, but maintained small discrete PFs not extending into other body parts). There were *no* significant differences in the representation of the other body parts in the 5 groups. In the leg-deafferented-only group, the deafferented cells responded to afferent input from an adjacent body part, yet retained their original connections to the cortical representation of the deafferented body part. In face-deafferented patients, deafferented cells ceased to respond to peripheral inputs, yet maintained their thalamocortical projections to the original body part representation. In some patients, deafferented cells could both stop responding to peripheral input and communicate meaningfully with their cortical target.

The Vc core (*but not* other nuclei more ventroposterior to Vc) was studied in 5 thalamic, 3 suprathalamic, 2 internal capsule and 3 cortical CP cases (versus 23 non-stroke pain and 24 movement disorder patients) with stereotactic micro-recordings (Davis *et al.* 1996). Microstimulation in the *tactile core of Vc* commonly evoked paresthesias, while threshold stimulation *never* or rarely (2%) evoked pain in non-stroke and movement disorders patients, respectively. By contrast, in CP, *28% of Vc sites microstimulated evoked painful sensations at threshold* (suprathreshold stimuli did so at 46% of Vc sites in CP versus 8% in other pains and 12% of movement disorders cases). There was no significant difference between the paresthesia thresholds of non-CP patients and motor patients, but these were *elevated two-fold in CP patients*, except 4 (2 patients with particularly small thalamic lesions and 2 patients with small cortical lesions). However, stimulation thresholds to elicit pain were similar in all patient groups. CP patients most often noted the stimulation-evoked pain as a *nondescript pain (33% of sites) or painful burning sensations (43% of sites)*, shocking (10%) or sharp (14%). In control groups, pain was elicited only with stimuli suprathreshold for paresthesias. Most common with suprathreshold stimuli was an unpleasant (or sometimes shocking) feeling in the non-CP pain group (61% of sites) and movement disorders (45%). The burning sensation so often reported by CP was never reported by the movement disorder patients and *at only two sites in the non-CP patients*. Interestingly, *qualities of evoked pain in pain patients did not necessarily relate to the quality of the patient's ongoing chronic pain*. Pain could be evoked at sites throughout tactile Vc, although most sites were located in the *ventral two-thirds*. Microstimulation within Vc almost always evoked a response, *even in the presence of suprathalamic infarcts* (and also with thalamic lesions). Vc stimulation in 62% of CP patients evoked pain: *this was not related to allodynia*, since pain was evoked in patients with (4/7) and without (3/6) it. In some CP patients, pain was evoked throughout the electrode trajectory within Vc, a clustering not seen in the other two groups. *At some Vc sites in CP patients, stimulation up to maximum current (up to 100 μA) did not evoke any sensation.* Suprathreshold stimuli in CP converted only a few responses from paresthesia to pain. In some patients with pain, there appeared to be a *decrease in cell density* in regions representing body parts whose afferents had been damaged. Although RF/PF mismatches in non-pain patients were noted for nearly half of Vc, they were minor or simple size discrepancies; stimulation at only 9% of Vc in these control patients resulted in gross mismatches. The total number of RF/PF mismatches was significantly greater *in both pain groups* compared with motor group, due to a greater increase in gross rather than minor or size mismatches in the pain patients. *The proportion of all mismatches was the same in the non-CP and CP groups and size mismatches were similar between CP and non-CP patients.*

In a major study, Radhakrishnan and colleagues (1999) compared the incidence of bursting in Vc of patients with neurogenic pain (including CPSP and SCI, whose numbers were not specified) and motor disorders. *The burst indices* (i.e., the number of bursting cells per track) *in the pain and non-pain groups were not significantly different from each other.* Low-threshold Ca^{2+} spike-evoked bursts (with shortening of the first interspike interval, an increase in the number of interspike intervals in the burst and progressive prolongation of successive interspike intervals) were identified in 57% of bursting cells in pain patients and 47% of non-pain patients, *suggesting no definite rapport with pain.* Only a few cells of the bursting kind were located in Vc, the majority being anterodorsally and ventroposteriorly to it (see also Ohye and Narabayashi 1972).

Finally, they (Manduch *et al.* 1999) did microelectrode recordings in 40 movement disorder and 37 chronic pain patients through Vc and regions ventroposterior to it. Stimulation evoked painful or innocuous thermal sensations at 2.9 and 4.7%, respectively (5023 stimulation sites). A total of 77% were located ventroposterior to Vc and of these 74% were located in or medial to the face/hand representation border in Vc. No significant differences were noted between controls and non-CPSP cases in the incidence of pain and temperature sites. Instead, the incidence of pain sites was higher in CPSP cases ($n = 11$) compared to the other 2 groups (9.5% versus 2.5% in the ventroposterior region of Vc and 15.1% versus 1.4% in Vc). In contrast, the incidence of thermal sites was lower below Vc in CPSP than in the other 2 groups, but *not different in Vc.*

5. Yamashiro and colleagues (1991) made microrecordings in the Vc of 2 patients with SCI, 1 with CPSP, 1 with MS-associated CP and 4 PNP cases. Epileptiform discharges from hyperactive neurons were recorded and two firing patterns seen. One showed regular firing which had 3–5 trains of epileptiform grouped discharges with a frequency of 4–5 Hz. The latter showed continuous firing. These hyperactive neurons were distributed in Vc, Vim and Vop and may have received facilitation from SI/MI.

6. Jeanmonod and colleagues (1996) recorded unit activities from the thalami of 74 patients with CP and PNP. Some 99.8% of their medial thalamic units did *not* respond to somatosensory stimulation (in contrast to a few other studies; see Lenz and Dougherty 1997). In addition to their unresponsiveness, half of the units showed a striking bursting (45.1%) activity (rhythmic: 25%; random: 30%) not due to sleep, as all patients were fully awake during surgery. The rhythmic-random low-threshold Ca^{2+} spike (LTS) bursting units were considered abnormal and were found distributed throughout the posterior half of CL. The rest of their sampled units displayed unresponsive sporadic activities. Many of them exhibited occasional LTS bursts. LTS bursts displayed a theta rhythmicity, with a mean interburst discharge rate of about 4 Hz. In patients with intermittent pain without steady component, they made recordings only during pain-free periods, and never showed a large amount of LTS bursts, as can be the case in patients with steady pain.

interpretation: Anomalous activity at several CNS levels is observed in CP patients. However, most anomalies are seen *both* in PNP and CP patients, making them *unspecific*; most importantly, they are not invariably found. Some findings involve the thalamus in the genesis of CP: (1) an increased incidence of pain evoked at threshold in Vc (core and shell) in CP versus PNP or other controls (see also Hassler and Riechert 1959; Levin 1966; Mazars *et al.* 1974); (2) a likely role of thalami ipsilateral to CP; (3) thalamic involvement in cold allodynia (see below). Different participation of *Vc, Vim and CL* may justify different qualities of CP. Interestingly, Lenz and Dougherty (1997) reported that sensations are more likely to be referred to deep structures at stimulation sites in Vc posteroinferior areas more than in the core. Along these lines, useful information should accrue by studying central pruritus patients: itch is a purely cutaneous sensation and might elucidate central mechanisms of cutaneous anomalous sensations (Canavero *et al.* 1997).

The reticular formation (and related propriospinal cells and fibers in the DREZ) is also likely involved (see Chapter 8). Somatotopic rearrangements (such as expansion of adjacent regions into denervated) and burst firing (Box 7.3) seem to be the result of denervation injury, and not a correlate of pain (unlike, possibly, phantom pain), since they can be observed in non-pain conditions (Jeanmonod *et al.* 1996; Tasker 2001b; see Chapter 8). Since Vc stimulation evokes tactile allodynia more commonly in CP than non-CP pains (Davis *et al.* 1996; Lenz *et al.* 1998), pain more frequently in those with hyperalgesia than in those without and in the representation of the part of the body where the patient experiences hyperalgesia than in the representation of other body parts (Lenz *et al.* 1998), the findings discussed may have a special relevance to allodynia (see Chapter 8).

2. Evoked potentials studies

1. Mauguière and Desmedt (1988) differentiated four types of CP of thalamic origin by somatosensory evoked potentials (SEPs), which explore dorsal column–medial lemniscal (DC/ML) function: group 1 had no CP, but complete hemianesthesia and loss of cortical SEPs on the affected side (analgic thalamic syndrome); group 2 had CP, severe hypoesthesia and loss of cortical SEPs; group 3 had CP and hypoesthesia, with cortical SEPs present, although reduced or delayed on the affected side; group 4 had CP with preserved touch and joint sensations and normal SEPs (pure algetic thalamic syndrome). All their 30 patients presented a thalamic lesion on CT. SEPs did not tell apart groups 1 and 2, but separated these two groups from group 3, in whom cortical SEPs were present.

2. Wessel and colleagues (1994) studied 18 patients with a single ischemic thalamic lesion, who had somatosensory disturbances and/or CP in the opposite hemibody, by correlating their clinical symptoms, SEPs and CT imaging findings. Patients were divided into three groups: (1) those with somatosensory deficits, CP, and abnormal SEPs, which comprised two thirds of the patients (classic thalamic pain syndrome); (2) those with somatosensory deficits, no CP and abnormal SEPs (analgetic thalamic syndrome), with a 1-year follow-up; and (3) those with almost normal sense perception, CP and normal SEPs (pure algetic thalamic syndrome). Six of the 8 patients with the analgetic syndrome had a posterolateral thalamic stroke in the territory of the geniculothalamic artery, which includes Vc, whereas groups 1 and 3 had CT evidence of paramedian or anterolateral thalamic lesions.

Box 7.3 Does bursting signal CP?

All thalamic relay (e.g., Vc) cells respond to excitatory inputs in one of two different modes: burst and tonic (Sherman and Guillery 2004). In burst mode, the inward T-type (IT) Ca^{2+} channel in soma and dendrites is activated and an inflow of Ca^{2+} produces a low-threshold spike (LTS) that in turn usually activates a burst (usually less than 25 ms long) of conventional action potentials. After about 100 ms or more of depolarization, the IT inactivates and the cell fires in tonic mode; after about 100 ms or more of relative hyperpolarization, inactivation of IT is alleviated and the cell fires in burst mode. Just like tonic, burst firing is an important relay mode during waking behavior and could play an important role in attention. Unlike single action potentials, which are very often filtered out, bursts – particularly coincident bursts – are reliably signaled, because transmitter release is strongly facilitated. In fact, single spikes are spontaneously emitted by neurons, creating "noise" (i.e., disinformation) (Lisman 1997). Bursts are particularly effective for synaptic communication in the cortex. Specifically, bursting can record significant, but possibly minor changes in specific afferent activity (initial stimulus detection) and use this to focus the tonic mode upon the causes of these changes for more accurate analysis. Also, rhythmic bursts may signal no transmission, while arrhythmic bursts may indicate sensory transmission. Switching between tonic and burst firing occurs irregularly every several hundred milliseconds to every several seconds, presumably reflecting slow changes in membrane potential that switch IT between inactivated and deinactivated. Only 5–10% of synapses on Vc TC cells come from the periphery: 30% are from local GABAergic neurons, 30% from cholinergic sources and 30% from SI layer 6. Thus the vast majority of inputs are modulating, controlling the state of IT and thus the response mode between burst and tonic (Sherman and Guillery 2004).

Despite several authors highlighting the importance of Ca^{2+}-related bursting activity (inside the more general phenomenon of sensitization) in the genesis of CP, several pieces of evidence nix this concept:

(1) Ca^{2+} LTS bursts in the thalamus (particularly Vc and CL) ("thalamic dysrhythmia") and supposed neurophysiological correlates thereof (i.e. theta/beta bands of juxtaposed cortical activity) are not specific to CP, and have been consistently observed in the same nuclei in PNP patients, as well as CNS disorders without a pain component (Jeanmonod et al. 1996; Llinas et al. 1999: no CP cases were studied in this latter paper). Also, loss of corticothalamic input (Llinas et al. 1999) believed by some authors to produce CP-associated electrophysiological anomalies, actually abolishes CP (see section on reports of sudden disappearance of CP).

(2) Although it seems more prominent in neurons with representation areas in the anesthetic part of the body, Ca^{2+}-related bursting is also found in normal awake controls, during slow-wave sleep and also during anesthesia. The proportion of intrinsically bursting cells in the intact cortex is about 15–20% (Steriade 1999; Sanchez-Vives and McCormick 2000) and many such bursting cells are found in the thalamus (Tasker 2001b). Most importantly, *there is no coincidence between pain sensation in CP patients and moment of burst discharge* (Ohye 1998) and following anterolateral cordotomy CP is not usually felt in areas of the body as surmised from, for example, Lenz's speculations (Beric et al. 1988).

(3) Bursting, as CP sensation-related activity, due to STT injury, cannot explain immediate-onset CP (is bursting immediate?) and also cases in which there is no clinically evident STT-mediated sensory loss (e.g., Stoodley et al. 1995).

(4) The balance of excitatory and inhibitory inputs leading to Ca^{2+} spike associated bursting is unclear (overinhibition? Loss of excitation?) and may depend on the presence or absence of RFs.

(5) Lenz's view that bursting and absence of RFs in the Vc BAA of SCI CP patients is due to decreased tonic NMDA excitatory drive with attendant hyperpolarization collapses on STT input being non-NMDA mediated. Also, the fact that Ca^{2+} bursting may be decreased by norepinephrine and increased by acetylcholine (i.e., amitriptyline's profile) is meaningless in view of poor efficacy in CCP (Chapter 5).

(6) In patients with spinal transection, the painful area overlaps with the area of sensory loss (Lenz et al. 1994), making bursting the result of sensory loss rather than pain.

(7) A 1 mm increment of electrode insertion in an area of spontaneous discharge can result in an artefactual temporary increase in activation of the existing discharge patterns (Andy 1983).

Models explaining bursting in relation to CP collapse for all these reasons (e.g., Jeanmonod et al. 1996). Moreover, those models, even in these authors' minds, have much more difficulty in explaining CP than PNP. The anatomical background too is unsupported: bidirectional TRN interconnections between pain-related CL and Vc cells, with back-and-fro exchange of waves of inhibition, starting from the less sensory-input-deprived CL exciting TRN, is presently unsubstantiated (Steriade et al. 1997).

Bursting can be a normal condition of thalamic functioning in awake humans. Possible increments of bursting in certain locations can be explained away as an injury-related disorder of normal thalamic oscillatory mechanisms (Ohye 1998; Tasker 2001b). On the other hand, Kim and colleagues (2004) proposed that it may be part of a robust pain-relieving mechanism. T-type Ca^{2+} channel activation in Vc can activate TRN cells, with subsequent hyperpolarization and rebound burst spikes again in TC cells through reciprocal Vc–TRN–Vc connections; hyperpolarization and/or burst sequences can contribute to sensory inhibition by reducing the responsiveness of TC neurons. Specifically, because a burst has a long refractory period (170–200 ms), bursting sequences might actually prevent rapidly recurring sensory signal inputs to TC relay cells. Inactivation of this Ca^{2+} channel and thus bursting interferes with sensory gating of pain. The nociceptive dampening/filtering role of the thalamus had been hypothesized by several past authors (e.g., "selective filter" [Lhermitte 1933]; "thalamic function . . . with . . . an inhibitory effect of normal afferent impulses" [Botterell et al. 1954]).

INTERPRETATION: Complete interruption of lemniscal transmission through Vc up to parietal cortex does not necessarily release the mechanisms underlying CP, refuting past theories of deficient lemniscal inhibition of nociceptive STT conduction. Most importantly, both series agree that complete destruction of Vc and possibly other nuclei may be incompatible with the occurrence of CP. Ohye (1998) reached the same conclusion. Thus, the sensory thalamus is necessary for CP to arise.

RESULTS OF NEUROABLATION

Current ablative techniques have no or only a limited role in the management of CP. On the other hand, they provide invaluable insight into the mechanisms subserving CP (see Table 7.1).

Interpretation

a. PRE- AND POST-CENTRAL GYRECTOMY (FIRST PROPOSED BY LERICHE 1937): Limited cortectomies relieved some cases for years, although others were failures. In the CP case reported by Lende and colleagues, cortical removal extended up to the border of the motor and sensory representation of the hand area and down to the sylvian fissure, with excision of the operculi of the pre- and post-central gyri, and exposing the insula. Thus, effective cortectomies should likely include not only SI, but also SII/insula and even MI. SI-MI coactivation in metabolic studies underlies the concerted effectuation of interrelated sensorimotor functions (see also Penfield and Jasper 1954; Libet 1973). At least some failures can be explained away by the wide variability in somatotopy in individuals and somatotopic differences not only

TABLE 7.1. Results of neuroablative procedures

Author(s)	Cause of central pain	Procedure	Efficacy/(follow-up)	Notes
Pre- and postcentral gyrectomies				
Dimitri and Balado (quoted by David et al. 1947)	Thalamic lesion (juxtainsular lesion affecting the corona radiata)	Cortectomy SI + large parts of superior and inferior parietal gyri	0%	At autopsy, iuxtainsular lesion in corona radiata
Horrax (1946)	CP, glioma of the left hemisphere	Corpus-callosectomy of parietal associative fibers	0%	
		Tumor excision	0%	
		SI gyrectomy	Relief at 14 mos, except arm/hand pain relapsed after 5 mos	
	CP, rolandoparietal glioma	SI gyrectomy	Relief until death mos later	
	SCI (bony spur at C6)	SI gyrectomy	0%	
Leriche (1949)	Thalamic lesion (1 pt)	Procaine injection into SI	Relief for 2 mos	
Stone (1950)	CPSP (1 pt)	Subpial section of the postcentral gyrus	Relief for at least 14 mos	No benefit from previous cervical cordotomy
Penfield and Welch (1951)	Thalamic lesion (1 pt)	SI gyrectomy	Relief for 18 mos, then relapse	SI stimulation triggered patient's pain
		MI (atrophied) gyrectomy	Relief, then relapse	
Lewin and Phillips (1952)	CP; brain injury (1 pt)	Excision of the cerebrodural scar + underlying subcortical cyst	Relief for 4 years	Convulsive seizures preceded by an aura including torturing, deep, gnawing pain in the wrist and hand, spreading to the left limbs and left side of the face
Erickson and colleagues (1952)	CP; thalamic (2 pts)	SI in toto gyrectomy	Relief for 2 years in both	
Spiegel et al. (1952)	CP (1 pt)	SI gyrectomy	No relief	
White and Sweet (1955)	CPSP (1 pt)	SI gyrectomy	Relief for 18 mos, then relapse	No benefit from previous cervical cordotomy
Biemond (1956)	CPSP (1 pt)	Limited (2 cm) SI cortectomy + insulectomy	Relief for months until relapse	At autopsy: softening in the parietal and insular cortex, degenerated fiber

Reference	Condition (patients)	Procedure	Outcome	Comments
Hamby (1961)	Pure cortical CP (1 pt)	Transpial incision five mm deeper than the gutters of the gyri along the posterior edge of SI and over three contiguous parietal gyri. Removal of the cortex and adjacent U-fiber areas of the white matter	Relief for 10 years	bundle tracing to thalamus (VPM) through the internal capsule, cell loss in VPM. Painful, prickling sensations in the arm and hand elicited from stimulation of SI
White and Sweet (1969)	CP, postcordotomy	SI gyrectomy (bar face sector) down to the sulcus cinguli	0%	Pain evoked by SI stimulation
Lende et al. (1971)	CPSP, brainstem (1 pt)	Cortectomy of SI–SII and MI	Relief for 20 mos	Pain not relieved by previous complete trigeminal rhizotomy
Psychosurgery				
Guillaume et al. (1949)	Thalamic syndrome (2 pts)	Frontal lobotomy	"Indifference" toward pain, which was still present and severe (one resumed some activity after surgery)	
Wertheimer and Mansuy (1949)	CCP (1 pt)	Frontal lobotomy	0%	
Freeman and Watts (1950)	CP, thalamic (1 pt)	Prefrontal lobotomy	Relief	
Scarff (1950)	CPSP (1 pt)	Left prefrontal lobotomy	Good relief, relapse at 4 mos	In other pains, unilateral lobotomy may relieve bilateral pains
Gaches (1952)	CP, brain (1 pt)	Frontal lobotomy	Improved, but not abolished	
Drake and McKenzie (1953)	Mesencephalotomy-induced CP (1 pt)	Frontal lobotomy	No	
Petit-Dutaillis et al. (1953)	CP, brain (1 pt)	Frontal lobotomy	Not available for review	
Le Beau et al. (1954)	CP (5 pts)	Bilateral BA 9–10 topectomy	Almost complete, but pain admitted on interrogation/ follow-up 4 years; 0%/follow-up 6 mos	

(continued)

TABLE 7.1 (continued)

Author(s)	Cause of central pain	Procedure	Efficacy/(follow-up)	Notes
Psychosurgery (continued)				
Le Beau et al. (continued)		Unilateral BA9–10 topectomy	Complete relief after 2nd surgery/follow-up not specified	
		Bilateral orbital gyrectomy	10–20% relief for 2.5 yrs	
		Unilateral frontal lobotomy	0% over 2 weeks	
Botterell et al. (1954)	CP; SCI (not available)	Prefrontal lobotomy	Gratifying (follow-up: not available)	
White and Sweet (1955, 1969)	CP (2 pts)	Bilateral orbital gyrectomy (BA 11–12)	Failure, then success at 2nd operation	
			0%	
	CPSP (1 pt)	Unilateral frontal leukotomy	Pain sometimes felt, but not bothering; total disappearance over 2 yrs until death another 2 years later (patient had neglect)	
	CCP, postcordotomy (4 pts)	Fractionated radiofrequency frontomedial leukotomy	Burning relieved, but PNP-associated hyperpathia 0% 100% immediate relief; total relapse at 2.5 mos 0% (2 pts)	
	CCP (1 pt)	Unilateral frontal leukotomy	Not complete relief, but no longer in need of analgesics for 16 years	
Constans (1960)	CP; brain (1 pt)	Frontal operation	Unsatisfactory	
Wycis and Spiegel (1962)	Tabes dorsalis (2 pts) CP (1 pt)	Bilateral prefrontal lobotomy	0%	Transitory relief with mesencephalotomy, then relapse
Foltz and White (1966)	SCI CP (3 pts)	Rostral cingulumotomy	1 fair at 4 yrs and 1 poor at 3 yrs (unilateral); 1 excellent at 1 yr, then fair at 2.5 yrs (bilateral cingulumotomy)	

270

Study	Patients	Procedure	Result	Comments
Porter et al. (1966)	CP; SCI	Prefrontal lobotomy	Gratifying	
Spiegel et al. (1966)	CPSP (1 pt)	Bilateral anterior capsulotomy	0%	
Nashold and Wilson (1970)	1 CPSP (brainstem)	Unilateral left frontal lobotomy	0%	
Turnbull (1972)	Tabes dorsalis (2 pts)	Bilateral cingulotomy	Relief	
Bouchard et al. (1977)	CP; brain (2 pts)	Ipsilateral cingulotomy	No benefit	
		Contralateral cingulotomy	Benefit	
Jefferson (1983)	CP; SCI (1 pt)	Bilateral stereotactic cingulotomy	"Reasonable relief"	Previous unsuccessful cordotomy
Ballantine and Giriunas (1988)	CP; brain (3 pts)	Bilateral stereotactic cingulotomy	No substantial relief	
Tasker (1990)	CP; SCI (1 pt)	Bilateral stereotactic cingulotomy	No relief	Followed by unsuccessful bilateral medial thalamotomy and mesencephalic tractotomy
Pillay and Hassenbusch (1992)	CP; brain (1 pt)	Bilateral stereotactic cingulotomy	No (VAS from 9 to 8); quality of life unchanged	
Mazars et al. (1976) cite two cases of thalamic pain submitted to frontal lobotomy by Siocet and Bartich with improvement, but not abolition				
Hypophysectomy–hypothalamotomy				
Mayanagi and Sano (1988, 1998); plus Amano et al. 1976 (in Japanese)	CP; brain and cord (at least 2 or more BCP pts)	Posterior hypothalamotomy (medial; III ventricle gray matter)	No (0–25% in one CPSP at max. follow-up 17 mos)	Pain increased by electrical stimulation in 2 pts
Levin (1988)	CP (7 pts)	Stereotactic chemical hypophysectomy	More than 50% relief in 6, 2 still relieved 2 yrs later; at least 2 relapses within a few mos	Several complications
Miles (1998)	CCP (1 pt) plus another CP?	Hypophyseal stimulation	0%	
Hayashi et al. (2005)	CPSP, thalamic (17 pts)	Pituitary gamma knife radiosurgery at the border between the pituitary stalk and gland (max. dose 140–160 Gy, 180 in 1 pt)	13/17 had pain reduction (within 48 hours): 76.5% At longer term (> 1 yr): 5/13 "effective relief" (in 1 pt >80% relief); 4/13 fully relapsed within 3 mos; 4/13 still relieved at 6 mos	Single 8 mm isocenter, 50% isodose line covered the border between the pituitary gland and lower part of pituitary stalk No complications Numbness not improved Neuromodulatory effect hypothesized

(continued)

TABLE 7.1 (continued)

Author(s)	Cause of central pain	Procedure	Efficacy//(follow-up)	Notes
Thalamotomies				
Hecaen et al. (1949)	CP (4 pts)	1 center median	Yes, immediate (4 mo)	Thalamic hand and clonus induced by Vc stimulation, no effect with DM stimulation
		1 center median + Vc	Yes, immediate and complete (f-up: 1 yr)	
		2 center median + DM	Yes, immediate and for at least 4 mos	
Talairach et al. (1949)	CP; thalamic (12 pts)	Vc (radioactive gold)	6, 75–100% reliefs; 2, 50% reliefs; 2, 25% reliefs; 2 deaths	
Baudoin and Puech (1949)	CP; brain (1 pt)	Local novocaine injection into Vc	0%	
Spiegel and colleagues (1952)	CP; brain (3 pts)	Vc	Temporary (max. 4.5 mos), in one relapse after a few weeks	
Talairach et al. (1955)	CP; brain (12 pts)	Vc	"Favorable" relief in 50% of pts	
Laspiur (1956)	CP; brain (2 pts)	Vc	Yes (in one, 100% relief, in the latter "spectacular" relief)/follow-up?	
Obrador et al. (1957)	CP; thalamic (2 pts)	Vc	0%	1 suicide
Hassler and Riechert (1959)	CP; brain (1 pt)	Vc	Relief, 5 weeks	
Hassler (1960)	CP; brain (4 pts)	Vc, limitans and CeM	Yes, lasting relief	
Bettag and Yoshida (1960)	CP; thalamic (4 pts)	Vc (3 pts) DM (1 pt)	In all, lasting relief	
Mark et al. (1960)	CP; SCI (4 limb burning dysesthesias) pts?	Vc	Partial pain relief, but recurrence after 6 mos	
Hankinson (1962)	CP; brain (2 pts)	CM and Vc	Yes (16–24 mos)	
Davis and Stokes (1966)	Neurogenic pains	Lateral plus medial nc	Immediate pain relief in 75% of pts, decreasing to 50–60% after 6–12 mos	

Reference	Pain condition	Target/lesion	Results
Bettag (1966)	Neurogenic pains	CM, DM	Persisting pain relief only in 6/31 pts. Pain relief only in 1/4 pts subjected to CM lesions, with or without DM
Spiegel et al. (1966)	CCP (1 pt)	Medial thalamotomy	100% relief; full relapse 1 wk later; 100% relief after reop. At 1.5 yrs, pain reduced
	CPSP (1 pt)	Medial thalamotomy	Partial relief. Late result: indifference to pain
	CPSP (1 pt)	Basal thalamotomy	100% relief for 3 wks, then partial relapse (superficial vs. deep pain) with allodynia, at 3 mos
	SCI pain (1 pt)	Bilateral basal thalamotomy	100% relief, full relapse at 4 mos
Kudo et al. (1968)	CPSP (6 pts) out of 17 with cancer or noncancer pain	Pulvinar	Whole series: 8 complete reliefs, 6 remarkable, 3 slight reliefs; pain remaining
White and Sweet (1969)	CP; brain (1 pt)	Pf (unilateral)	Poor result
	CP; MS (1 pt)	Pf (unilateral)	Good relief
	CCP (cervical) (1 pt)	Vc	Fair relief
	CCP (conocaudal) (1 pt)	Pf (bilateral) and ant. Nc. (unilateral)	Good relief
	Tabes dorsalis (1 pt)	Vc and DM (unilateral)	Poor relief
Sugita et al. (1972)	CP; brain (unspecified)	CeM, Pf, intralaminar, MD	No effect
Siegfried and Krayenbuehl (1972)	Neurogenic pain	Vc, intralaminar system plus DM	No. 1 of 9 pts with Vcpc thalamotomy relieved. Not available for review
Cooper et al. (1973)	Burning hypesthesia and spastic hemiplegia (3 pts)	LP-pulvinotomy	Relief in 3. No relapse. *Acute pain sensation not affected*

(continued)

TABLE 7.1 *(continued)*

Thalamotomies *(continued)*

Author(s)	Cause of central pain	Procedure	Efficacy/(follow-up)	Notes
Amano et al. (1976) (and Sano et al. 1966)	Thalamic CP (10 pts) Other CP (14 pts)	Thalalaminotomy (i.e., CM-Pf and CL)	Thalamic CP: follow-up 1–24 months. At discharge: 100% in 3, slight residual but tolerable pain in 6, 0% relief in 1. At follow-up: 100% in 3, tolerable pain in 4, tolerable pain with drugs in 2, 0% in 1. Other CP: at discharge: 100% in 2, slight residual but tolerable pain in 6, tolerable with drugs in 3, some relief but intolerable in 1, 0% in 2. At follow-up: 100% in 2, tolerable in 4, tolerable with drugs in 3, some relief but intolerable in 2, 0% in 2	
Mayanagi and Bouchard (1976–77)	CP (thalamic: 3 pts)	Basal: CM +/− pulvinar	Follow-up: 6 mos CP "difficult to control"	
Mundinger and Becker (1977)	CP	Medial nc	40% good; total relief up to 14.5 yrs	
Siegfried (1977)	CP + neurogenic pain (13 pts)	Pulvinar	Yes, dramatic initial relief in several. Recurrence within 1 yr in several	*Some had subtle sensory alterations*
Pagni (1977)	CP; brain CP; SCI	Intralaminar nc (including CM/Pf), sometimes extending to Vc and DM	Total or partial long-term relief in 12 BCP and 3 CCP Pagni's experience with CP: 30% relief	Survey. Dysesthesia can persist unmodified. Multiple thalamic (CM-VPL/VPM-pulvinar) and mesencephalic coagulations may be necessary if lesions to a single structure are unsuccessful. Center median lesions "very effective" for thalamic pain, with long-lasting results. Basal thalamotomies for

Reference	Diagnosis	Procedure	Result	Comments
Yoshii and colleagues (1980)	CP (14 pts)	Pulvinar (bilateral if needed; supranucleus pulvinaris medialis nc lesion in all cases)	Yes, *immediate complete* in 6 pts, almost complete in 7 pts, good in 1 pt. At 3.5–10 yrs: 4 pain-free, 4 almost pain-free, 3 sufficient pain relief, 3 failures. Cases with follow-up > 5 yrs: 1 pain-free, 2 almost pain-free, 3 sufficient pain relief, 2 failures	brainstem lesions. Long-term results with CM-Vc, intralaminar and DM lesions generally unsatisfactory. No bearing on final outcome from bilateral lesions
Hitchcock and Texteira (1981)	CP, brain (3 pts) Postc ordotomy/thoracotomy dysesthesias (5 pts); CP, brain (6 pts). Postcordotomy dysesthesias (1 pt)	Basal (including Vcpc and n. limitans portae); Medial (CM), some bilateral	Yes (2/3 pts); Yes (5/5 pts); Yes (5/6 pts); Yes	CM thalamotomies deemed superior, particularly if bilateral, to basal thalamotomies (better pain relief and fewer side effects). Very high rate of complications
Niizuma et al. (1982) Includes Niizuma et al. (1980)	CPSP (17 pts, one of which cheiroral)	Unilateral/bilateral center median	Relief (1, 100%) in 56%, then full relapse within 7 mos in all	
Barcia Salorio et al. (1987)	CPSP (2 pts)	LINAC radiosurgical Vc thalamotomy	Burning paroxysms abolished, background pain diminished/follow-up 6 mos	
Laitinen (1988; see also 1977)	CPSP (2 pts)	CM thalamotomy	Yes (6–24 mos)	CM-intralaminar and pulvinar lesions highly effective for CP. However, in a mixed series of cancer and neurogenic pain, only 29% were pain-free after 2.5 yrs
	CPSP (3 pts)	CM-intralaminar thalamotomy	Yes, *immediately* (8–18 mos)	
	SCI (1 pt)	CT-guided pulvinarectomy	Good early result	
Ohye (1990, 1998)	CPSP, mainly deep muscle pain (about 40 pts)	Vim (a part)-Vcpc (deep portion) thalamotomy (i.e., coagulation of the isolated hyperactive area around the thalamic stroke lesion)	Deep pain of compressing, burning or sometimes squeezing nature considerably ameliorated	*No true effect on paresthesia and numbness*

(continued)

TABLE 7.1 (*continued*)

Author(s)	Cause of central pain	Procedure	Efficacy//(follow-up)	Notes
Thalamotomies (*continued*)				
Jeanmonod *et al.* (1996, 2001)	CP, parietal cortex (5 pts), thalamus (3 pts), brainstem (4 pts), spinal cord (12 pts)	Medial thalamotomies (if necessary, lesion ipsilateral to pain)	Yes, 50–100% relief in 40% of BCP pts and 38% of SCI pts. Relief was best for evoked and intermittent pain and superficial pain, poorer for steady pain (which lingered on in more than half the cases) and deep pain	*Relief only of deep pain and not superficial or dysesthetic pain* Satisfactory relief in 4/9 Generally without postop. somato-sensory – including pain – deficits; in several, postop. improvement of somatosensory deficits
	CPSP (9 pts)	Vim and/or CL thalamotomy	Satisfactory relief in 4/9	
			One CCP patient referred by us: 0% relief (+ complications)	
Hirato *et al.* (1995)	CPSP (thalamic and putaminal) (2 pts)	Radiosurgical Vim thalamotomy	A: Vim thalamotomy: some relief, relapse, radiosurgical Vim thalamotomy, relief B: Vim thalamotomy: poor relief, gamma thalamotomy good relief (not abolition) for 3 mos	Relief seen in both after 3–6 mos (!?)
Young *et al.* (1995)	CP (thalamic) (3 pts) SCI pain (1 pt)	Gamma knife medial thalamotomy	Median follow-up for whole group of 20 mixed pains pts; about 1 yr relief seems to have been obtained in at least some	
Frighetto *et al.* (2004)	CPSP (MCA stroke and thalamic stroke) (2 pts)	Radiosurgical CM/Pf thalamotomy	A: immediate relief, relapse at 4 mos (relieved by MCS) B: some drug reduction, allodynia improved, 3 yrs later drugs only twice a week	No 100% abolition; effect on pain before onset of necrosis (!); necroses 3.5 × 5 mm and 8.5 × 7 mm (too large to have exclusively targeted CM-PF)

Mesencephalotomies (STT tractotomies and reticulotomies) and other brainstem procedures (coagulations)

Walker (1942)	Thalamic pain (1 pt)	Open lateral	Death after 26 h	
Torvik (1959)	CP (2 pts)		Not available for review	
Wycis and Spiegel (1962) *Including patients reported in previous series*	CPSP (14 pts)	Spinothalamic tract plus reticular formation at midbrain level	11 initial pain disappearances or abatements, 3 failures, 2 deaths	3 mesencephalotomies plus thalamotomies: 1 complete relief for 10 yrs, 1 partial relief, 1 transient indifference
	CP due to parietal lesions (2 pts)	As per above, plus possible thalamic impingement	Follow-up: 4 full relapses (1-5 mos), 2 partial relapses (1-5 mos), 5 long-term good reliefs	
	1 (pontine lesion)		Pain relief (6 mos)	
	1 (ACoA aneurysm)		0% relief	
Helfant et al. (1965)	CCP (3 pts)	Mesencephalotomy	1 complete relief for 1 yr, 1 transient relief, 10%	
	CPSP (thalamic) (1 pt)	STT	0%	
Orthner and Roeder (1966) *Includes Roeder and Orthner (1961)*	CPSP (1 pt)	Lateral plus medial lesions	*Almost complete relief for 26 mos up to death*	
Gioia et al. (1967)	CP + neurogenic pain (2 pts)	Medial lesion	Poor	
Turnbull (1972)	Tabes dorsalis (1 pt)	Combined mesencephalotomy-thalamotomy-cingulotomy	1 modest relief	
Schvarcz (1977)	CP (5 pts?)	Mesencephalotomy	4 pain reliefs at 6-24 mos	Not available for review
Amano et al. (1980, 1986, 1992)	CPSP (25 pts) CP; tumor (1 pt) Postcordotomy dysesthesia-PCD (1 pt) Tabetic pain-TB (1 pt)	Rostral mesencephalic reticulotomy (highly selective lesion in the medialmost portion of the midbrain reticular formation, medial to the STT which is not lesioned unlike Nashold's procedure) contralateral to pain in all cases	Group 1: 2 complete reliefs, 3 partial reliefs at 50-70 mos Group 2: 6 complete reliefs, 9 almost complete reliefs, 6 partial reliefs at <50 mos PCD 0% relief. TB almost complete relief at 57 mos	Results confirmed in 1992. 64% complete or near complete pain relief. No postop. dysesthesias One of the pts relieved 100% at 11 yrs noticed at year 7-8 tactile-thermoalgesic anesthesia of left hemisoma

(continued)

TABLE 7.1 (continued)

Mesencephalotomies and other brainstem procedures (continued)

Author(s)	Cause of central pain	Procedure	Efficacy/(follow-up)	Notes
Shieff and Nashold (1988) (includes all patients from Nashold's previous publications on this treatment) (1963–1985)	CPSP, brain (20 pts); CPSP, brainstem (7 pts)	Lesion at: 1. medial lesions at superior colliculus level	14 early pts: 5, 100% reliefs; 6 fair (minimal residual pain, non-opioids required); 3, 0% reliefs	4 pts with repeat early surgery, 6 reoperated for late relapse and 1 pain-free after 4 procedures
			12 late pts (+ 1 death + 1 lost to follow-up): 7, 100% reliefs; 2 fair, 1 poor (significant residual pain), 2 0% (follow-up: 3–60 mos)	*Unilateral lesions relieved bilateral pain*
		2. lesions at inferior colliculus level	13 early pts: 5, 100% reliefs, 5 fair; 1 poor; 1, 0% (1 moribund); 12 late pts: 4, 100%; 3 fair; 2 poor; 3, 0%	*Gradual disappearance of pain* *Lesion impinging on reticular formation*
Laitinen (1988)	Thalamic pain (2 pts) Paraplegia pain (1 pt)	STT	? ?	Whole neurogenic pain group: 25% relieved at 3 yrs. Complications in half, including new dysesthesias
Sampson and Nashold (1992)	CPSP (brainstem) (2 pts)	Caudalis DREZ	1 complete relief, 1 partial relief (4–48 mos)	Arm ataxia
Gorecki and Nashold (1995)	CPSP (4–5 pts?)		50% relief at 3 mos?	
Tasker et al. (1991)	Brain CP (11 pts)	Mesencephalotomy with/without medial thalamotomy	Steady pain relieved in 3 (plus other 3 temporarily) and failed in 5; intermittent pain relieved in the only pt who had it; evoked pain relieved in 3 and unrelieved in 2	Evoked pain more responsive than steady pain
Bosch (1991)	Thalamic pain (2 pts)	Rostral mesencephalotomy	0% relief at 1 yr	

Teixeira *et al.* (1998, 2003)	CP, Wallenberg (7 pts)	Bulbar trigeminal stereotactic nucleotractotomy	Orofacial pain <VAS 3 in 85.7% of pts immediately and at follow-up (2 yrs)	1 pt full relapse in 4 weeks and one partial relapse in 6 mos. One repeat procedure
	CP, brainstem	Caudalis DREZ	Failure	
Midline commissural myelotomy (and stereotactic central C1 myelotomy)				
Sourek (1969)	2 MS and 1 tabes dorsalis (pain at L2-S2 in both MS and L1-S1 in tabes)	Commissurotomy at D10-11/12 in MS and D11-L1 in tabes	All 3 immediately relieved after surgery. 1 MS case had no relapse at 1 yr (at 6 mos girdle pinprick analgesia disappeared). No follow-up in other 2 due to poor general conditions	
Lippert *et al.* (1974)	1 paraplegia pain at T11	Surgery at T12-S4	Over 7 mos relief from 80 to 20%	Follow-up: NA
	1 MS paraplegia pain	Surgery at T12-S2	Relief over 6 mos	
	1 transverse myelitis with girdle pain	Surgery at T5-8	Much relieved	
King (1977)	1 gunshot wound to L1	Commissurotomy at T11-S1	Total relief (26 mos, until death)	
Schvarcz (1978)	1 MS	Stereotactic trigeminal nucleotomy	Details as of CP not given	
	3 spinal lesions	Stereotactic extralemniscal myelotomy	0.5-6 yrs follow-up	
Anterolateral cordotomies (spinothalamic tractotomies)				
Frazier *et al.* (1937)	CPSP (1 pt)	Right, then left cordotomy (C5 and C3)	Relief for 6 mos, then for 2.5 mos until death	Facial pain treated by gasserian ganglion alcohol injection
Turnbull (1939)	CP, brain (1 pt)	C3 anterolateral cordotomy	*Immediate abolition of pain* *Follow-up: 1 yr*	No relief from previous sympathetic block
Kuhn (1947)	CP, cord	Cordotomy	Partially effective	
Freeman and Heimburger (1947)	SCI CP (45 pts)	Cordotomy	Partially effective; 96% relief at 18 mos	
Davis and Martin (1947)	SCI pain (18 pts)	Cordotomy	1 lasting relief, 2 for 1-2 wks with full relapse, all others failures	

(continued)

TABLE 7.1 (continued)

Author(s)	Cause of central pain	Procedure	Efficacy/(follow-up)	Notes
Anterolateral cordotomies (continued)				
Stone (1950)	CPSP (1 pt)	Cervical anterolateral cordotomy	0%	
Pollock and colleagues (1951)	CP, cord (16 pts)	Cervical anterolateral cordotomy	2 total pain reliefs 9 abolition of end-zone pain (but not diffuse pains) 5 failures	
Drake and McKenzie (1953)	CP after lateral mesencephalotomy (1 pt)	Spinothalamic tractotomy at bulbar level	100% relief	Temporary relief from cortectomy (see Table)
Botterell et al. (1954)	CP; complete SCI (5 pts)	Bilateral high thoracic cordotomy	3 excellent or good pain reliefs (2, 3, 8 yrs); 1 early failure, 1 late failure (6 yrs)	In each case, pain was sharp, cramping, stabbing and episodic. Burning pain in saddle area present in 2 cases, eliminated in 1
White and Sweet (1955)	CP, brain (1 pt)	Anterolateral cordotomy at C2	No pain relief	Electrical and burning sensations, allodynia
Krueger (1960)	CP; postcordotomy (1 pt)	Higher cordotomy	Pain abolition	Not available for review
Bohm (1960)	CP; cord	Cordotomy	Partially effective	Previous bilateral thoracic cordotomy. Burning pain
	CP; postcordotomy (1 pt)	Lower bilateral cordotomy	0%	
Porter et al. (1966)	SCI CP and root damage (34 pts)	Bilateral T1-T3 cordotomies	0% for burning pain in the legs	Shooting or electrical-like pain relieved at least partially in 87% at 1–3 mos and 62% at 8–20 yrs (cauda pain) Rhizotomy unsuccessful in cases subsequently relieved by cordotomy *Burning leg pain not an indication*
Waltz and Ehni (1966)	CPSP (1 pt)	Unilateral C2 anterolateral cordotomy	*100% relief, full relapse at 6 mos*	

Study	Patients	Procedure	Results
Joyner et al. (1966) (Freeman coauthor: see above)	CP, cord	Cordotomy	Partially effective
White and Sweet (1969)	Paraplegia pain (12 pts)	High thoracic cordotomy	8 late reliefs (9 early)
	Tabetic crises (6 pts)		5 late reliefs (6 early)
	Paraplegia pain (2 pts)	High cervical cordotomy	1 early plus 1 late failure
	Tabetic crises (3 pts)		2 reliefs (plus 1 early failure)
	Thalamic pain (1 pt)		1 early failure
			Follow-up: up to 12 yrs
Sweet (1991)	CP, brain (1 pt)	Cervical anterolateral cordotomy	*Pain relief*
Tasker et al. (1992)	34 (cord CP)	Percutaneous cervical cordotomy	Steady pain: c. 75% of pts unrelieved; 20% of pts relieved 25–50%; the rest relieved >50%
			Intermittent pain: c. half the pts relieved >50%; c. one third relieved 25–50%; the rest unrelieved
			Evoked pain: half the pts relieved >50%, one-fourth 25–50% and the rest unrelieved
			Results at 1 year
Parent et al. (1992)	CPSP (1 pt)	Cordotomy	0%
Cordectomies			
Armour (1927)	SCI pain	Cordectomy at the lower end of the cord and adjacent cauda equina (T12–L2)	Complete pain relief in thighs and lower abdomen. War conocaudal injury
Davis and Martin (1947)	CP; cord (1 pt)	Cordectomy	0%
Freeman and Heimburger (1947)	CP; cord	Removal of a 2–3 cm cord segment at T3–4	Unsuccessful. Leg pain

(continued)

TABLE 7.1 (*continued*)

Author(s)	Cause of central pain	Procedure	Efficacy/(follow-up)	Notes
Cordectomies (*continued*)				
McCarty (1954)	Traumatic T7 total transverse lesion; pain at T5–6 (1 pt)	Removal of the lower 21 cm of the cord from T5 down to the conus	Narcotics stopped/follow-up: 6 mos; Annoying girdle pains relieved 6 mos later and occasional root pain at T5	
Botterell *et al.* (1954)	SCI (thoracic gunshot) pain (1 pt)	Excision of the damaged cord up to grossly normal cord +T4–5 rhizotomy	Girdle pain at lesion level totally relieved for 8 yrs; Burning pain in the feet arising after cordectomy	
Smolik *et al.* (1960)	SCI pain (4 pts), including 1 pt with anterior spinal artery syndrome – ASAS	Cord removal from the T10 level down through conus medullaris and upper cauda equina	Pain and spasm relief in 2 pts; Unsuccessful in ASAS pt despite flaccidity	
Werner (1961)	SCI pain (1 pt)	Cordectomy	Pain persistence after first myelectomy. Pain relief after a 2nd myelectomy	End-zone pain. First resection left the scarred proximal cord stump adhering to the dura
Druckman and Lende (1965)	SCI pain (1 pt)	Cordectomy just above trauma level (T11 vertebra); Second higher cordectomy 3 cm above previous one in normal tissue	No pain relief; Complete pain relief. Follow-up: 18 mos. Persistence of mild burning in legs	Conocaudal injury. Pain in lower abdominal and inguinal areas + mild burning in legs + girdle pain. No pain relief from a previous bilateral T11–12 rhizotomy
Druckman (1966)	SCI pain (1 pt)	Cordectomy above injury through normal cord	Pain relief. Follow-up: 12 mos	
White and Sweet (1969)	SCI pain (2 pts)	1. Limited cordectomy; 2. Cordectomy up to T11	No pain relief; Pain relief. Follow-up 4 yrs	Severe burning pains in legs
Melzack and Loeser (1978)	SCI pain (5 pts) with complete transection	Cordectomy at various levels	2 unsuccessful (burning pain in legs, abdomen, buttocks); 1 partial (1st cordectomy at T9–12 abolished part of the	Sympathetic blocks ineffective

Reference	Patients	Procedure	Outcome	Comments
Nashold and Bullitt (1981)	SCI pain (2 pts)	Cordectomy of tethered cord	pain for 2 yrs with worsening at 3rd year; 2nd one at T4-5 ineffective	T4 fracture; severe pain in legs only upon head flexion
		1 cm long low thoracic cordectomy	2 pain reliefs (paroxysmal shooting pains in legs abolished for 11.5 yrs with full relapse; thoracoabdominal pain abolished by T8-9 operation with gradual full relapse by 5 yrs)	T12-L1 fracture; pain in both legs
Durward et al. (1982)	SCI pain (6 pts), in 5 also posttraumatic syringomyelia	Cordectomy somewhat above the area of trauma at T6-8 (upper level of transection below the upper level of the syrinx) in 3 (1-4 yrs after CP onset)	Pain abolished; Pain relief. Follow-up: 12 yrs; Pain relief of arm pain in 3	
		Cordectomy at various thoracic levels (T2 for a C6 lesion, T4-5 for major injury at T7 plus syrinx, T10-12 for same level injury)	No pain relief of leg-buttock pain in 3	
Jefferson (1983, 1987)	SCI pain (19 pts), diffuse to legs in 15	Cordectomy at T11 and/or below	Pain relief: 70-100% in 14/15 pts (100% in 7/14 pts); Partial (leg pain abolished, abdominal-genitals-buttocks pain unrelieved) in 1	Lesions at/below T11 with episodic, electric shock/spasm non-burning pain more likely to respond to cordectomy immediately, completely and permanently
		Cordectomy at T10-11 and T3-7 (+ limited rhizotomy)	0-25% relief	In some cases cured of their pains, there was still severe widespread cord damage at the upper incision level

(continued)

TABLE 7.1 (*continued*)

Author(s)	Cause of central pain	Procedure	Efficacy/(follow-up)	Notes
Cordectomies (*continued*)				
Tasker et al. (1992)	CP, cord (12 pts)	Cordectomy	Steady pain relief: none in 70% of cases, 25–50% in 30% of cases	
			Intermittent pain relief at 1 yr: >50% in 60% of cases, 25–50% in 40% of cases	
			Evoked pain relief (>1 yr): >50% in 80% of cases, 25–50% in 20% of cases	
Pagni and Canavero (1995b)	CP, cord (2 pts)	Cordomyelotomy (T5–SI myelomeres)	Shooting pain/spasms abolished; moderate burning to legs and perineum lessened	Long-lasting (10 yrs) pain relief
DREZ lesions				
Samii and Moringlane (1984)	SCI pain (5 pts)	DREZ lesions	Pain relief: 70–100% in 2/5, 50–70% in 2/5, <50% in 1/5	Pain at T2–3; burning pain in 1, burning and needles in 1, in 3 unspecified
Dieckmann and Veras (1984)	SCI pain (2 pts)	DREZ lesions	0%	
Richter and Seitz (1984)	SCI pain (2 pts)	DREZ lesions	0% benefit	
Thomas and Jones (1984)	SCI CP (1 pt) Tumor CCP (1 pt)	DREZ lesions	Poor relief Good relief	
Wiegand and Winkelmueller (1985)	SCI pain (20 pts)	DREZ lesions	Pain relief (5–34 mos): 100% in 9, 80% in 1	At follow-up, 10 had maintained their early postoperative relief and moved from 80 to 100% relief
Friedman and Bullitt (1988)	SCI pain (56 pts): end-zone pain (31 pts); burning dysesthesic pain (25 pts)	DREZ lesions (lesions from a few segments above to a few segments below)	Pain relief end-zone pain: 74% good (100% relief and/or no analgesics needed OR residual discomfort not interfering with daily living	Bilateral pain resistant, but 9 of 10 with unilateral pain had good relief

Reference	Patients	Procedure	Results	Notes
			activities), 6% fair (still requiring some analgesics), 20% no result	
Powers et al. (1988) (also includes Powers et al. 1984)	CCP (9 pts)	DREZ lesions, laser	Pain relief diffuse dysesthetic pains: 20% good, 12% fair, 68% no results	
	SCI pain (cauda) (2 pts)		5 successes, 4 failures / 0% / Follow-up: 4–63 mos	End-zone pain in 4: all relieved / Below-level pain: relief in 2/8 / Midline (perineal, scrotum) pain: relief in 0/3
Sweet and Poletti (1989)	SCI pain (1 pt), trauma	DREZ lesions at T3–5 +posterior poliotomy (LX ablation)	Complete relief of thoracic end-zone pain and coccygeal/foot pain for 3 mos. At 13 mos, >50% relief	
	CP (1 pt), T12 AVM	Extensive DREZ lesions	0% of diffuse bilateral pain from lower abdomen downwards	
Kumagai et al. (1990)	SCI pain (4 pts)	DREZ	50% relief at 11–30 mos	Not available for review
Young (1990)	SCI pain (26 pts)	DREZ lesions (standard and laser)	55% of pts relieved. Follow-up: up to 5 yrs / 83% of pts with cauda equina lesions relieved	*Midline pain, especially in mid-lumbar area or genitalia, unrelieved*; end-zone pain benefited
Tasker et al. (1992)	SCI pain (4 pts)	DREZ lesions	No effect on steady pain / 25–50% relief on evoked pain present in 2 pts (>1 yr)	
Edgar et al. (1993)	SCI pain and other pains (120 pts)	Computer-assisted DREZ lesions / Standard DREZ lesions	End-zone pain relieved in 92% of pts; follow-up: 2–96 mos / End-zone pain relieved in 58% of pts	93% had diffuse pains and/or sacral pain
Rath et al. (1996)	Paraplegia pain (22 pts)	Junctional DREZotomy	Diffuse burning: 5 failures of 6 / Spinal cord cyst: 5 failures of 7 / End-zone pain relieved in most who had it / Follow-up: mean 54 mos	

(continued)

TABLE 7.1 (continued)

Author(s)	Cause of central pain	Procedure	Efficacy/(follow-up)	Notes
DREZ lesions (continued)				
Nashold and Pearlstein (1996) (includes all previous papers of the Duke's group on this procedure)	Conocaudal pain (39 pts)	DREZ lesions	Pain relief at a mean of 3 yrs: good (no analgesics required) in 54% of pts; fair (nonnarcotics still necessary, but pain not interfering) in 20% of pts 100% relief in 35% of pts at 10 years	Narcotics down from 90% of pts to 12%. Conocaudal pain relieved in 60% *Best results in electric shock pain and end-zone pain* Facial pains abolished in 40% at 10 yrs
Sampson and Nashold (1992)	Pontine CPSP (1 pt) CP, mesencephalic AVM (1 pt)	Caudalis DREZ	100% relief 2 days later over 4 yrs 50% relief 8 days later (death 4 mos later during surgery)	
Sindou et al. (2001) (includes all previous papers of Sindou on this procedure)	SCI (44 pts)	Radicellotomy	>50% pain relief in 14/16 pts (6 mos–7 yrs) Long-term good results in 68% of pts	Below lesion pain not favorably influenced, particularly perineosacral; radiculometameric pain responsive
Prestor (2001)	SCI CP (1 pt) Syrinx CP (6 pts)	Junctional DREZ	0% Excellent relief (83.3%) Good (16.7%) at 6–48 mos	
Falci et al. (2002)	SCI pain (41 pts), generally at T10–L1, but 6 cases at T4–9	DREZ lesions guided by multiple electrophysiological techniques	Group A (9 pts): 100% relief in 56% of pts (50–100% relief in 78%); follow-up: 6–7 yrs Group B (32 pts): 100% relief in 84% (50–100% relief in 88%); follow-up: 1–6 yrs *End-zone pain (present in 6 of 32): 100% relief in all. Below-level pain (present in 26 of*	15% of repeat surgeries 4.7% of pts developed a new permanent pain of low intensity (VAS 1–3) Evaluation: telephone interview and/or outpatient evaluation (VAS/verbal scales)

Reference	Condition	Procedure	Results	Comments
Spaic et al. (2002)	SCI pain (T9–L4) (26) pts	DREZ lesions	32 pts): 100% relief in 81% of pts (50–100% relief in 85%) Thermal pain (burning and similar), steady pain and diffuse infralesional pains: 0% long-term relief. Shooting, cutting, stabbing, sharp, cramping, constriction, throbbing end-zone pains: 100% relief in 70% of pts and >50% relief in 20% at 13–50 mos	
Rogano et al. (2003)	SCI pts (complete/incomplete) (11 pts)	DREZ lesions	VAS from 9.7 to 1.9: end-zone pain only	

Spinal rhizotomies, peripheral blocks, sympathectomies and sympathetic blocks

Reference	Condition	Procedure	Results	Comments
Garcin (1937)	CP (including syringobulbia)	Alcohol injection of the gasserian ganglion	Failure in 2 cases	Review of cases reported by Foix, Foerster, Schaefer, Ravina and Haguenauer, Parker
		Retrogasserian neurotomy	Good-total control of pain	
Frazier et al. (1937)	CPSP (1 pt)	Bilateral cordotomy, alcohol injection of the gasserian ganglion and radicotomy of C2–3	Good results	
Slaughter (1938)	SCI pain, conocaudal, burning	Sympathectomy	Relief	
Turnbull (1939)	BCP (1 pt)	Sympathetic block	Failure	
Hecaen et al. (1949)	CPSP (1 pt)	Sympathetic block Stellectomy.	Failure	
Pollock et al. (1951b)	SCI pain	Sympathectomies	Failure	
Spiegel et al. (1952)	CP (face only) (1 pt)	Trigeminal rhizotomy Stereotactic mesencephalotomy	Failure Benefit	Subsequent unsuccessful cortectomy and lobotomy
Bonica (1953)	CPSP (1 pt)	Repeated paravertebral pantocaine blocks and later subarachnoid alcohol block	Good results for 2 mos, relapse and again benefit from a new block	Peripheral blocks eliminate normal afferent stimuli

(continued)

TABLE 7.1 (continued)

Author(s)	Cause of central pain	Procedure	Efficacy/(follow-up)	Notes
Spinal rhizotomies, peripheral blocks, sympathectomies and sympathetic blocks (continued)				
Rowbotham (1961)	CP, brain (1 pt)	Retrogasserian neurotomy	Failure	
		Stellectomy	Failure	
Campanini and De Risio (1962)	CP, brain (1 pt)	Stellectomy	Good pain relief	
Porter et al. (1966)	SCI pain	Sympathectomy	Failure	
Waltz and Ehni (1966)	CPSP (1 pt)	Sympathetic lidocaine block	Failure	
White and Sweet (1969)	CPSP, Wallenberg (1 pt)	Alcohol injection of III branch of trigeminal n. and later gasserian ganglion	Failures	
		Retrogasserian rhizotomy		
		Alcoholic injection of the thoracic sympathetic chain		
		Sympathectomy		
	CP, syringobulbia	Trigeminal rhizotomy	Failures	
	CP (several pts)	Sympathectomies	Failures	
	CCP, postcordotomy (1 pt)	Rhizotomy	Failure	
Nashold and Wilson (1970)	CPSP, brainstem (1 pt)	Peripheral blocks (local anesthetic, alcohol) in trigeminal branches	0% relief	
Hannington-Kiff (1974)	CPSP (6 pts)	Guanethidine sympathetic block	6/6 pain relief	Placebo (saline) or bupivacaine ineffective
Melzack and Loeser (1978)	SCI pain (5 pts) with complete transection	Sympathetic blocks	Failure	
Loh et al. (1981) (likely includes almost all pts previously published in Loh et al. (1980) and Loh and Nathan (1978), where apparently a	1. CP, brainstem (no confirmatory CT scan)	1. Guanethidine block (leg)	1. Complete permanent relief	All pts had burning pain plus several kinds of allodynia/hyperpathia
	2. CPSP	2. Sympathetic chain block	2. 50% 1 h relief	*No placebo injections!*
	3. CPSP	3a. Guanethidine block 1	3a. Pain and allodynia much	Only pts with hyperpathia-allodynia

further tumor CCP case and a postcordotomy CP case were also included)

Condition	Treatment	Result	Comments
	3b. Guanethidine block 2	improved for 5 days 3b. No effects	
	3c. Guanethidine block 3	3c. Pain almost gone, allodynia much improved for 40 h	Also, guanethidine infusion did *not completely* block sympathetic control of digital blood vessels.
4. CPSP (negative CT scan)	4a. Sympathetic chain block	4a. Complete relief for 2.5–48 h	No effects on sensibility of normally innervated regions, but pts may notice an area of diminished sensibility and numbness restricted to the territory of the damaged nerve
	4b. Guanethidine block	4b. Complete relief for 12 h	
5. CCP (Schneider's syndrome)	5a. Sympathetic chain block	5a. 50% relief of burning and allodynia improved for 20 h	
	5b. Guanethidine block	5b. Slight relief of pain, allodynia slight or moderate relief for 24 h	
6. CP, multiple sclerosis	6a. Guanethidine block 1	6a. Burning improved (?), allodynias removed or much improved for 4–6 h	Pain relief beyond area of block in 2 cases. Case 4: stellate block *also blocked leg pain*; case 3: neck-ear pain relieved, *plus shoulder pain*
	6b. Guanethidine block 2	6b. Burning abolished, allodynias abolished or much improved for 60 h	
	6c. Guanethidine block 3	6c. Burning 75% reduced, allodynias abolished or much improved for 20 h	Stellate block: local anesthetic; IV guanet: 15 mg in 30 ml saline
	6d. Guanethidine block 4	6d. Burning 50% reduced, allodynias improved or much improved for 20–24 h	
	6e. Guanethidine block 5	6e. Burning abolished, allodynias abolished or improved for 4–6 h	
	6f. Iontophoretic guanethidine 1 and 2	6f. Pain reduced in fingers	
7. CP, multiple sclerosis	7a. Guanethidine block 1	7a. Slight effect on burning and allodynia for 2 h	

(continued)

TABLE 7.1 (continued)

Spinal rhizotomies, peripheral blocks, sympathectomies and sympathetic blocks (continued)

Author(s)	Cause of central pain	Procedure	Efficacy/(follow-up)	Notes
Loh et al. (continued)		7b. Guanethidine block 2	7b. Burning halved, allodynia much improved or abolished for 60 h	
		7c. Guanethidine block 3	7c. Burning halved, allodynia modestly improved for 3 h	
	8. CP, cervical astrocytoma	8a. Left sympathetic chain block	8a. Burning almost abolished and allodynia improved for 1 h	
		8b. Right guanethidine block 1	8b. Burning halved, allodynia improved for 1 h	
		8c. Guanethidine block 2	8c. Burning halved, allodynia improved for 1 h	
		8d. Iontophoretic guanethidine 1 and 2 in phalanges	8d. Tenderness improved, allodynia gone	
Tasker et al. (1992)	CCP (5 pts)	Rhizotomy (L4, T12–L1, L1–2 bilaterally, intercostal nerves)	Pain relief in 2/5 (C4, T5–12) (hyperpathia only)	Rhizotomy only transiently effective for steady pain and then worsening
D. Long (comment to Milhorat et al. 1996)	Syringomyelia CP	Sympathectomy	Most failures	
Milhorat et al. (1996, 1997)	Syringomyelia SCI CP (2 out of 15 pts)	1. Sympathetic block with 10 ml of 0.25% bupivacaine, then stellate ganglionectomy	1. Prolonged relief, then 100% relief at 5 mos	
	Syringomyelia CP (1 pt)	2. Similar blocks sympathectomy	2. Relief 100% relief 22 mos later	
Yamamoto et al. (1997)	CPSP, thalamic and suprathalamic (39 pts)	Stellate ganglion block	Failure	Stellate ganglion block with 10 ml of 0.5% mepivacaine and to cervical or lumbar epidural block with 5 ml of 0.5% mepivacaine

290

between individuals, but also between hemispheres in an individual (Penfield above). Anyway, SI cortectomies have a better track record than, for instance, frontal operations, including cingulectomy/cingulotomy and focal lesions of SI can indeed abolish CP in a somatotopographical fashion (Canavero *et al.* 2001). As suggested by electrophysiologic data (section on neurophysiology above), cortical stimulation studies (Chapter 6) and sudden disappearances of CP following lesions ipsilateral to pain (section on reports of sudden disappearance of CP below), *some failures of cortectomies and thalamotomies to relieve CP – but also cases of CP with apparent total destruction of SI – can simply be chalked up to lesioning the wrong side, as the corticothalamic loop we posit at the basis of CP has shifted ipsilaterally to pain* (Chapter 8). After SI damage, input may also be rechanneled to *surviving areas of SI* or other sensory zones (e.g., SII) (see Bittar *et al.* 2000). In sum, SI is involved in the mechanism of CP.

A considerable amount of evidence suggests that SI has a pivotal role in sensory discrimination/localization of pain (reviewed in Willis and Westlund 2004). The inconsistency of results of early lesion and functional imaging studies (only half reported SI activation) on the role of SI in pain processing has been explained: the probability of obtaining SI activation appears related to the total amount of body surface stimulated (spatial summation) and probably also by temporal summation and attention to the stimulus (see Schnitzler and Ploner 2000). Anatomically, SI consists of four cytoarchitectonically defined areas, each with a representation of the body surface; unlike the tactile modality (reviewed in Iwamura 1998), pain processing appears to be less hierarchically organized, with *BA1 as main focus of nociceptive* processing with nociceptive neurons clusters in layer III–IV (Schnitzler and Ploner 2000; Willis and Westlund 2004).

Unlike all other cortical areas (including SII and ACC), SI is the *only one with a clear somatotopic organization* on neuroimaging studies (Coghill *et al.* 1999), an essential pathophysiologic consideration. Actually, *SI does not truthfully map the body surface (somatotopic homunculus) on all occasions* but, depending on the stimulus, may represent an internal brain image that is linked to subjective perception, rather than to objective sensory input, being activated in a manner that corresponds to the perceived stimulus. Thus, representations on SI may both reflect integrated higher brain functions and simple topographic representations of physical stimuli detected by the periphery. The degree of SI activation enabling emergence of a perceived image is related to the type of information that generates the illusion. In many cases, the image of the world within the brain is congruent with neither the "real" nor the perceived world (Eysel 2003).

SI may be directly involved in elemental awareness with a role of 40 Hz coherence in conscious perception at 150–300 ms (Meador *et al.* 2002) (but not at 40 ms; Preissl *et al.* 2001). However, conscious awareness of a stimulus location on the body likely involves the interaction of other brain regions along with SI, including BA40 (inferior parietal lobule) and portions of the dorsolateral prefrontal cortex (DLPFC). Moreover, pain is highly intrusive, attention-grabbing and is widely distributed (SI, PCC, DLPFC, ACC).

Human evidence indicates that SII is involved in recognition of the painful nature of the stimulus (particularly if moving) and may play an attentional role (hence, its bilaterality of activation), but is clearly not essential for stimulus localization/discrimination (see Schnitzler and Ploner 2000; Fujiwara *et al.* 2002); in humans, it receives few fibers from Vc (Kaas 2004). Unlike tactile input, noxious input simultaneously activates SI and SII (see Schnitzler and Ploner 2000; see also Hobson *et al.* 2002). First pain is particularly related to SI activation, second pain to ACC activation; both are associated with SII activation (Ploner *et al.* 2002). Actually, SII and the (right) posterior insula may be considered as a unique structure (and cannot be separately resolved by present day PET) (see also Frot and Mauguiere 2003). The insula may integrate pain-related input from SII and the thalamus with contextual information from other modalities before relaying this information to the temporal lobe limbic structures (pain-related avoidance memory/learning) and to autonomic stations (amygdala, brainstem, etc.). Patients with insular lesions recognize a stimulus as painful, but exhibit absent or inappropriate affective responses (Berthier *et al.* 1988), as early stages of affect are mediated in the insula.

The posterior parietal cortex (PPC, BA5-7) may play a role in conscious pain perception and body awareness (Witting *et al.* 2001) and in the initial stages of cortical motor planning (Driver and Mattingley 1998). PPC receives input from SI and SII, while the DLPFC and the PPC are the most densely connected areas of the association cortex (and may actually process attentional-orientation toward incoming sensory input). Lesions to PPC produce multisensory (body schema) neglect syndromes. Nonetheless, a role in CP is questioned by Hoogenraad and colleagues (1994), who described a 46-year-old man with ischemic infarction of the right parietal cortex following carotid dissection and, among others, left hemianesthesia with almost complete loss of all sensory modalities. MRI disclosed an infarction involving the *posterior part of the postcentral (SI)*, supramarginal and angular gyri plus inferior and superior parietal lobe. Over the next month the patient was unaware of his left arm, had no feeling in the arm, could not use it, but when he saw the arm being approached by someone it would suddenly move sideways as if it had been stung; simultaneously, he experienced a burning pain. The involuntary withdrawal movements of his left arm were so embarrassing that he tied it to his belt. Eight months later, with eyes closed, he showed loss of superficial sensation (pain and touch) in the left side of his body, more severely in the arm than in the leg, trunk and face, the distal parts of the extremities being affected most. No delayed pain reaction occurred. There was also complete loss of postural sense, which resulted in sensory ataxia and pseudo-athetoid movements. Vibration was not perceived. There was lack of awareness of the left half of his body and inability to move his left hand and fingers without visual control. With his eyes open and his gaze directed at his left hand, the patient was able to open and close the hand very slowly. There were no sensory abnormalities on the right side of his body. On seeing that the left part of his body was approached for sensory testing, the patient invariably made a brisk withdrawal movement; at the same time he felt a burning pain that was accompanied by grimacing. On moving about, an incidental contact that was *not anticipated* did not result in pain and withdrawal. When the patient himself approached his left arm with his right hand there was neither pain nor withdrawal (suggesting that attention activates CP).

b. FRONTAL (PSYCHIATRIC) SURGERY (LOBOTOMY, TOPECTOMY, CINGULECTOMY/
CINGULOTOMY, LEUKOTOMY): Unlike other chronic pains (Bouckoms 1989), results
are generally disappointing for CP. In rare cases in which it was deemed effective,
the pain was simply less distressing and bothersome (pain indifference), the patient
less anxious or depressed by pain; spontaneous complaints about pain are diminished
and a patient's ability to appreciate the meaning of the pain may be disrupted.
According to Turnbull (1972), "bilateral cingulotomy alone is ineffective when pain
is caused by a major organic disease" (p. 962), including CP.

Bilateral cingulotomy/capsulotomy (but also some psychiatric conditions) result
in decreased pain tolerance and *hyperphatic-type* responses to acute painful stimuli
following frontal surgery (e.g., Davis *et al.* 1994; Talbot *et al.* 1995). This is the reverse
situation expected from some theories (Craig 1998), in which interruption of the
thalamocingular path or destruction of cingular areas may actually relieve CP.
Contrary to some speculations (Pattany *et al.* 2002), frontal lobes are not essential
to CP generation. However, prefrontal activity may lead to an *increased salience
of pain* at the cost of other cognitive and emotional behavioral abilities, with pain
constantly interfering with attention to other tasks.

In humans, the anterior cingulate cortex (ACC) may be divided into a caudal
region, showing increased activity during *pain* per se (from STT input), an
adjacent part preferentially involved in *general attention* (alerting/orienting attention
[at 125 ms] and [escape] response competition monitoring [at 200 ms] to pain;
Dowman 2002) and a rostral region involved in *pain affect* (i.e., unpleasantness
of pain). Rostral ACC (and/or underlying cingulum) tonically suppresses pain,
with opposite effects on pACC and insula (reviewed in Petrovic and Ingvar 2002),
but chronic pain engages both ACC and mid-cingulate cortex (MCC) (which also
includes cingulate motor areas) (Vogt *et al.* 2003); differential involvement of MCC
in pain may result in different outcomes in cingulotomy analgesia. Interestingly,
differences between physically and psychologically induced pain may be quantitative
rather than qualitative, with a role of rostral/perigenual ACC and pericingulate
areas in source monitoring (Raij *et al.* 2005).

The significant involvement of CC in pain processing may be an evolutionary relic
from a distant past when the prefrontal neocortex had not yet evolved and hippocampus, cingulate cortex, cingulate and brainstem motor areas/nuclei and amygdala
represented the highest order cognitive, afferent and efferent levels (McCrone 1999).
In humans, the assembly of information and motor-autonomic response to a painful
experience may depend largely upon the evolutionarily late PFC and its extensive
output to multiple brain sites, with a particularly important role for late cognitively
driven stages of pain affect and for the sharp consciousness of a mental event
(McCrone 1999). According to Freeman and Watts (1950), "the frontal lobes are
important structures, not so much for the experiencing of pain as for the evaluating of the sensation, the estimation of its significance in terms of the self and
of the future." However, this network plays clearly no *primary* sustaining role in
chronic CP.

Finally, Guiot's group is said to have temporarily relieved CP by bilateral ablation
of BA6 (Garcin 1968), but stimulation in these areas never provided a benefit (one
personal case plus others from a Japanese group; see Chapter 6).

c. HYPOTHALAMOTOMY AND HYPOPHYSECTOMY: Amano (1998) concluded that, unlike cancer pain, posteromedial hypothalamotomy is not effective at all for neurogenic pain, including CP, thus disproving the theory of Spiegel and colleagues (1954) and Spiegel and Wycis (1962) of CP arising from diversionary impulses on the hypothalamus. Interestingly, no postoperative sensory deficit is apparent; chronic cancer pain disappears, but pain can still be induced by pinprick. This dissociation after posteromedial hypothalamotomy is similar to that seen after medial thalamic lesions.

Why pituitary lesions can temporarily allay some CP patients is a matter of speculation. While a placebo effect cannot be excluded in reported studies, according to Levin (1988)

> Pain relief may result from excitation of central pain-suppressor mechanism by means of either a humoral agent distributed by the CSF...or by a direct neural stimulus. Hypophysectomy...either eliminates a hormone responsible for pain augmentation produced by the pituitary or induces (possibly by elimination of feedback suppression) a neural or humoral response, originating from the hypothalamus, which is responsible for pain suppression.

This humoral factor could be arginine-vasopressin, with involvement of a hypothalamo-thalamic antinociceptive pathway (Fujita and Kitani 1992) or corticotropin releasing factor (CRF), a peptide secreted from the hypothalamus throughout the brain with significant analgesic effects by the IT route.

d. THALAMOTOMIES: The literature is for the most part too old to be significant and many series of thalamotomies did not differentiate results according to pain category and are not available for discussion; most are pre-CT and MRI. Importantly, there is poor agreement on thalamic nomenclature among series. With older technology, it is difficult that lesions may have been limited to Vcpc and also other nuclei are difficult to evaluate.

Thalamotomies for CP aimed at lesioning the entrance point into the thalamus of quinto and spinothalamic pain fibers, limitans nucleus, Vc or nonspecific nuclei (CM-Pf, CL, DM, pulvinar and anterior nuclei) were believed to involve the spino-reticulothalamic (polysynaptic) pain pathways or thought to modify the emotional response to pain. Paradoxically, therapeutic lesions in Vc resulted in CP (White and Sweet 1969; Siegfried and Krayenbuhel 1972). Cassinari and Pagni (1969) concluded that only large thalamic lesions centered on CM-limitans-CL nuclei would completely interrupt spinoreticular pathways (partial lesions would be only temporarily effective by a temporary suppression of hyperactivity of thalamic or cortical neurons, for lack of facilitation). Lesions centered on Vc always encroached on the nuclei of the diffuse projection system of the thalamus immediately close by, and this might have either promoted or limited CP onset. Mazars (1976, p. 141) stated that all posterior thalamotomies are followed, after a more or less long time, by CP. Basal thalamotomies, placed above the midbrain at the base of the medial thalamus, extended laterally to interrupt both specific and nonspecific pain afferents, and exactly enclosed Vcpc: results have been similar to other sites. *Independently of the targeted nuclei*, initial results of thalamotomies are positive in most cases, with immediate relief of CP after Vc, CM and pulvinar lesions in some patients (see Table 7.1). Results appear to be *modestly better* (and complications lower, with no or little sensory loss) with medial (particularly bilateral) than with Vc thalamotomies (see also Tasker 1990). Bilateral medial lesions, though, increased the risk of cognitive impairment, by interfering with attentional processes. Few CP patients appear to have benefited in the long term. The great variability of response, relapse rate of pain (up to 50%), non-negligible operative mortality, dysphasia and severe dysesthesias make stereotactic thalamotomy a poor option for CP. Bilateral lesions produced many more complications and deaths and bilateral extensive destruction of thalamus is incompatible with life; severe, permanent complications and deaths have been reported with all thalamotomies. Interestingly, *some unilateral lesions relieved bilateral pain.*

Recent image-guided series provide some additional data. Jeanmonod and colleagues (1996, 2001) found 50–100% improvement in 40% of CP – much less than for PNP – at 2 years, in line with the experience of Tasker (1990) and Young and colleagues (1995), after medial thalamotomies (see also Ohye 1998). The lesions centered in CL, where most bursting units were found, revealed themselves to be the most efficient. Next, in descending order of efficiency, came Pf, PO, PuO and PuM nuclei. Results after lesions in CM and midline nuclei were the least efficient. However, *steady pain with thermal qualities proved the most resistant pain profile than intermittent pain and allodynia, deep (proprioceptive) pain more resistant than superficial pain.* Magnin and colleagues (2001) observed that in neurogenic pain (including CP) CL stimulation leads to paresthesia, in motor disorders to motor reactions and in psychiatric disorders to emotional feelings, i.e., CL is a supporting nucleus, not specific to CP. It should be noted that pulvinotomy, like medial thalamotomies, can reduce chronic, but not acute, pain (Richardson 1974). Tasker (2001a) concluded that there may be a place for medial thalamotomy for evoked-intermittent pains. On the other hand, Ohye (1998) found Vim thalamotomies *effective for deep pain only* in about 40 CP cases. He also concluded that CM-Pf used as a target in the past may have been the wrong target (Ohye 1990; but see Weigel and Krauss 2004). This is interesting, as old series did not distinguish the various components of CP sufficiently. Excellent results for CP have been reported after pulvinotomy by some (Yoshii *et al.* 1980; Laitinen 1988), but these are difficult to analyze (Tasker 1990).

Taken together, available data suggest involvement of several thalamic nuclei in the genesis of CP. Certainly, unlike medial lesions, Vc lesions add to denervation, perhaps resulting in less long-term relief due to shift of the CP generator contralaterally (see Chapter 8). VMpo plays no role in the genesis of CP (Montes *et al.* 2005).

The puzzling efficacy, at least in the short term, of lesions of different nuclei may be explained by invoking current anatomical concepts. Cortical areas can speak to each other through higher order thalamic nuclei, with one thalamocortical (TC) pathway reporting to its own cortical area the major (layer 5) output of another cortical area (i.e., higher order TC cells have a role in corticocortical communication) in tonic mode. Through their layer 6 corticothalamic (CT) connections, they can in turn modify the report of a cortical output, as this is passed through the thalamus, by promoting burst or tonic mode. Higher order nuclei receive from layer

5 pyramidal cells about the cortical output (versus first order nuclei). Within each sector of the reticular nucleus (TRN), cortical areas with the same spectrum of function (e.g., pain) may influence each other through the action of TRN on sensory or associative thalamic nuclei. Cortical areas receiving thalamic afferents from higher order relay nuclei may well be dominated by that input, rather than by other direct cortical connections (explaining, for example, pulvinotomy effects on CP: pulvinar is a higher order nucleus projecting to SI, but without STT input). Neurons in separate somatosensory nuclei of the dorsal thalamus influence (excite or inhibit) one another's activity through the TRN (Crabtree *et al.* 1998), further contributing to efficacy of different thalamotomies.

Interesting cytoarchitectonic data strengthen the concept. The spread of coherent activity across ensembles of cortical neurons has traditionally been ascribed to intralaminar nuclei (Castro-Alamancos and Connors 1997), but in fact this 40 Hz synchronization can be the sole result of a matrix of calbindin-immunoreactive (CAL+) neurons *present in all thalamic nuclei* and projecting *diffusely* to superficial layers of several adjacent cortical areas (Jones 2001). In some nuclei, a core of parvalbumin-immunoreactive (PA+) neurons is superimposed upon the matrix. Core neurons project in a topographically ordered fashion to middle layers of the cortex in an area-specific manner. Matrix neurons, recruited by corticothalamic connections, can *disperse* activity across cortical areas and thalamic nuclei. Their superficial terminations can synchronize specific and nonspecific elements of the thalamocortical network in coherent activity (perhaps also explaining bilateral recruitment during allodynia). Subcortical inputs too (e.g., the STT) adhere to this scheme, being less precise to matrix and more focused on the core. Thus, after a population of cortical cells is activated by whatever stimulus, it feeds back onto the matrix cells of its thalamic relay neurons, engaging, via the diffuse projections of the matrix cells, other adjacent populations of cortical cells. These cells (layer VI) in turn would feed back to the matrix cells of their thalamic relay nuclei, and so on, forming links between distant neurons. *Multiple thalamic nuclei could be recruited by corticothalamic fibers returning from the first area to nuclei other than that from which that area receives its principal thalamic input and might be a key element in binding together the activities of multiple cortical columns in the generation of a sensory percept.* If sufficiently widespread, it could provide a basis for interactions between distant cortical areas in uniting perception with planning strategies for action, but also explain effects of thalamotomies.

The terminations in superficial layers of matrix neurons, together with those of PA+ cells in middle layers, form a coincidence detection circuit. The vertical integration of coincident matrix inputs to apical dendritic branches of cortical pyramidal cells in upper layers and of PA+ core inputs to their dendrites in middle layers should promote *oscillatory* activity in these cells. This would be reinforced by the projections of cells in layers V–VI back to the thalamus, first engaging core and matrix cells that are topographically related to an activated set of cortical columns, but soon spreading across more widespread areas of thalamus and cortex. In this way, *transient links* would be formed between discrete populations of cortical and thalamic cells with different relationships to a cognitive event. Attention would modulate this synchronized neuronal activity and affect intensity of CP.

e. MESENCEPHALOTOMIES: These have been performed both to interrupt the STT or the reticular formation. At rostral mesencephalic level, the medial lemniscus, neospinothalamic tract, reticulothalamic tract and PAG lie contiguously adjacent to one another (from lateral to medial, respectively). Since STT lesions – but not coagulation of the termination site of the paleospinothalamic path – triggered new CP (Cassinari and Pagni 1969), most surgeons treating CP attempted larger medial lesions impinging on the reticular formation, thus including the paleospino-reticulo-thalamic pathways (often combined with medial thalamotomy). The "larger lesions appeared more effective for relief of central dysesthesia" (Nashold *et al.* 1969). However, Tasker (1989), reviewing 92 published protocols of patients with CP/PNP, showed that only 27% gained satisfactory long-term relief, from mesencephalotomy, with several complications and operative deaths. Laitinen (1988) concluded that "mesencephalotomy has no place in the treatment of chronic pain. The efficacy of this approach is no better than that of nonspecific thalamotomies, but side effects are more frequent and more serious" and Bosch (1991) also concluded against the use of mesencephalotomy in CP. There are more than 70% postoperative dysesthesias after open and 15–20% after stereotactic mesencephalotomies, with 5–10% mortality in stereotactic series (Tasker 1989). However, Amano and colleagues (see Table 7.1) achieved complete or near complete long-term relief in almost two thirds of their CP patients, with no postoperative dysesthesias or deaths, by aiming only at the reticular formation ("pure" rostral medial reticulotomy). Their target was located at the border between the PAG and the medial end of the mesencephalic reticular formation (RMR) at the level between the superior colliculus and the posterior commissure (Amano *et al.* 1980). The pretectal area was avoided by burring at 30% of glabella-inion distance. Microrecording showed nociceptive neurons in the RMR, characterized by large RFs and delayed firing in response to pinprick stimulation. *High-frequency stimulation produced severe pain mostly contralateral to the side of stimulation in a very restricted area.* Similar results were reported by Shieff and Nashold (1988; see Table 7.1). These latter authors observed how CP resolved *gradually*, never suddenly (unlike subparietal lesions), after mesencephalotomy (Amano *et al.* did not discuss this point); also, *unilateral lesions relieved bilateral pain.* In any case, somatotopographical constraints exclude a primary role of the reticular substance in the genesis of CP, since the spinoreticulothalamic system has very large and/or bilateral RFs, while CP is generally unilateral (references in Willis and Westlund 2004). Thus, the reticular formation may be involved in modulating a rostral generator and/or conscious experience of CP (Chapter 8).

f. OTHER BRAINSTEM PROCEDURES: Trigeminal nucleotomy and DREZ exert their effect by interruption of the intranuclear polysynaptic trigeminal pathway. Midline myelotomy may act by interrupting multisynaptic midline pathways and pontine lesions spinoreticular pathways.

The open caudalis DREZ operation has been successful in relieving the facial pain of pain resulting from damage to the trigeminal pathways in the brainstem. Pain due to brainstem involvement was reduced in 67% of cases (Nashold and Pearlstein 1996). However, the number of patients receiving this and similar interventions is too small to afford conclusions.

g. ANTEROLATERAL CORDOTOMIES (SPINOTHALAMIC TRACTOTOMIES): According to Joyner and colleagues (1966), 103 reported cordotomies have successfully relieved paraplegia pain (CP not broken down), and only 27 of the 154-strong group were unrelieved. On the other hand, White and Sweet (1969) reported that, despite an initial 56% incidence of pain relief in paraplegics, only 33% have remained pain free in the long term. Low cordotomies have been much less successful than higher ones, all at the expense of significant sensory loss. Davis and Martin (1947) found cordotomies ineffective in several cases of CCP.

The pain that responds to cordotomy is not the steady pain. White (1963) stated that "when the spinal cord is involved rather than its sensory roots, spinothalamic tractotomy, or even a complete myelotomy, is not likely to eliminate pain in the back and legs." Botterell and colleagues (1954) stated: "in complete lesions...burning pain has proved a problem difficult of solution in cases of injury to the...spinal cord," but "by contrast, jabbing, shooting, crampy, gripping, colicky and vice-like pains, have been regularly relieved by satisfactory bilateral tractotomy" (i.e., open cordotomy). Porter and colleagues (1966) stated that "cordotomy has...no effect...on the frequently encountered burning pain in the lower extremities (in traumatic paraplegia)." According to Lipton (1989), cordotomies "should not be used (for denervation pains) because when pain returns it may have dysesthetic qualities and the patient is worse off than previously." Rosomoff (1969) considered cordotomies futile for CCP and found a high incidence of associated dysesthesias in this group. Tasker (1990) too stated that long-surviving cord CP patients often relapse, or new pains emerge and/or the analgesic levels achieved by cordotomy fade with time. By interrupting the spinothalamic fibers, this obviously sets the stage for further later different pains (although it was suggested that bilateral cordotomies may lessen this risk). According to Tasker and North (1997), postcordotomy dysesthesias typically take time to develop and occur in 1–1.5% of cordotomized patients, in about 4% being long lasting and severe. Other series provide higher figures (6–20%), but data in many series are difficult to interpret. Tasker (1997) operated on 23 CCP patients with percutaneous, plus 8 with open cordotomy. Pain recurred in 8 after 1–21 years with gradual fading of analgesia. Repetition of cordotomy in 6 restored the level of analgesia in all, but pain relief was recaptured in only 3. He (Tasker *et al.* 1992) relieved spontaneous pain in 27%, intermittent spontaneous pain in 86% and evoked pain in 75% of his SCI CP cases, showing how intermittent/evoked pains were dependent upon transmission in STT paths. Thus, STT-tomies may relieve some cases of CCP (and exceptionally BCP); in the majority, CP relapsed shortly contralaterally (White and Sweet 1969), ipsilaterally (Bowsher 1988) or bilaterally (Graf 1960).

Thus, MS CP, CPSP, postcordotomy burning pain and pain due to scarring of the upper thoracic spinal cord are poorly responsive to anterolateral cordotomies (but also cordectomies and traditional DREZ lesions), with some exceptions (single cases of, e.g., Botterel *et al.* 1954; Davis and Martin 1947; Pollock *et al.* 1951a). Hyperactive spinal cells may feed the brain generator; reduction of this bottom-up barrage in some patients (obtained by cordotomy, cordectomy and DREZ lesions) may at least transitorily interfere with supraspinal mechanisms, as discussed above.

h. POSTERIOR CORDOTOMIES AND COMMISSUROTOMIES: Patients with clear-cut CP are not on record or are just a handful.

i. CORDECTOMIES: Cordectomies relieved the same types of pain that respond to cordotomy and DREZ surgery.

j. DORSAL ROOT ENTRY ZONE (DREZ) LESIONS: The first drezotomy ("*Radicellotomie*") for paraplegia pain was done in December 1972 by Sindou, consisting in incomplete section of the dorsal root plus a small 1.5–2 mm section cut into the lateral portion of the dorsal horn. Nashold did his first DREZ lesion in September 1974, with the aim to destroy the damaged dorsal horns, where hyperactive secondary nociceptive neurons were thought to generate the pain state. The DREZ operation in the paraplegic is generally done bilaterally (unilaterally in case of one-sided pains), beginning at the level of the traumatic transection of the spinal cord and extending rostrally over the next three dorsal roots and caudad over two levels; laminae I through V are ablated. Complications are common and include a rise in sensory level in all, partial or complete loss of pinprick and light touch sensation in 70–80% of patients, motor deficits (up to 14%), CSF leaks, worsening of bowel–bladder–sexual deficits, epidural and subcutaneous hemorrhages. These are more frequent in patients with spinal cord damage and those with bilateral DREZ. In patients with incomplete paraplegia, DREZ lesions must not extend too deeply to avoid additional neurologic deficits. By contrast, in patients with complete motor and sensory deficits below the lesion, this can be done extensively on the selected segments. In the series of Falci and colleagues (2002), in 2.3% of patients a temporary pain developed at their new postoperative level of sensation. A permanent pain (VAS 1–3) developed in 4.7% of the patients at their new level of sensation at a follow-up of up to 7 years.

In Nashold's series (Nashold and Pearlstein 1996), long-term relief (pain-free) of chronic pain from SCIs was obtained in 35% of his patients, with burning pain and electrical shocks being most responsive. Favorable categories included patients with incomplete neurological deficit, blunt trauma and conocaudal lesions with predominant leg pains. Approximately 70% of the paraplegic patients reported good pain relief immediately after the procedure, although half experienced some recurrence of the pain postoperatively, usually within the first year. In these patients the recurrent pain was usually described as less debilitating than the original pain. Pain in dermatomes at or just below injury (burning, shooting or electrical), radiating down into the legs and activated by stroking/touching the skin over the adjacent dermatomes, and unilateral pains *usually responded* to surgery, but *sacrococcygeal and vague diffuse burning pains did not or poorly so* (Nashold and Pearlstein 1996). Another favorable group were those who proved to have nerve root avulsions at operative exposure. Sindou and colleagues (2001) came to similar conclusions. Radicellotomies performed for pain associated with below-T10 spinal cord lesions are effective only in patients whose pain has a radiculometameric distribution, i.e., the pain corresponding to the level and extent of the spinal cord lesion (end-zone pain). *Pain in the territory below the lesion, especially in the perineosacral area, is not favorably influenced* (while leg pain after caudal lesions is). Nashold also noted that in

18 cases with an intramedullary cyst (syrinx), drainage of the cyst alone did not suffice, whereas in 18 in whom this was combined with DREZ lesions, 12 good and 2 fair results were achieved.

As mentioned, hyperactive STT and propriospinal cells may contribute to feed the supraspinal generator (see Chapter 8).

k. SPINAL RHIZOTOMIES: Dorsal rhizotomy is unsuccessful in relieving CP and can trigger anesthesia dolorosa (Pagni *et al.* 1993).

l. SYMPATHECTOMIES AND SYMPATHETIC BLOCKS: Alajouanine and Brunelli (1935) and other authors (reviewed in Garcin 1968, but also recently Falci *et al.* 2002) thought that sensory afferents may traverse the sympathetic trunk and have a role in CP. A few patients with BCP and CCP have been temporarily – and on occasion for prolonged periods – relieved by sympathetic blockade, whether complete or not, whether by local anesthetic or guanethidine. This relief appeared to depend on hyperpathia. When relief occurred, hyperpathia, steady burning and intermittent shooting spontaneous pain, *but not usually deep pain, disappeared*. Occasionally, hyperpathia was relieved but not spontaneous pain, or hyperpathia longer than steady pain, but *spontaneous burning pain was not relieved independently of hyperpathia*. However, those studies generally lacked a placebo control and it is not clear why sympathetic fibers should have a role in CP with allodynia, but not without: likely, the block reduced sensory barrage tout court, also explaining why not all the peripheral nerves of the affected region had to have their sympathetic nerve supply blocked (cases 3–4 of Loh *et al.*; see Table 7.1).

The existence of sympathetically maintained pain appears to be more fiction than scientific fact (Ochoa 1999; Schott 2001) and peripheral blocks, including sympathetic blocks, are flawed (Bonicalzi and Canavero 1999a, b, 2000). Direct recordings from human sympathetic nerve fibers have failed to substantiate the notion of an increased sympathetic outflow in patients with neuropathic disorders (Blumberg 1988; Jänig and Koltzenburg 1991). C-fibers (visceral) are found in sympathetic nerves, where "private" lines in the sympathetic nervous system have been characterized (Hallin and Wiesenfeld-Hallin 1983); occasional positive effects in CP could be mediated through effects on these fibers (Schott 2001).

The vast majority of authors report no benefit from sympathetic block and/or sympathectomy in CP (Nashold 1991; Sjolund 1991; Bowsher 1994; Tasker 2001). The vasomotor, sudomotor and trophic disorders observed in certain cases may just be reflex phenomena induced by pain (Garcin 1957) secondary to change in mobility.

REPORTS OF SUDDEN DISAPPEARANCE OF CP

"Vis sanatrix naturae"

There are a few cases of CP which *suddenly* vanished after long-standing disease. Nature is teaching us a valuable lesson we must learn from.

Case 1 (Spiegel *et al.* 1954; Hassler 1970). They observed sudden disappearance of thalamic hyperpathia due to a lesion of the posterior portion of the thalamus after a new larger lesion in the posterior ventral nucleus of the thalamus.

Case 2 (Gybels and Sweet 1989, p. 342). These authors treated one patient with pain in the right leg of 12-year duration after a left cerebral stroke. Several neurosurgical operations (not specified) had no effect, but morphine (0.05 mg) administered via a ventricular catheter was followed by a 1–2 day long complete pain relief and severe paraparesis; 0.025 mg relieved the pain for 12 hours without motor deficits. Satisfactory relief continued for 7 months, at which time "a major left cerebral infarct produced a right hemiplegia and complete relief of her pain."

Case 3 (Soria and Fine 1991). Their 62-year-old patient developed an acute stroke with a right hemisensorimotor syndrome, including pain and temperature hypoesthesia. Typical CPSP with allodynia developed over 12 months. The threshold for pain, temperature and light touch was increased, but, when exceeded, the pain resulting was intolerable. One year following the stroke, a CT revealed a small lacunar infarct of the left thalamus. Somatosensory evoked potentials revealed absent N18, N20 and P27 components. Several drugs and other kinds of treatment had no enduring, satisfactory effect. However, 7 years after the original episode, a second stroke produced sudden right hemiplegia, motor aphasia and complete disappearance of both the pain and the allodynia. At follow-up, 5 months later, there was pain and temperature hypoesthesia in the right half of the body. A late CT scan revealed a well-demarcated, low-density lesion in the left parietal lobe, deep in the centrum semiovale, adjacent to the body of the lateral ventricle. Pain was still *absent 1 year later* (Figure 7.3).

Case 4 (Hirato *et al.* 1993). These authors reported a patient with CP after a putaminal lesion, in whom many irregular burst discharges were encountered in the thalamus (Vim-Vc). PET revealed thalamic hypoactivity and cortical hyperactivity. CP disappeared after a small subcortical hemorrhage had accidentally occurred near the cerebral cortex around the central sulcus during surgery.

Case 5 (Canavero *et al.* 2001). This woman developed disabling left hemisoma (C4 sensory level) CP following surgery for a C4–5 herniation, with prominent thermomechanical allodynia in involved regions. She was refractory to multiple drug therapy. During MCS, a microdialysis catheter was inserted into right SI arm area. Within 48 hours of surgery, the patient started to complain of a "dead flesh" sensation to the left arm distal to the deltoid. A CT scan showed a

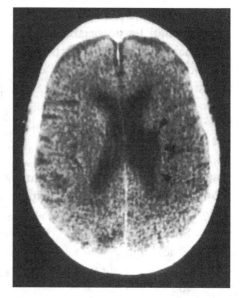

Figure 7.3: This patient developed CP after a pure thalamic stroke (not shown). A further stroke along the parietothalamic axis abolished the pain. (Adapted from Soria and Fine [1991], with permission from the International Association for the Study of Pain.)

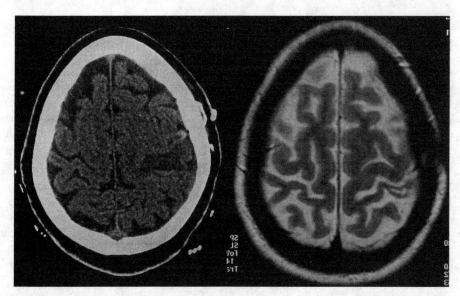

Figure 7.4: CT scan of a SI stroke selectively abolishing arm cord central pain (left). MR image showing resolution of the stroke at a time when central pain had relapsed (right). (From Canavero *et al.* [2001], with permission.)

right SI infarction and the catheter was removed. *For 20 days*, the patient complained of her previous pain, *except for the left arm.* Thereafter, her CP returned with the same intensity and characteristics as per before the stroke. During those 20 days there was complete dense anesthesia of the limb with no sign of allodynia (mechanical and thermal). Burning pain was absent (VAS/NRS: 0). MRI 8 months later showed a normal-appearing SI with only a serpiginous area inside (Figure 7.4).

Case 6 (Helmchen *et al.* 2002). In June 1999 this 58-year-old man experienced sudden stroke with left-sided sensorimotor symptoms (bar face and neck), with both lemniscal and spinothalamic deficits. CT showed a hemorrhage in right thalamic Vc. Three months later, he noticed the gradual onset of a throbbing, burning, aching, dysesthetic pain on his left side (maximal in the arm) (VAS 8) which became disabling and was aggravated by movements and cold stimuli. Ten months later, hemihypesthesia and hypalgesia were unchanged (movement was improved), but there was mechanical and thermal (cold and warm) allodynia; on CT, a circumscribed hypodense lesion was seen in the posterior right thalamus. MRI also showed a few subcortical parietal and frontal infarctions in the centrum semiovale not involving the ACC. Drugs were ineffective. In April 2001, while washing his hands, he could no more appreciate warm temperature on his right hand, although being able to differentiate between warm and cold water on his left arm; allodynia on the left was *gone* and the spontaneous aching CP on his left side *disappeared.* He presented sensory deficits on the right side, particularly severe thermalgesic hypesthesia. On the left, he could differentiate warm and cold stimuli in his hand, without a trace of allodynia. There was still hemidysthesia and hypesthesia, particularly in the arm. Simultaneous tactile, but not thermal, stimulation was localized to the right arm. There was no thermal or algesic sensation in his right hand, while in his left it was practically normal. Over the following 2 months, sensory deficits largely improved on the right side, bar position sense. Concomitantly, spontaneous CP and – to a smaller degree – cold thermal allodynia redeveloped on the left side and still increased over the following months. *Almost 1 year later*, left CP still persisted, but *without warm thermomechanical allodynia*. No CP had yet developed on the right side. On SSEPs there was prolonged P40 latency on right tibial nerve stimulation. MRI showed *left* hemispheric postcentral parietal ischemic infarction (5 × 4 × 5 cm) that involved *SI, supramarginal gyrus, SII*, external capsule and a very small portion of the posterior insula, sparing the anterior insula, internal capsule and the left thalamus.

Case 7 (Daniele *et al.* 2003). A hypertensive 68-year-old woman developed acute left hemiparesis with mild–moderate motor impairment, hypoesthesia and tingling sensation which increased over the days. CT showed a *right* thalamic hemorrhage. Several days after discharge, she began to complain of spontaneous pain in her left limbs, sometimes described as burning and excruciating, and tactile allodynia. Carbamazepine at 800 mg was only partially effective. Three years later, the pain was unabated, with partial reduction of hypesthesia. Then, she suddenly developed acute aphasia. A CT showed a *left* frontoparietal ischemic lesion plus bilateral lacunar infarcts. For the next 3 years (until death) her pain and allodynia were completely gone.

Similar cases of disappearance without pathologic confirmation are on record. For instance, White and Sweet (1955) reported a woman suffering from thalamic CPSP. Two-staged bilateral orbital gyrectomy gave no relief of pain. However, four months after operation the pains *inexplicably disappeared* and the patient was well. Patient 2 of Michel and colleagues (1990) developed *"douleur fulgurante en coup de couteau"* to the left hand, plus brachial paresis and tactile and pinprick hypesthesia. CPSP worsened, but 3 weeks later it disappeared with onset of brachiofacial left hemiplegia, only to be replaced by cheirooral paresthesias; a CT scan showed a superficial cortical hypodensity straddling right SI/MI. Young and Rinaldi (1997) state that in one patient, who experienced a right-sided thalamic hemorrhage, neglect of the left side of the body developed that relieved the patient of her pain, but they do not state if it was CP. Franzini and colleagues (2003) reported disappearance of CPSP partially relieved by MCS after an undetailed "brainstem stroke."

Finally, there is one single case report (Koszewski *et al.* 2003) of full CP relief following thalamoparietal radiation lesioning. Three years previously, a 72-year-old man developed a right hemispheric stroke. Immediately after the stroke he was hemiplegic and hemianesthetic. Then sensibility renormalized and his plegia became a nondisabling hemiparesis. Three months after stroke, he developed burning pain and allodynia in the left hemibody and became suicidal. In 2002 an MRI showed a right lesion covering most of the putamen, claustrum, external capsule and part of the insular cortex; the internal capsule was at least partially damaged. He was submitted to stereotactic anterior capsulotomy *for no clearly explained reason*. During surgery, stimulation of the border between the internal pallidum and posterior limb of the internal capsule diminished, but not fully abolished the pain. Two large lesions were done covering the whole border *between the posterior limb of the internal capsule and the lentiform nucleus*: in this area only, stimulation controlled

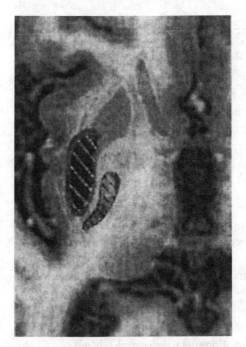

Figure 7.5: Brain MRI scan depicting surgical lesion in the posterior limb of the internal capsule abolishing central poststroke pain. (From Koszewski *et al.* 2003, with permission from VSP, an imprint of Brill Academic Publishers.)

the whole left side of the body. The whole CP syndrome disappeared *immediately* after lesioning. Right after surgery, there was motor worsening which slowly resolved to previous levels; nociceptive sensibility was fully preserved (*implying that a descending input was interrupted*) and no emotional change was noted. Five months later the patient was still pain-free (Figure 7.5).

There are many reports of mostly *sudden* disappearance of CP after treatment of the triggering lesion, so called *reversible CP*.

1. Michelsen (1943) reported four cases of meningiomas impinging upon the parietal cortex, in which pain and associated sensory phenomena in the involved extremities were present. In his *case 4*, the pain was completely relieved by removal of the lesion, and in his *case 3* it was relieved for 4 years before it reappeared. His *case 5*, with a depressed skull fracture over the anterior and posterior central gyri with cerebral contusion, exhibited paraplegia and bilateral hyperpathia and hyperesthesia. Position sense was absent in the right leg and diminished in the left, while pain and touch were recognized and localized. After debridement, the pain gradually cleared, hyperesthesia receded and sensation improved.

2. Silver (1957) reported a patient who had a stroke, with hemiplegia and aphasia. Eight years later, he gradually developed very severe paroxysmal burning pain in the right arm. An AVM of the left parietal area was diagnosed at angiography and completely removed in two stages. Under local anesthesia, *manipulation, traction upon and clipping of the component blood vessels reproduced the pain*. The pain was abolished *almost immediately* and relief maintained for the 5 years of observation.

3. Di Biagio (1959) totally and permanently relieved a CP patient with steady and intermittent paroxysmal, but no hyperpathia or allodynia, components following extirpation of a right subcortical parietal tuberculoma.

4. Hamby (1961) reported on a young man who developed severe burning pain with allodynia in the left upper limb following a car accident. Two years later, at surgery, the parietal cortex was found to be covered by extensive pools of subarachnoid fluid. Drainage of these pools revealed yellow, atrophic, leathery looking cortex resembling that following an old infarct. This area was sharply separable from normal cortex and extended from the sylvian fissure upward almost to the interhemispheric fissure, and apparently was limited anteriorly by the postcentral gyrus. Stimulation over the postcentral gyrus behind the motor points elicited painful prickling sensations in the upper limb. Stimulation in the normal-appearing postcentral gyrus above the arm area elicited painless prickling sensations in the foot. A transpial incision was made 5 mm deeper than the gutters of the gyri along the posterior edge of the postcentral gyrus and over three contiguous parietal gyri. The cortex and adjacent U-fiber areas of the white matter were easily removed. On the next day the patient had no subjective pain or dysesthesia or allodynia. The patient remained pain-free *10 years* after surgery.

5. Retif and colleagues (1967) reported on a patient (their case 3) who had an anterior parietal meningioma with purely paroxysmal fit-like pain and a jacksonian march. Removal was followed by a complete recovery. EEG showed an irritative pattern.

6. Stoodley and colleagues (1995) reported a 63-year-old woman who gradually (over many years) developed constant dull pain to the whole right hemisoma (worse in the face) and an unpleasant tingling sensation on being touched on those areas. There was *no* sensory deficit. Neuroradiologically, she harbored a saccular aneurysm of the bifurcation of the left internal carotid artery extending up to the left thalamus. There was complete resolution of all her sensory symptoms *immediately* following surgical clipping and for a follow-up of *18 months*.

7. Potagas and colleagues (1997) described a patient with intermittent pain in the right arm caused by an otherwise asymptomatic low-grade glioma of the white matter of the parietal operculum whose pain stopped after excision of the tumor.

8. Fukuhara and colleagues (1999) reported on a woman with a 9-year story of progressively worsening of episodic deep aching/burning CP to the right hemisoma. *No* sensory deficit was present. Neuroimaging disclosed an arterovenous malformation in the corona radiata of the parietal lobe, along the posterior horn of the lateral ventricle. Embolization achieved *complete* remission. Transient sensory hypesthesia was seen (postembolization subparietal ischemia?).

9. Albe-Fessard (personal communication to Barraquer-Bordas *et al.* 1999) had a woman with CP in an anesthetic facial area. She had a huge parietal meningioma with maximal compression on face area. Removal led to CP disappearance and renormalization of sensibility.

10. Tasker (2001) operated on a patient with a right parietal hemispheral meningioma presenting with contralateral dysesthetic causalgic pain, which *disappeared* after removal of the tumor.

11. We observed several cases ourselves. Pagni and Canavero (1993) reported on a woman suffering paroxysms of pain, described as "burning," "lancinating" or "electric shock-like," which increased in frequency over the months. MRI disclosed a posterior T6–7 meningioma. Extirpation resulted in total remission over 24 hours, without any further recurrence. Canavero and colleagues (1995) described a man who developed acute Schneider's syndrome and hyperacute allodynia to the limbs (worse in the arms in C6–8 dermatomeres bilaterally) within 30 minutes of a fall. Allodynia was so intense to make sensory examination impossible. On MRI, there was spondylotic narrowing of the vertebral canal with large osteophytes at C4–7, particularly on the posterior aspect. A voluminous spur jutted out of the right posterior aspect at C7; the C5/6 disk was posteriorly excluded, impinging upon and nicking the anterior surface of the dural sac, with greatest narrowing at C4–6. Upon reawakening from surgery (C5/6 discectomy plus stabilization), the allodynia had *completely disappeared*. Sensory examination at this time showed thermoalgesic hypesthesia in the four limbs. Two weeks later, typical CCP involving the four limbs appeared and gradually worsened. Pagni and Canavero (1995) relieved CP involving one leg after aspiration of a benign intramedullary cyst (follow-up 10 years; unpublished observations). Canavero (1996) reported on a woman who developed burning pain in her left arm and, episodically, in the whole hemibody due to a bleeding cavernoma in the white matter deep to the inferior parietal lobe. CP totally regressed after the bleeding cleared, only to return with a new bleeding years later (unpublished observations). Canavero and Bonicalzi (2001) reported on two patients. The first suffered from severe burning pain and allodynia to one leg which totally vanished within 24 hours of extirpation of a cystic tumor at conus level (follow-up: 3 months). The second was immediately relieved of her intermittent CP following embolization of an aneurysm at the vertebral–PICA junction impinging on the medulla (follow-up: 2 months). Finally, we relieved a 54-year-old woman of her pain to the left leg, misdiagnosed as sciatic pain, after shunting a large parietooccipital arachnoidal cyst. Another woman with a meningioma compressing SI had painful fits to the hemibody, abolished after surgery (Canavero and Bonicalzi, unpublished observations).

CP associated with MS may often present during acute relapses and spontaneously vanish as the relapse clears (e.g., Portenoy *et al.* 1988). Some cases of CP receded after shunting for syringomyelia (e.g., Suzuki *et al.* 1985; Milhorat *et al.* 1996; Attal *et al.* 2004; see also Chapter 8) and it is reported that type I Chiari malformation-associated neurogenic pain (but not particularly sensory loss) responds well to surgery (Meadows *et al.* 2001; Bejjani and Cockerham 2001).

However, generally speaking, CP is a chronic pain, which usually stays with patients for the rest of their lives. On rare occasions, it may gradually subside even after prolonged periods (CPSP; Greenspan *et al.* 1997; Kim 1999). According to Schott (2001), CP can disappear spontaneously even after many years, temporarily or permanently, generally slowly, but he does not back up this assertion with personal or published evidence; however, he had a patient with unremitting CPSP for 15 years except for 8 hours of 100% relief during a flight (similar to cases of causalgia and Parkinson's disease). Slow disappearances would feature ever longer pain-free intervals, although, when present, pain would be as severe as ever. Andersen and colleagues (1995) reported that in two patients CPSP disappeared spontaneously: one had evoked dysethesia and shoulder pain at 1 month and another, with a lower brainstem infarction, complained of ocular pain with a Horner syndrome. The CPSP case 1 of Michel and colleagues (1990) simply reported an abatement of his pain. Garcin (1968) stated that regression of brainstem CP is exceptional, but a few cases were seen.

8 PIECING TOGETHER THE EVIDENCE

"... in the light of knowledge finally achieved, deductions seem almost obvious and can be understood by any intelligent student; but the experience of research, gropingly in the darkness, with its profound anxiety to succeed and its alternating character between certainty and discouragement, can only be understood by him who has experienced it." (**A. Einstein,** 1935)

The evidence reviewed strongly suggests that CP may be understood as the result of a localized reverberation loop between the parietal cortex (SI, and perhaps SII) and the sensory thalamus (Vc, core and shell) with a supporting role of Vim, CL and its SI projections, and pulvinar (Canavero *et al.* 1993; Canavero 1994), as this is the only mechanism able to explain pain disappearance following lesions limited to the subcortical white matter (see Box 8.1). This dipole is exquisitely adjusted to explain somatotopographical pain distribution in CP (Canavero 1994). The loop, with its descending excitatory arm, is engaged bilaterally, with contralateral — or, in some cases, ipsilateral — predominance. In those rare cases with complete SI or thalamic destruction (e.g., maxithalamotomies), the reverberant loop can be activated contralaterally. CP appears to be more frequent after right-sided lesions, perhaps due to lateralization of norepinephrine. Since the evidence points to a major role of this arm in CP sustenance (see also Yamashiro *et al.* 1991), we propose that STT lesions (or simple interference, without actual sensory loss) unbalance the normal oscillatory corticothalamic "dialogue," starting in SI, where GABA levels drop acutely, and induce changes caudad along a diffuse spinotruncothalamic reticular core (see in Gybels and Sweet 1989; Nandi *et al.* 2004), which becomes hyperactive. The end result is bilateral facilitation from multiple top-down ("locked SI") and bottom-up (cord and brainstem reticular) sources. Intrathalamic activity hinging on TRN can be entrained by corticothalamic oscillations and drive, in turn, the cortex.

The substratum of release is speculated to be a genetically defective GABA A receptor at cortical sensory level, which may be present in about one-fifth to one-third of the population (see the speculation of Zimmermann [1991] of a molecular defect at the level of inhibitory synapses as the underpinning of neurogenic pain).

Box 8.1 Historical note

Livingston (1943) proposed that chronic pains following peripheral neural injury were the result of "a vicious cycle" set up as a "central perturbation of function" in the "internuncial neuron centers of the spinal grey matter" by an irritant focus. He wrote:

> once the central process is started it assumes the major role... If the trigger point is removed early, the process may subside spontaneously. If the process is permitted to continue... even a removal of the original irritant may not be sufficient to establish a cure... the central disturbance is the essential factor in many diseases, and that there should be better means for eliminating pain than by a chordotomy or posterior root section or other anatomic interruptions of nerve continuity.

Building on the work of Lorente de No' in the 1920s on the concept of closed self-reexciting chains within neuronal pools, Von Hagen (1957) wrote:

> chronic pain syndromes, i.e., sustained pain after the disappearance of the original impetus, cannot develop unless cortical components are involved ... [it] is the product of reverberating circuits in the nervous system of which the cortical components are of great importance... the various emotional reactions related to this state, namely, preoccupation with symptoms, introspection concerning among other things the memories of the pain and anticipation of the future, depression, and anxiety, as well as emotional stress brought on by other conflicts, also serve to reinforce the reverberating circuits and further perpetuate the disability.

Likewise, Talairach and colleagues (1960) believed that:

> Certain factors favorise the concepts of the cerebral cortex taking part in the elaboration of the painful sensations, the parietal lobe being directly involved... it seems proved that there are reverberating thalamo-cortico-thalamic circuits, capable to modify at any time the modalities of the afferent impulsions and their non specific incidences.

Thus, they coagulated the white matter beneath the parietal lobe in four causalgic, two phantom pain and two facial pain patients, as

> a sub-cortical lesion localised at the cross-road of thalamo-cortical paths should achieve a sufficiently generalized section of the painful afferences, and disturb in the same time this modulating system of thalamic activity or more generally the regulation of the areothalamic couple.

In particular, they wanted to interrupt the path to SII. Sano and coworkers (1966) hypothesized that CP due to thalamic lesions might be due to a reverberating circuit between hyperirritable cells of the lateral and medial thalamic nuclei. Emmers (1981) speculated that peripheral nociceptive sensory input may impinge upon a preexisting low-threshold thalamic discharge system to activate a self-sustained reverberating system of parallel facilitatory feedback loops. The reverberating system between the lamellar, CM-Pf and SII neurons would sustain a more or less constant level of centrally activated pain referred to a given body part, depending upon the somatic representations of the involved SII neurons.

The reticular formation (RF) becomes bilaterally "primed" right after injury; one possible role, besides "feeding" the loop, could be to engage a dedicated pain-coded sensory loop contralaterally (this may also occur by corpus callosum-mediated transfer of anomalous oscillatory activity to the opposite side). Since the switch from unconscious to conscious state likely correlates with the strength of activation in a given area (Zeki and Ffychte 1998), a hyperactive RF feeding on the cortico-thalamic loop may contribute to the conscious feeling of CP. Thus, in "patients with deafferentation pain the medial midbrain tegmentum becomes hypersensitive to stimulation, and that along with posterior thalamus, thalamic radiations and somatosensory cortex, acquires the property, absent in somatic pain syndromes, of generating not only a painful conscious awareness but also a reasonably accurate reproduction of the patient's pain," but only in the already painful sites; "due to deafferentation, mesencephalic reticulo-thalamic-cortical circuits become sensitive not only to electrical stimulation but also to natural neural input" (Tasker *et al.* 1980).

That the cortex (above all SI) plays a leading role is supported by this being the initial target of IV propofol and IV ketamine, which effectively relieve CP. Lack of opioid efficacy (and CS superiority on other neuromodulatory techniques) in CP may be due to this highly corticalized mechanism, notably to a dearth of opioid receptors in SI. Even in some studies of acute pain, cortical activity can be detected before subcortical responses appear (Casey *et al.* 2001). Rosso and colleagues (2003) recorded SEPs 2 hours before and 3 after percutaneous cordotomy in 7 cancer patients and found that *nociceptive STT denervation may induce a rapid modulation of cortical (SI), but not spinal or brainstem, neuronal activity along the lemniscal pathway.* On the other hand, CP usually requires an at least partially intact thalamus, ipsi- or contralaterally, as proved by too massive a thalamic destruction being incompatible with CP (see SEPs data and Spiegel's case of remission in Chapter 7). Ohye (1998) found that, in CP, the initial hemorrhage or infarction in the thalamus is rather small (less than 1 cm in diameter), in cases that developed CP within 1 year; patients with massive thalamic involvement following initial stroke did not manifest CP, but only hypesthesia in general.

Absence of pain is a homeostatic, dynamic condition between pro- and anti-nociceptive CNS activities. Malfunction (even at a molecular level) of inhibition (including transformation of inhibitory synapses into excitatory ones), possibly on a genetic basis, with changes in dynamic cortical network strength, may allow pathologic sensory deprivation or alteration of ascending sensory or descending modulatory fibers to disrupt the normal, homeostatic pattern of neuronal activity of sensory systems. This alters the network functional mode to the point that a *dedicated* oscillatory (resonant) pain loop (perhaps seen as coherent theta activity) is switched on in the thalamocortical axis responsible for subjective states indefinitely (Canavero 1994), with other brain areas playing a corollary role. In other words, the same mechanism responsible for the genesis of consciousness can generate CP when its organization and timing are altered by disrupted inhibitory dynamics.

Different qualities of pain, but also different neurometabolic findings, may be explained by individual degrees of activation of the same cells or activation (frequency discharge/oscillatory changes) of several sets of cells, in different cortical layers and thalamic nuclei, depending on site and extent of damage. The loop would be under the influence of cognitive, emotional and attentional networks, explaining fluctuations in time of CP. This mechanism would apply to all CP conditions, from dorsal horn to cortex.

One consequence of the establishment of such loop would be the functional dissolution of processing circuits, with loss of information, triggered by stable neural anomalies that hinder correct data estimation. The thalamocortical system becomes less flexible (efficient) in sampling inputs and evaluating information both from evoked and spontaneous sensory stimuli, flexibility implying the capacity to occupy different bands of discharge frequencies. In the cortex, stimuli are coded with a loosened information exchange and peculiar sparse clusters of connectivity (Biella *et al.* 1999), i.e., information processing decorrelates. Loss/distortion of proper spatiotemporal sequence/somatotopy of incoming impulses at cord, brainstem or thalamocortical levels in CP has already been entertained by past authors (e.g., Foix *et al.* 1922; Zuelch and Schmid 1953; Donovan and colleagues 1982).

Thus, we may now have a cure for CP, i.e., a stereotactic lesion in the subparietal white matter, in some cases bilateral, targeting the descending facilitatory arm of the loop. Neurosurgical experience shows that, once the sensory component of chronic pain is abolished, pain affect also is renormalized (not vice versa) and this would be the case for the proposed intervention. Of course, this intervention, carrying the same morbidity/mortality of, for example, deep brain stimulation, should be reserved to patients refractory to therapies detailed in Chapters 5 and 6. The proposed scenario also would explain successes with electroconvulsive therapy (Canavero 1994; Chapter 6).

Importantly, the present framework nixes the idea that *in chronic pain*, the widespread nature of pain (*matrix*) processing precludes effective focal treatment by neurosurgical means (Melzack 1991): CP can be reversed (Chapter 7, Section 4). Also, the vast majority of proposed theories, including exclusively based thalamic theories of CP, collapse on such clear-cut observations.

EXPLORING THE THEORETICAL FRAMEWORK

Classic neurophysiology has focused on the encoding of information through changes in the firing rate of neurons, but measuring mean discharge rates may not yield the full information transmitted. When networks of neurons interact, the result is often rhythmic activity within defined frequency ranges that can engage in temporal synchronization and de-synchronization ((de)correlation), i.e., changes in the bands of oscillations convey additional information to neuronal firing rates. Neurons fall into step with one another forming ensembles firing in relative synchrony for brief periods, before some neurons drop out of synchronization to join another ensemble. Synchrony between trains of action potentials has both oscillatory and non-oscillatory components (Jones 2001). Importantly, they cannot be detected as CBF changes, since sensory discrimination, for one, may require a limited fraction of neuronal population and a change in synchrony may suffice. These assemblies are dynamic and shifting and are associated with perception.

According to Llinàs and Parè (1991, 1997): "only a minor part of its connectivity is devoted to the transfer of direct sensory input. Rather, most of the connectivity is geared to the generation of internal functional modes, which may, in principle, operate in the presence or absence of sensory activation [p. 521]... the number of cortical fibers projecting to the specific thalamic nuclei is larger than the number of fibers conveying the sensory information to the thalamus. Thus, a large part of the thalamocortical connectivity is devoted to re-entrant or to *reverberating* activity...the insertion of neurons with intrinsic oscillatory capabilities into this complex synaptic network allows the brain to generate global oscillatory states [i.e., population coding] which shape the computational events evoked by sensory stimuli" (p. 526).

Oscillations are generated in different sectors of the thalamus or cerebral cortex, even if they are disconnected from other structures; in the intact brain, these coalesce within complex wave sequences owing to neuronal interactions. Large ensembles of cortical and thalamic neurons discharge synchronously at stereotyped frequencies associated with different conscious states. During alert wakefulness, high-frequency oscillations occur spontaneously or as part of sensory-elicited events in the relay nuclei of the thalamus and the cortical areas to which they project, "binding" distributed aspects of sensory perception (consciousness). Thus, "disruption of oscillation and/or temporal synchronization may be a fundamental mechanism of neurological disease" (Farmer 2002). Stochastic oscillating or clustered discharges with the same mean discharge rate may have very different effects on transmitter release, temporal summation of postsynaptic potentials, long-term changes of synaptic strength and second messenger effects (Sandkuehler 1996; but see critique in Pareti and De Palma 2004) (Box 8.2).

CP can be understood inside this framework: CNS lesions are not simply depriving the brain or parts thereof of afferent input; they are disrupting an ongoing pattern of neuronal activity.

TRIGGERING PERSISTENT OSCILLATION

Three approaches appear promising in the present context and these will be briefly discussed. The gist is bistability, i.e., the property of switching between two stable states (e.g., pain–non-pain).

1. **Neural networks.** Neural networks are dynamically regulated entities, constrained by their anatomical connectivity and membrane properties of the component neurons. They can be "tuned" and *configured* into several operational modes, each depending upon the expression and modulation of the constituent cellular, synaptic and network building blocks, and in accordance with the conditions of the moment. *By changing the properties of selected synapses, cells or pathways, the operation of a network can be dramatically altered, e.g., from mutual inhibition to mutual excitation*; controlling inputs may turn an oscillatory circuit on and off, and the functional connectivity can be reconfigured by ascending and descending CNS influences, i.e., a radical rewiring. Control systems able to switch the operational mode of nociceptive cells exist in the CNS (Willis 1985). Also, a single network can participate or generate a large repertoire of outputs, which may be determined, among others, by sectorial damage to targets of innervation (e.g., Selverstone and Moulins 1985; Getting 1989). Persistent activity can arise from a large neural network that involves recurrent excitatory loops through reciprocal excitation between the

Box 8.2 Thalamocortical rhythmicity

The neocortex and thalamus are a unified oscillatory (reverberant) machine and they work in concert (Jones 2001). The main cortical projections from Vc end in layers IV and III forming dense, topographically organized arbors that synapse mainly with dendritic spines, plus some branches ending in layer VI. Synapses formed by Vc TC axons in layer IV are less than 10%. Possibly, individual TC synapses produce a stronger synaptic drive than intracortical synapses. CT fibers go back to correspondent TC neurons only to a limited extent. Anatomically and functionally, feedback connections are quite different from feedforward connections: although much more numerous than the latter between the same structures (Ullman 1995; Sillito et al. 1994), individual feedback projections mediate less powerful effects, having more sparsely branching, widespread arbors, with fewer less effective synapses largely on distal dendrites (versus proximal dendrites of feedforward fibers), and also being less precisely focused within a sensory representation, reaching a larger proportion thereof (see references in Kaas 1999; Ergenzinger et al. 1998). Overall, top-down feedback connections seem better designed to stimulate weakly larger groups of neurons and modulate ongoing activity (versus feedforward connections creating activity in smaller groups of neurons). Following, for example, NMDA block of corticothalamic (CT) SI cells, these fibers might focus transmission (small RFs), via GABA interneurons in Vc and TRN (and eventually other thalamic nuclei), thus placing thalamic plasticity under cortical SI control (Kaas 1999). Also, top-down influences may alter the overall functional nature of SI and layer-specific mechanisms of sensory processing (Krupa et al. 2004). On the other hand, intranuclear inhibition through the TRN may affect RFs of cortical neurons.

Thalamocortical rhythmicity is driven by the thalamic GABAergic reticular nucleus (TRN) that projects to almost all thalamic relay nuclei (Shepherd 2004). It receives excitatory glutamatergic inputs from axon collaterals of thalamocortical (TC) fibers that traverse it on their way from thalamic relay nuclei (including Vc) to cortex and of corticothalamic glutamatergic fibers that project back from cortical layer VI to thalamic relay nuclei. However, it is possible that not all TC/CT axons give off collaterals to TRN. TRN cells are highly interconnected through inhibitory, mainly GABA A, dendrodendritic or axodendritic synapses: they can generate rhythmic sequences of LT Ca^{2+} spikes (through an interaction between the LT Ca^{2+} current and a Ca^{2+} activated K^+ current), which, through activation of GABA A receptors, generate similar bursting in TC cells. These in turn excite TRN cells, closing a disynaptic loop. TRN cells show the highest levels of tonic activity during heightened vigilance. Some GABA TRN cells also project to local inhibitory neurons located in different dorsal thalamic nuclei. Thus, some TC cells may be disinhibited inside a surrounding core of inhibition. In primates, the TRN can be divided into a number of sectors each concerned with a different function. Each sector is connected to more than one thalamic nucleus and to more than one cortical area; each sector has topographically mapped connections with the thalamus and cortex. For instance, Vc relates to one sector of TRN, bidirectionally, and TRN also receives from SI. Connections are not the same for each sector: TRN acts as a nexus where several functionally related cortical areas and thalamic nuclei interact modifying TC transmission through the inhibitory connections that go from TRN cells to TC relay cells. In the somatosensory system, both first- and higher-order nuclei project to the same sector (e.g., Pom — higher order — relays to SII; Vc — first order — to SI). Although complete human data are not available (Guillery et al. 1998), humans appear to have a network of intrinsic thalamic and cortical GABA interneurons. A mutual inhibitory coupling exists between TRN cells, responsible for nuclear oscillation, synchronized by CT input. TRN cells may also project to *contralateral dorsal thalamus* in the intrathalamic commissure, potentially influencing the cerebral cortex and basal ganglia of *both* hemispheres (Steriade et al. 1997).

The cortex has a powerful role in controlling the coherence of thalamic oscillations. CT synaptic volleys succeed in synchronizing pools of thalamic cells by activating GABA TRN cells that project to thalamic relay cells and hyperpolarize them. Slow cortical oscillations initiated apparently in layer 5 as an excitatory interaction between pyramidal neurons propagate through the neocortex. This generates a depolarized state through recurrent excitation regulated by inhibitory networks, thus allowing local cortical circuits to enter into temporarily activated and self-maintained excitatory states. At each step of the pathways that link various neocortical areas, CT neurons impinge on TRN cells that in turn produce inhibitory rebound sequences in dorsal thalamic relay neurons projecting in the reentrant corticopetal systems, thus changing the time course and synchronization of intracortical events. Short-term plasticity processes, i.e., persistent and progressive increases in depolarizing synaptic responses and

BOX 8.2 Thalamocortical rhythmicity *(continued)*

decreases in inhibitory responses, can lead to self-sustained oscillations owing to resonant activities in closed loops. *The repeated circulation of impulses in reverberating circuits could lead to synaptic modifications in target structures* (Steriade 1999; Sanchez-Vives and McCormick 2000). *Under certain physiological conditions one neuronal neocortical electrophysiological type can be transformed into another by small changes in membrane potential or synaptic activities inside thalamocorticothalamic loops* (Steriade 1999; Sanchez-Vives and McCormick 2000).

Neurons with intrinsic oscillatory properties (cell-drive oscillators), networks of non-intrinsically oscillating GABA interneurons (network oscillators based on reciprocal inhibition, recurrent cyclic inhibition, but also on recurrent excitation), driven by tonic metabotropic glutamatergic input or (more often) mixed oscillators and long loop thalamocortical interactions all contribute to both the occurrence of oscillatory activity and their frequencies. Longer range synchrony in the neocortex could occur by resonating with the thalamocortical loop (Jefferys *et al.* 1996). Recurrent processing may have a specific role for perceptual awareness (Supèr *et al.* 2001).

Individual neurons can have frequency preferences that enable them to generate spontaneous oscillations or respond best to inputs within a narrow frequency window (low- and/or high-pass filtering behavior creating a notch filter leading to resonance), with a role in determining the dynamics of coherent brain activity. Resonance and spontaneous oscillations can coexist in the same system, being two aspects of the same basic phenomenon of frequency preference. A resonant system evolves continuously into a spontaneously oscillatory system as the amplifying conductance is increased. The frequency of the oscillations of the resonance is set by the properties of the resonant conductance. There are three classes of frequency-dependent mechanisms in central neurons: solitary resonances, resonances arising from interaction with amplifying mechanisms (e.g., NMDA mediated) and spontaneous oscillations caused when a resonant current interacts so strongly with an amplifying current that the resting membrane potential becomes destabilized. In other words, slowly activating currents that actively oppose changes in membrane voltage produce resonance: the frequency of resonance is voltage-dependent. The scope of resonance may be to help integrate inputs to neurons (Hutcheon and Yarom 2000).

The overall setpoint of the thalamocortical system is modulated by several inputs from brainstem, hypothalamus (activating) and cortex (layer 6) (Shepherd 2004). Thus, there is a high concentration of 5HT/histamine input in CL and related nuclei, while TRN cells are excited by NE and 5HT (inhibiting TC output) and inhibited by Ach (M2) from Meynert's nucleus (during novelty or danger) and GABA (e.g., from basal ganglia or other TRN or inhibitory interneurons) (facilitating TC output): the process can be highly selective, creating foci of inhibition or disinhibition, e.g., in Vc. The GABAergic projection from basal forebrain may target TRN, but not Vc. Transition from burst to tonic mode in TC cells results from 5HT, NE, Ach, histamine, nitric oxide and glutamate input, vice versa only from glutamate input. NE/DA fibers modulate the loop, by acting on layers 5 (thalamoreceptive) and 1 (where dendrodendritic synapses between TC projections from CL and those from bursting pyramidal cells in layer 5 exist).

cortex and thalamus (Wang 2001), but can also be produced locally within a cortical area from reverberatory excitation, stimulus selectivity being formed by recurrent inhibition within a columnar cortical network (Goldman-Rakic 1995). Persistent activity can also be maintained by reciprocal loops between cortical areas (see references in Wang 2001); extensive horizontal excitatory connections are known to exist, especially in layer 2–3. Feedback excitation can also originate from regenerative membrane dynamics of single neurons: voltage and Ca^{2+} gated ion channels could in principle generate bistability between a resting and an active state, sustained by a plateau potential. Activation of relevant ion currents could require neuromodulatory signals such as acetylcholine. Also, the coupling strength of the neural network of the brain changes periodically, with a cyclic alteration from a central to a parallel processing mode of information, reflecting state transitions from synchronized, low complex EEG activity to desynchronized high complex activity and vice versa, with a disturbance of temporal order (Tirsch *et al.* 2004).

2. **Nonlinear dynamics.** The emergence of patterns in open, non-equilibrium systems (e.g., the brain) is governed by their stability in response to small disturbances and predicts macroscopic transitions between patterns of differing stability (Meyer-Lindenberg *et al.* 2002). Using ergodic nonlinear dynamics, discharge patterns can be represented by an attractor (Stewart 1997). The emergence of a persistent "attractor state" (attractors with non-integer dimensions are called fractals) requires that excitatory connections in a recurrent network are sufficiently strong; when the strength of excitatory connections between neurons within each subpopulation is increased beyond a critical threshold, *persistent activity appears as an all-or-none phenomenon.* Below the critical threshold, only the spontaneous state exists; above it, the spontaneous activity state is still dynamically stable to small perturbations, because at low firing rates excitation is effectively counteracted by feedback inhibition. However, if a stimulus generates a transient high activity in a neural subpopulation, recurrent reverberation is now sufficiently powerful to drive this group of cells to "escape" from the spontaneous state. A higher firing activity leads to an even larger recurrent synaptic excitation, which becomes sufficient to sustain a persistent active state after the stimulus is withdrawn. The firing rate is eventually stabilized by negative feedback. As a result, a stable attractor of *persistent* activity with an *elevated firing rate* is realized, which coexists with the stable spontaneous state, i.e., chaos can synchronize. Among possible contributors to control of firing rates are outward ion currents in the cell, feedback inhibition, short-term synaptic depression and saturation of the synaptic drive at high frequencies. A prediction from attractor models is that persistent activity depends on the strength of recurrent excitation in an abrupt manner, so that *activity could disappear suddenly when excitatory synaptic transmission is gradually reduced by pharmacological means.* Through a complex mechanism involving temporal filtering of rhythmic signals through resonance, subthreshold oscillations and bursting (Izhikevich *et al.* 2003), *the brain can reorganize itself dynamically within a few milliseconds, without changing the synaptic hardware.* Structured excitatory connectivity can arise from a columnar organization or through hebbian long-term plasticity (but synaptic reverberation is also possible). Persistent activity can be stored in the form of a "bump attractor," a spatially localized persistent activity pattern naturally arising from a network connectivity under certain conditions and sustained by recurrent synaptic excitation within a local group of pyramidal cells. *Stable bump attractors typically require that lateral inhibition is spatially more widespread than excitation with interneurons with broader tuning curves and/or projecting widely to their targets.* A loop is more stable if the network's recurrent synapses are primarily mediated by NMDA receptors.

3. **"Small world" networking.** The brain has a mixture of order and chaos, with local thick connections and more random global connections. This paves the way to small world networks (Strogatz 2003): regardless of its size, any two points within neurons are always linked by only a small number of steps. When 10–20% of

neurons participate in shortcuts, the network forms self-sustaining loops of activity. For instance, following an activating pulse, region A may activate region B through a shortcut that would similarly trigger C; a shortcut from C sparks A again, completing the loop. A second strong activating pulse may shut the whole system down again. This conceptual approach directly leads to bistability (Roxin *et al.* 2004). In this scenario, shortcuts are fast relay channels that allow reciprocal influences to spread rapidly in the entire population. A small world architecture entrains a more efficient global coordination (Buchanan 2002; Strogatz 2003).

WHAT RELEASES CP?

While a variety of cultural, psychological and physiological factors contribute to variability in both clinical and experimental contexts, the role of genetic factors in human pain sensitivity is increasingly recognized as an important element, notably genetic predisposition acting, for example, at receptor level (Mogil 1999; Kim *et al.* 2004). Women, despite possessing an adjuvant nicotinic spinal anti-nociceptive path locally mediated by estrogens, are known to be more responsive to noxious stimuli (Woodrow *et al.* 1972) and to be at much greater risk for developing a large number of pain syndromes. Pain thresholds increase with age (Schludermann and Zubeck 1962), due to an apparent age-related change in the central primary afferent response to peripheral insult (Friedman 1991). PET studies reveal that humans widely differ in baseline and pain-induced levels of endogenous opioids (Zubieta *et al.* 1999, 2001), with larger activation of the opioid system correlating with lower sensory and affective ratings to the sustained pain stimulus. Pain sensitive persons show more frequent and more robust pain-induced activation of SI, ACC and PFC than "stoic" ones (Coghill *et al.* 2003). We proposed that there may be a genetically determined "oscillation threshold" of pain-coded thalamocortical neurons, which may be particularly low in CP patients (Canavero 1994).

If we consider single diseases originating CP, it is difficult to say whether CP is truly more frequent in one or another, due to a lack of epidemiological evidence. For instance, there may be a difference among compressive (e.g., meningiomas) versus disruptive (e.g., ischemia) lesions. On the other hand, purported rarity of tumor-associated CP may either depend on underdiagnosis, infrequence of parietal lobe lesions compared to all possible brain sites or be related to the fact that many tumors displace, rather than destroy, neural tissue during the early stages of their development; however, compression can be enough to trigger CP. What is now clear is that the incidence of CP at thalamic, brainstem and cord (too few epidemiological data are available for the cortex) differs little (Chapter 1): after thalamic stroke with sensory symptoms, mesencephalic stroke, spinal cord injury (below-level pains only) and MS, this runs at, respectively, 17–18%, 15–25%, about 25% and about 18%. It might seem that STT damage leads to CP in a similar percentage of patients, regardless of level. This would nix older theories that differential incidences of CP are due to anatomical proximity rather than not of different pain bundles (STT versus SRT) at cord, brainstem and thalamic levels (e.g., Cassinari and Pagni 1969; Nathan and Smith 1984), an anatomically moot observation. This population of patients must have something in common besides anatomical damage (idiosyncrasy), since STT damage alone is necessary, but not sufficient to release CP.

During the past 100 years or so, several theories have been proposed to justify CP release. Following the original proposal of Head and Holmes (1911) to explain the thalamic syndrome ("exaggerated responses in cases where the thalamic centre has been freed from control" of descending cortical origin), imbalance/disinhibition ("escape") theories prevailed, in light of their explicative potential (Botterell et al. 1954).

1. STT inhibits ML. According to a theory (Beric 1993, 1999, and references therein), stroke or SCI patients with complete sensory ascending dysfunction (STT, perhaps also SRT, and DC/ML) do not — bar rare exceptions — develop CP (however, this does not mean that 80% of sensory stroke patients who do not have CP have complete destruction of sensory pathways, which is not the case). Instead, dysesthesias are reported in incomplete SCI patients, all with mild, moderate or severe disruption of STT modalities and partial or complete preservation of A-beta mediated (DC/ML) modalities, with movement, gait and even, in some instances, SCS (e.g., in one ASAS case; see also Cole et al. 1987) exaggerating the dysesthesias. TENS, SCS, thalamocapsular DBS and even CS may worsen CP in some patients (see Chapter 6). Triggs and Beric (1994) found that 6 (1 thalamic lesion, 2 a brainstem lesion and 3 a cortico-subcortical lesion) of 48 stroke patients had functionally limiting dysesthesias induced in the setting of dynamic mechanical allodynia or by neuromuscular electrical stimulation (NMS). All these had relatively preserved sensibilities attributable to DC/ML function. Even during remission, dysesthesias and pain could be triggered by additional afferent input to the DC/ML system; gentle touching of partially deafferented dermatomes evoked dysesthesias in two of their anterior spinal artery syndrome (ASAS) CP cases. Since dysesthesias usually appear at the time when dorsal column modalities of sensations can again be elicited, in the face of severe and still complete interruption of STT functions, the recovery and activity in the DC/ML system may be surmised to set off a chain of events at thalamocortical levels. In fact, CP often arises as sensory (and motor) loss improves (Schott 2001a). One exemplificative patient (case 22, Mauguière and Desmedt 1988) showed an aggravation of the pain, as lemniscal transmission improved and cortical SEPs partially recovered. None of 4 patients with combined lateral and medial medullary stroke developed CP (Kim et al. 1995b), nor did ASAS patient 3 of Triggs and Beric (1992), who had the most severe anterolateral system dysfunction. These authors (Triggs and Beric 1993) also reported disinhibition of somatosensory evoked potentials in a patient with ASAS. On the other hand, cordectomies which completely destroy all ascending afferences should quench below-level CP and do not. SCS actually relieves, at least initially, a minority of incomplete SCI CP patients and so does TENS (see Chapter 6). CP occurs in cases with complete spinal transection or following supratentorial lesions affecting both STT and ML sensibilities. Benefit is also seen after electrophysiology guided DREZ lesions for both at- and below-level pains. Cordotomy can relieve evoked pains (without worsening spontaneous pains) in several patients. In light of these objections, Beric concluded that the suggested

mechanism is only responsible for dysesthesias and *not* pain. Actually, lemniscal fibers do play a role in tactile allodynia (see below).

2. ML inhibits STT. Fabritius (1907) believed that it was damage in the posterolateral columns of white matter of a corticofugal pathway that was correlated with the appearance of the spontaneous pains that beset some of his patients after SCI. Förster (1927, 1936) observed that, after division of the posterior columns or the medial lemniscus, normally painful stimulation becomes excessively painful, stimuli normally painless become painful and, above all, spontaneous unpleasant dysesthesias and more or less severe spontaneous pains in those parts of the body corresponding to the lesion in the posterior column may occur. After weeks to months, symptoms gradually disappeared, but in some cases persisted for years. Förster (1927) wrote: "in the area of the posterolateral columns, possibly in the boundary zone with the gray matter, a corticofugal pathway runs which exerts a damping influence on the pain system associated with neurons of the posterior horn whose loss leads to increased excitability of these posterior horns" (see also Riddoch 1938; Frazier *et al.* 1937). Pool (1946) noted in his posterior cordotomies that "The application of cool or warm objects to the skin produced an exaggerated and disagreeable sensation of cold and warm respectively, causing the patient to flinch." Orthner and Roeder (1966) believed that CP resulted from lesions of the ML (but not of the SRT) tract. The patients reported by Nathan and colleagues (1986) with posterior column lesions

> had an abnormally increased sensation with pricking, warm and cold stimuli, with rubbing the skin and with any stimuli that caused tickle. Pain on pressure had a lower threshold than in the normal; and painful stimuli felt more unpleasant and more painful than in normally innervated regions. In fact, all forms of sensibility relying on impulses in the spinothalamic complex were increased. When the lesion had been made in one posterior column, these effects were ipsilateral to the lesion and occurred in the segments deprived of posterior column fibers. That this increased sensation is accompanied by an increased discharge in the relevant neurons is suggested by the fact that "in one patient the threshold of the flexor response to noxious, warm and cold stimuli was lowered."

Sweet (1991) believed that "it seems possible that the pain following posterior column lesions ... is due to elimination of tonic suppressor impulses in this same region." One of his patients with bilateral cancer pain in the torso had a bilateral cordotomy in two stages at high dorsal levels. Both incisions accidentally generously incised both posterolateral columns. Months after the second operation, CP developed first on one side, then on the other, in analgesic areas. The only type of posterior column sensory deficit was a loss of vibration sense in the right leg. Autopsy revealed extensive demyelination of the ventral 70% of the posteromedial columns of white matter and less intense degeneration of the ventral part of the posterolateral columns of white matter. A second patient developed CP and spasticity in all four limbs since birth, from a central cerebral lesion. He underwent a two-stage bilateral upper thoracic cordotomy, which relieved the pain in both legs. At autopsy, there was an even greater posterior, but a lesser anterior, extension of the lesions on both sides. There was no involvement of the posterior horns or posterior columns on either side.

The differing incisions in these two cases "intimate that the pain suppressor function in the posterior columns was destroyed in the first case." Actually, posterior cordotomies never gave rise to persistent pain (Chapter 2) and posterior columns are intact in cases of CP following anterolateral cordotomies and ASAS. SCS, which should engage this tonic suppressor mechanism, is ineffective even in the majority of patients with retained DC function (see Chapter 6) and can even worsen CP (Triggs and Beric 1994). The impairment of touch processing seen in CP patients can be normalized by pain relieving procedures (e.g., propofol, TMS and CS), so that the patient can feel touch normally (see also Nathan 1960). Actually, lemniscal activity in BA3b and STT pain related BA3a are mutually inhibitory by intracortical connections (Tommerdahl *et al.* 1996; see also Apkarian *et al.* 1994; Schnitzler and Ploner 2000). In the human Vc, STT terminal clusters appear to be relatively separated from lemniscal terminal areas, with some overlap (Lenz and Dougherty 1997). This notwithstanding, the strongest opposition to a role of DC/ML fibers in CP comes from several CP patients having intact epicritic conduction.

3. STT inhibits SRT. A slow multisynaptic spinoreticulothalamic pathway (SRT) is strongly suggested by neurosurgical evidence (see King 1977; Gybels and Sweet 1989, p. 192), but also by current clinical (medial medullary infarctions; Bassetti *et al.* 1997) and neurophysiological data (Rousseau *et al.* 1999). According to several authors (e.g., Noordenbos 1959; Hassler 1959; Cassinari and Pagni 1969; Nathan and Smith 1984; McGowan *et al.* 1997), damage to STT weakens this damping on SRT (slow multisynaptic ascending system) at all levels of cord and brainstem and CP arises (i.e., *local disinhibition* of the polysynaptic system which becomes hypersensitive): "The more the lesion spares the paleospinothalamic afferents, the greater the chances of occurrence of central pain." (Lhermitte also postulated a damping of the SRT by the ML.) At least one report (Mikula *et al.* 1959, 25 mesencephalotomies) concluded that sparing the reticular system reduces the incidence of dysesthesias. On the other hand, Amano's group (Table 7.1) abolished CP in many cases by selective destruction of the reticular formation, with no new CP arising (unlike STT mesencephalic interruption): this is the strongest evidence up to now of a role of the reticular formation in CP.

4. Descending fiber damage. Some believe that the simultaneous involvement of multiple different descending inhibitory fibers and ascending pathways may be more important than denervation singly. An imbalance of descending modulating pathways, affected at sites remote from the injury, is thought to be a mechanism of release. It should also be recalled how there not only exist antinociceptive systems, but also pro-nociceptive systems, so that different degrees of injury may tip the balance toward one of them, favoring, or not, hyperexcitability and the onset of pain (Millan 2002). Since the brainstem analgesia systems have bilateral effects, damage thereof is unlikely to explain a unilateral pain syndrome; besides, it is not clear what would predominate in CP, excitation or inhibition (Sandkuehler 1996; Porreca *et al.* 2002). Others find that initiation (but not maintenance) of CP is independent of reduction or loss of descending or propriospinal inhibitory fibers.

5. Thermosensory disinhibition. According to this hypothesis (Craig 1998), a cold signaling enteroceptive A-delta STT path from spinal LI to thalamic nucleus VMpo to (purported) thermosensory (cold-recipient) dorsal mid/posterior insula (which then modulates brainstem thermoregulatory stations) normally inhibits a medial heat-pinch-cold nociceptive (HPC) STT path (from multimodal cells receiving input from C fibers) passing from LI through thalamic nucleus MDvc en route to ACC. In CP patients, a lesion of the cold path disinhibits the medial path, with cold allodynia and deep burning pain being selectively felt in the ACC, with activation of homeostatic behaviors. Cold allodynia would be due to impairment of thermal sensibility. This theory is *totally refuted* by an impressive number of observations: (1) not all patients with CP complain of burning or thermally described pain; (2) a minority only complains of cold allodynia, in the face of frequent (but not universal) impairment of thermal sensibility, and actually the most extreme cold allodynia occurred in a patient with normal cold detection thresholds in one study (Greenspan et al. 2004); (3) disrupted thermal sensation in CPSP is not associated with a corresponding relationship between altered cold perception and spontaneous pain (Jensen et al. 2002); (4) CP may be felt superficially and in depth; (5) unexplained (by the theory) nonthermal allodynia; (6) heat or increases of body temperature during exercise or fever do not allay CP (as suggested by this theory), but in some cases (e.g., Romanelli and Heit 2004) may well worsen it (e.g., MS CP, plus heat allodynia in some BCP/CCP cases): cool air actually temporarily reduced the intensity of CP in at least one of our patients; (7) contrary fMR evidence of thermal coding in the insula (Brooks et al. 2002); (8) no ACC activation during cold allodynia in CP patients (Chapter 7, Section 1); (9) no unequivocal metabolic evidence for a role of ACC in perceived unpleasantness of pain (Casey et al. 2001) and cold pain tout court; (10) inefficacy of cingulotomies to relieve CP, but not other chronic pains; (11) clear-cut anatomical evidence contrary to the existence and/or importance of the cold and HPC paths (see complete list in Wall 1995); although a segregated warmth spinal path exists in humans (Iannetti et al. 2003; Friehs et al. 1995). Lahuerta and colleagues (1994) noted how surgical interruption of the STT does not abolish pain sensation completely: only 1500 STT fibers reach the cortex, and other paths are required; (12) non-exclusive role of VMpo as a thermal-specific thalamic relay and ample doubts about its existence (Percheron 2004; Willis and Westlund 2004); (13) failure of elicitation of painful or unpleasant sensations by electrical stimulation, even with high currents, at sites in the ACC, where pain-sensitive. neurons can be recorded in human patients (Hutchison et al. 1999), as pain-related activity in the ACC may represent descending modulation rather than perception of pain; (14) a metaanalysis of all chronic pain imaging studies found that a decreased incidence of activity in ACC and thalamus, coupled with decreased coding for perceived pain in ACC, as well as an increased incidence of activity in the prefrontal cortex, all contradict the thermosensory hypothesis (Apkarian et al. 2005).

6. Injury discharges. Rare patients have no sensory deficit, even with laser SEPs. Frank injury is not necessary to induce the pain state: "Indeed, the process we call 'central sensitization' may not require that a nerve be injured at all, but only that a noxious stimulus be delivered" (Devor et al. 1991). Enhanced patterns of

electrical discharges can alter central processing of sensory input without actual damage, provided an acute, severe pain stimulus is given. Even when injury occurs, the first signals to reach the CNS and notify that it has taken place are so-called injury discharges, short high-frequency signals lasting several minutes at most transmitted along nociceptive fibers. It is speculated that a rapid depolarization ensues in dorsal horn inhibitory neurons, disabling them via an excitotoxic mechanism, with attendant long-lasting disinhibition of primary afferent input to the dorsal horn (the basis of preemptive analgesia: Bonicalzi *et al.* 1997).

7. Different side of injured brain. Right thalamic lesions are more likely to originate CP (see Chapter 2). Increased frequency of chronic pain (including CP) after right-sided lesions may be due to right hemisphere's specialization for negative high-arousal emotions (including pain) and for monitoring of somatic state. In normal subjects, pain threshold and pain tolerance are lower on the left hemisoma than the right for electrical thermal and focal pressure stimulation; patients with right hemisphere injury lesions tolerate pain longer than those with left hemisphere lesions and show reduced galvanic skin responses to ipsilesionally administered painful stimuli; there is greater alpha EEG suppression in the right compared to the left hemisphere during exposure to thermal pain (see references in Nasreddine and Saver 1997). This may be due to cortically mediated attentional factors (Meador *et al.* 1998, and references therein). Also, the human thalamus shows a strong right lateralization of norepinephrine, which has a role in somatosensory information processing (Oke *et al.* 1978; Canavero and Bonicalzi 1998b).

8. Intensity of STT damage. Since lesion location is not predictive of CP, as lesions may be found at all levels from brainstem to cortex (opposite to speculations of other authors, e.g., Sweet (1991), who believed the site of the lesion, rather than the presence of the deafferentation, is the most critical factor determining pain onset), it is speculated that the important factor in releasing CP is the degree of pain and temperature loss and "the level (concentration) of transmitter receptors in these pathways" (Bowsher *et al.* 1998). However, cordotomy severely or completely interrupts STT, but CP follows in only a minority of cases, and so ASAS. Specularly, CP patients with minimal damage to the STT exist.

9. Wrong temporospatial integration of sensory input (Kendall 1939: injury to fast, but not slow, pain fibers eliminates refractoriness of end-stations to slow fiber input; Walker 1955: greater interruption of STT fibers bound for Vc than for CL, with diffuseness of output; Nathan and Smith 1984: massive cortical activation by impulses traveling along the reticulothalamocortical paths of the diffuse projection system). Subliminal impulses may become supraliminal, but since nociceptors do not fire tonically (Ochoa 1993), only tactile stimuli should be involved.

10. Engagement of latent pathways. Injury appears to lead to the *unmasking of latent pathways*: supposedly, central connections display a continuous adjustment between activated and latent states, offsetting too much excitation or inhibition. This may depend on inhibitory interneurons, keeping "fringe inputs" from being effective. This unmasking would basically consist of a rapid reorganization due to rebalancing of excitation/inhibition. According to Nathan and coworkers (1986),

"the sudden onset of a lesion must alter the activity of the CNS...The usual organization of facilitation and inhibition will be changed...The organization of descending control is bound to be altered drastically. That there are possible pathways constantly closed by inhibition was shown by Kirk and Denny-Brown (1970) and Denny-Brown et al. (1973)." In patients with complete section of the spinothalamic complex and dense and persistent contralateral analgesia, immediate onset of allochiria is seen in the previously analgesic area after cordotomy. Although allochiria is not CP, it has supported speculations that CP may be subtended by an already existing, but unavailable, subsidiary pathway (Nathan and Smith 1979; Nagaro et al. 1993) localized in the posterior third of the cord (posterior horns or Lissauer's tracts), as reference of pain and CP may be observed following complete destruction of the anterior two thirds of the cord (like in ASAS). This *mirror pain (or reference of pain or allochiria)* occurs in 9–63.3% of cordotomized patients and in some can be severe (Tasker and North 1997). Nagaro and colleagues (1993) found that in 7/66 patients undergoing percutaneous cordotomy, allochiria appeared immediately after induction of analgesia and disappeared when analgesia faded. It was elicited only from analgesic areas and was experienced either *at the same or a more cephalad dermatomal level* on the contralateral body (only in one patient in the literature it was more caudad). Each patient with allochiria also developed new contralateral, usually mirror, pain after cordotomy and, in one patient in whom mirror pain appeared 6 hours after the cordotomy, subarachnoid phenol block temporarily relieved both, suggesting a spinal mechanism. The fact that allochiria is observed after destruction of the anterior two-thirds of the spinal cord (also in ASAS) supports the idea that the pathways responsible for reference of pain, normally silent, are found in the dorsal horn (lamina II) and connecting fibers (propriospinal) including the tract of Lissauer. The disappearance of referred pain with contralateral cervical cordotomy shows that the impulses causing reference of pain reach the dorsal horn neurons which have a receptive field where the pain is felt and go up the contralateral anterolateral column (Nagaro et al. 1993). Thus, allochiria and new mirror pain may depend on loss of feedback inhibition from second-order neurons and/or more central neurons of the nociceptive pathway of an already existing subsidiary pathway, i.e., a network of short neurons which connects dorsal horn neurons longitudinally and latitudinally. Destruction of tonic descending inhibitory pathways is excluded, as reference of pain occurs only from the region rendered analgesic by cordotomy, while disinhibition would occur more widely than this region. Despite the interest of such rapid appearance of mirror pain, this is a completely different phenomenon than acute-onset CP.

DISSECTING THE ROLE OF GABA

GABA is the most important inhibitory neurotransmitter in the human CNS. Of three classes of receptors (A, B, C), GABA A receptors are foremost in the regulation of brain excitability, timing-based signaling, setting the temporal window for synaptic integration and synchronizing neural networks. However, it has become clear that *there is no unique GABA A (and possibly also B) receptor in the CNS, instead there is great heterogeneity, with a large number of different GABA A receptor subunits with distinct regional distribution*; also, individual GABA A receptor subtypes are associated with distinct neuronal structures and subcellular distributions. Thus, *composition differs not only in different parts of the brain or in different cells, but also in the same cell at different synapses,* and *their differential activation is correlated with distinct pharmacological and behavioral phenotypes. The same GABAergic axon can form distinct types of synapses onto different classes of target neurons* (Markram *et al.* 2004). While synapses at the soma control action potential generation, synapses at distal dendrites control incoming input and propagation of Ca^{2+} currents. Each receptor subtype (more than 20) has its own target identity depending on the subunits.

GABA receptors are pentameric heterooligomers; 19 distinct GABA A receptor subunit genes are known, classified into 8 classes (α 1–6, β 1–3, γ 1–3, δ, ε, θ, π and ρ 1–3). GABA A receptor assembly can be derived from a permutation and combination of two, three, four or even five different subunits, with the majority of subtypes in the brain composed of assemblies of alpha, beta and gamma subunits. Distribution of the major subunits in various regions of the brain varies: e.g., the cerebral cortex has intermediate levels of α 1–4 subunits and low levels of α 5 subunit, whereas the thalamus contains high levels of α 4 subunits and intermediate levels of δ subunit (Olsen and Avoli 1997; Sleghart and Sperk 2002; Kittler and Moss 2002; Rudolph and Antkowiak 2004; Olsen and Betz 2006). The number of synaptic GABA A receptors can be dynamically modulated and the modulation of 5HT and dopamine receptor function also hinges on modification of GABA A receptor activity (Sleghart and Sperk 2002; Kittler and Moss 2002). Finally, inhibitory interneurons are heterogeneous (about 50 types), some long-ranging, some also displaying bursting patterns; their role at both cortical and thalamic levels may vary greatly among various types of processing streams (reviewed in Markram *et al.* 2004).

The consequences of GABA A receptor activation on active membrane properties is context-specific, depending on the history of the membrane (the ratio of activated to inactivated to closed voltage gated channels at the time of GABA A receptor activation), the spatial location of GABA A receptors and the distribution of voltage gated channels along the somatodendritic axis. *GABA neurotransmission can be excitatory in basal conditions, also in adult tissue,* so that "hypofunctionality" of a GABAergic pathway can in reality decrease the global excitability of the network. Unlike cationic glutamatergic synapses, GABA synapses have a unique feature resulting from their chloride permeability that enables them to shift from an inhibitory mode of operation to one that mainly excites (Cossart *et al.* 2005).

What happens following injury (for simplicity, we assume no fundamental difference among trauma, ischemia and compression)? Considerable and rapid plastic changes in the amount and distribution of many CNS receptors take place: neurons can alter their chemical code and increase, decrease or change the expression of neurotransmitters; intense electrical activity may in itself affect the concentrations of some peptides (see Bullitt 1991). However, data strongly suggest that the key to CP lies in GABA receptors, specifically GABA A receptors. Given its clear-cut profile of action at subhypnotic dosage, propofol provides an important window, much more than barbiturates or benzodiazepines (see Chapter 5). GABA A modulation affords the strongest levels of CP relief (particularly propofol) — while ketamine, less potent, would point to NMDA receptors — and appears to be more effective than GABA B modulation (although this assumption is based on incomplete evidence).

Following injury, not only the number of GABA A receptors can change, but even, and perhaps more importantly, the subunit composition (*subunit switch*) — as also seen in epilepsy — perhaps as a result of aberrant compensatory plasticity (i.e., a new receptor isoform that is less functional might become relatively more abundant). Intracellular changes other than subunit switch can also change GABA A receptor function: receptorial or release mechanisms are primary candidates to explain those alterations, e.g., phosphorylation processes or anchoring of the receptors by gephyrin, GABA receptor-associated protein and others. Uncoupling may be rapidly produced and reversed, without alteration of gene expression. The result may be altered, *persistent*, regulation of inhibitory function, i.e., hypo-functionality. The process of subunit switch is clearly *dynamic* (Cossart *et al.* 2005).

Both SI and sensory thalamus show a tonic inhibitory tone, modulated by sensory input: this has important consequences on stimulus localization and receptive fields (RFs), but also for compensatory adjustments following injury. In the cortex, GABA has a particularly high density in layer 4. Prolonged or overactive GABAergic synaptic transmission (or chronic high doses of GABA agonists such as benzodiazepines and baclofen) can lead to *decreased* (downregulated) GABAergic function (A and B). This plasticity may occur *over a few seconds* (e.g., during modestly enhanced glutamate activity) — up to years in other contexts. *GABA levels in the human SI are reduced within minutes of deafferentation* (Levy *et al.* 2002) and propofol data point to a disrupted GABA A inhibition. *Subtle reductions in GABA inhibition result in large changes in excitatory conduction and spread of activity to distant cortical sites* (even in the face of paradoxical increases in evoked polysynaptic inhibition due to enhanced excitatory drive onto GABA interneurons) and local changes in GABA activity may lead to temporary associations between adjacent cell groups, enabling reorganization (Jacobs and Donoghue 1991). Also, a deficit in dendritic (versus somatic) inhibition (from dendritic projecting interneurons) can reduce the excitability threshold (Cossart *et al.* 2005). Inhibition is carefully modulated at several levels, including specific transporters and "tonic" spill-over currents (Semyanov *et al.* 2004) in a dynamic balance.

The β subunit (β 2-3) is key to the direct actions of propofol (reviewed in Rudolph and Antkowiak 2004). Low versus high doses differentially activate different sub-units, and propofol may directly activate GABA A receptors in the absence of GABA (reviewed in Olsen and Avoli 1997). Barbiturate and benzodiazepines action, in contrast, hinges on α subunits (Olsen and Avoli 1997; Rudolph and Antkowiak 2004). These data may guide the search of — possibly — altered genes in CP patients.

Exceptional cases of patients worsened by GABA agonists (Chapter 5) are not in contradiction to the above discussion. Inhibition is not always reduced: for instance, in a few brain regions of some epileptic patients it can be *increased* as a compensatory mechanism to hyperexcitation (Brooks-Kayal 1998; Nusser *et al.* 1998). Moreover, GABAergic activity may be excitatory depending on local circuitry through a disinhibition (Koehling 2002); also, when GABA B receptors are located at inhibitory terminals (autoreceptors), their activation will decrease GABA release and may result in excitatory influence (Olsen and Avoli 1997). Hyperactivity at GABA synapses leads to an increased number of postsynaptic GABA A receptors and an *alteration in their subunit composition* (Olsen and Avoli 1997). Paradoxically, small decreases in glutamatergic excitation within cortical circuits which may decrease excitation of interneurons might also lead to a relative disinhibition of pyramidal neurons and hyperexcitability (Salin and Prince 1996). More simply, in propofol non-responders (generally patients with ischemic/mechanical disruptive rather than compressive lesions), the hypothesized glutamatergic hypertonus may be too intense to be swamped (see in Canavero *et al.* 1996).

In sum, following injury, alterations occur rapidly, do not necessarily require neuronal damage, may become long-lasting; an inhibitory-to-excitatory shift of GABA actions can even become permanent (Cossart *et al.* 2005).

WHICH ROLE FOR NEUROPLASTICITY?

Neuroplastic changes are at the basis of much current thinking on the pathogenesis of chronic pains of different kinds and these will be shortly discussed.

That injury may cause hyperactivity has been known since Hall (1841) and Claude-Bernard (1880). A supersensitive state of denervated neural structures was postulated by Cannon and Rosenblueth (1949), who, even though they did not mention pain, recognized the fact that reorganization of the CNS follows denervation, discussed "plasticity" of the neurons, the interchangeability of the nervous pathways and influences, "the functional opening of new vicarious pathways determined by training" and the onset of "initiative foci."

Supposed animal models of chronic neuropathic pain evidenced a smorgasbord of plastic alterations, all apparently important in their genesis, that are rather difficult, even for proponents, to integrate in a coherent picture, including possible pre-emptive manipulation (e.g., Juliano *et al.* 1991).

One commonly discussed entity is so-called *central sensitization*, which follows prolonged or repeated noxious stimulation of STT neurons at the time of the pain-inducing lesion, possibly due to loss of effectiveness of inhibitory mechanisms within the spinothalamocortical pathway. This consists of a spectrum of derangements which include increased spontaneous discharge, evoked pains, but also denervation supersensitivity (an enhanced response of neural cells to the transmitter lost, and then reexpressed) and RF expansion, due to loss of sensory input. It is considered to be a form of long-term potentiation. So-called *wind-up*, a progressive increase in neuronal excitability akin to sensitization, observed in a minority of spinal cells only and some, but not all, chronic pains, follows repeated stimulation of nociceptive C fibers (Baranauskas and Nistri 1998). Although the NMDA receptor is considered pivotal to such changes, long-term sensitization actually requires co-activation of several receptor systems and possibly complicated unsus-pected mechanisms, depending on species and cell type, among others (Baranauskas and Nistri 1998); NMDA receptors are involved in many forms of synaptic plasti-city, so that additional mechanisms are necessary to impart specificity to pain-induced sensitization (making prevention of sensitization through NMDA block impractical).

Another plastic change which has been amply discussed as a possible contributor to chronic neuropathic pain is *sprouting*, a hierarchical and lesion-specific, non-random phenomenon, which follows injury. It includes *collateral sprouting* from uninjured neurons with variable restoration of anatomy (rapid: days, complete in days or months; extent: 40 micra), *ingrowth* from healthy, but functionally distinct neurons (1 month after injury), *pruning* (with growth of new axons from injured cell) with a more normal anatomic restoration (4 months after injury, lasts 2, extent up to 1 mm). Sprouting can lead to *rewiring*: e.g., intracortical sprouting can lead to generation of powerful monosynaptic excitatory feedback and intraspinally Aβ fibers may retarget STT neurons, or non-pain-relaying neurons, in LII and even switch neurochemical profile and function as C fibers. At the end of a literature review, Tasker and Dostrovsky (1989) concluded that, if sprouting occurs, it is of very limited extent and probably limited to a subpopulation of primary afferents and/or axons of CNS neurons, playing no role in receptive field expansion.

We have already discussed *decreased inhibition from lesions of descending or segmental pathways*, with changes in facilitation and inhibition (see above).

A fundamental role is attributed to somatotopographical rearrangements (repre-sentational remodeling), with expansion of RFs at all CNS levels, supposedly due to changes in synaptic efficacy, disinhibition with unmasking or strengthen-ing of latent, but ineffective, excitatory and convergent synaptic inputs, changes in intracellular processes leading to altered neuronal excitability, sprouting with creation of new synaptic connections. Acute lesions as well as manipulation of sensory inputs, can lead to rapid reorganization of the cerebral cortex, occurring within minutes to hours (references in Levy *et al.* 2002), through a rapid reduction of tonic GABA inhibition. Somatotopic rearrangements (up to 2−3 cm in cortex) have been reported in human pain states, namely phantom pain, and widely believed to correlate directly with painful sensations, particularly at cortical levels (Flor 2003). The more extensive SI reorganization after injury may depend in part on the activation of the widespread network of horizontally connecting axons within cortical areas − a feature missing in subcortical areas (e.g., the thalamus); the immediate expansion or new expression of RF in SI (disinhibition of silent inputs from body areas adjacent to denervated areas) may be subserved by the wide arboriza-tion of TC afferents. Cortical layers contribute differently to plasticity: cells in supragranular and infragranular layers respond rapidly to changes in sensory experience and then contribute to modifications in Layer 4 (Diamond *et al.* 1994). Yet, short-term dynamics of horizontal pathways in the middle of uniformly deprived SI change only modestly and vertical intracortical pathways are unaffected following loss of input. Thus, uniform loss of sensory activity has a limited effect on short-term synaptic dynamics and competition between deprived and spared sensory inputs is necessary to produce large-scale changes in synaptic dynamics after sensory deprivation (Finnerty and Connors 2000). Human evidence disproving the role of somatotopic rearrangement has been published (e.g., Moore and Schady 2000; Vega-Bermudez and Johnson 2002) and referred sensations/ mislocalization do not appear to be a direct perceptual correlate of cortical reorganization (Knecht *et al.* 1996). Knecht and colleagues (1998) report that phantom sensations can be evoked even in normal persons *without deafferentation* and pain itself in chronic pain patients can lead to representational reorganization (references in Knecht *et al.* 1996).

Generally discussed with injury-related neuroplasticity is *neuronal degeneration*, including inhibitory cells, and shrinkage, along with substantial dendritic atrophy, loss of dendritic spines and truncated dendrites and/or loss of the proximal axons and perikaryo-nuclear alterations. However, transneuronal degeneration with neuronal loss may be incompatible with concurrently extant central sensitization, and acute loss of GABA cells, for one, is excluded by the timeline of GABA decrease (although GABA cells appear to be particularly sensitive to disruptions of blood flow to the brain: over time these effects might kill them or reduce their ability to make and release GABA).

Truth is, neuroplasticity is something intrinsic to the nervous system, independent of injury. For instance, cortical maps express experience-dependent plasticity and SI normally reorganizes during various tasks; after injury, it serves a purpose of recovery.

All the discussed neuroplastic changes simply cannot sustain irreversible changes during CP, because CP can be promptly reversed (Chapter 7). This is not unique to CP. Cases of years-long neuropathic pains, including trigeminal neuralgia and carpal tunnel syndrome pain, resolve immediately after pain relieving surgery (Schott 2001a). Just as chronic pain is so often entrenched, changes in the nervous system following injury and disease (central sensitization) might be envisioned as irreversible. Abolition of chronic pain resulting from gross structural nerve damage sustained over many years is difficult to explain by current views on the major and extensive peripheral and central somatosensory changes thought to occur after nerve lesions. Interestingly, reversible epidural blocks of the nerve roots result in the *acute* appearance of new RFs that are lost and replaced by the original RF after the peripheral nerve recovers (Metzler and Marks 1979), pointing to great flexibility. Thus, either that they can be rapidly reversed or not, such changes would be inconsequential. Instead, they might play a role in the initial stages of CP: a GABA A receptor subunit switch was previously suggested. Further, loss of sensory input cannot explain immediate and delayed-onset pains, which are clinically identical: in the former, processes involving slowly developing, continually progressive neuronal changes cannot be essential for the generation of pain; likewise, loss of sensory input produces an *immediate and simultaneous* change in neuronal activity at multiple CNS levels — for instance, human thalamic neurons develop novel RFs within minutes (5–15 minutes) of lidocaine block (Kiss *et al.* 1995) and SI rapidly reorganizes during acute cluster headache attacks (Soros *et al.* 2002), with dendritic filopodia appearing within minutes (Maletic-Savatic *et al.* 1999). Thus, it is difficult to understand the progressive "entrenchment" (Schott 2001) some believe to exist. Further, denervation supersensitivity is present in both pain and non-pain cases.

In the nontraumatic cervical anterior spinal artery syndrome, a relatively rare anterior myelopathy with severe, practically complete interruption of the STT at the spinal level, STT fibers cannot be involved in any kind of transmission from the periphery, and thus maintain sensitization (Beric 1993) (however, uninterrupted SRT projections might play this role).

According to Tasker's group (Kiss *et al.* 1994), *the role of somatotopic reorganization in the genesis of CP — but also PNP — is entirely speculative.* Unlike animal models, there appears to be different patterns and degrees of somatotopic reorganization in the human, all (or none) of which may be associated with a pain syndrome. They conclude: "Although in some cases changes in somatotopic representation were observed, these changes were not consistent in all the groups and therefore unlikely to be the common cause of pain in these patients." Ojemann and Silbergeld (1995) found that "adult human sensory cortex retains its somatotopy even after two decades without conscious perception of that body part," after major peripheral denervation — unlike MI. Woolsey and colleagues (1979) also found maintenance of cortical sensory maps. Experience with extradural cortical stimulation in CP (see Chapter 6) confirms that sensory maps (the "homunculus") are stable. Unlike many, but not all, primate models of SI plasticity, humans display a relative preservation of the cortical sensory homunculus. Thus, in humans, *deprived, but reactivated neurons do not take on new and appropriate functions, but carry out their original roles long after they have had time to adopt new ones* (Davis *et al.* 1998). In a study of 12 thoracic SCI patients, 9 reported phantom sensations and 2 referred phantom sensations. In these 2, fMRI showed a relation between SI activation and the percept of referred phantom sensations. The authors concluded that, instead of somatotopical cortical reorganization, cortical plasticity may be the expression of co-activation of nonadjacent representations even distant between them, supported by somatotopic subcortical remapping projected to the cortex (Moore *et al.* 2000). Turner and colleagues (2003) examined with fMRI a group of SCI patients versus healthy controls. Unlike amputation, no evidence of expansion of the hand representation into nearby cortical areas was found, with hand sensory representation undergoing a much smaller posterior shift of hand motor representation. Reorganizations in the order of those seen in phantom sensation simply lack in CP. However, those few cases of CP regressed after stopping MCS (see Chapter 6) have been explained with some kind of reverse neuroplasticity in SI.

BILATERALITY OF CENTRAL PAIN

Although individual brain regions and networks of brain regions exhibit some degree of functional specialization, acute pain is processed by a highly distributed, redundant and resilient brain system, with — unlike other sensory modalities — detailed information about the intensity of a painful stimulus being conserved at multiple levels in both hemispheres — an arrangement that would justify the difficulty of eliciting painful sensations by cortical stimulation, as simultaneous activation of several regions may be necessary (Willis and Westlund 2004, and references therein). In other words, there is no "unique" pain center. Acute pain is essential for survival: individuals born without the ability to perceive pain frequently die from injuries and infections they have never felt. The distributed processing of pain within the human brain ensures that this critical ability to detect tissue injury can be spared in the face of extensive CNS damage. On such grounds, Melzack-Casey's hypothesis of sensory discriminative and affective motivational components of pain being processed in parallel by distinct neural systems fatally collapses, all the more so since it has never been seriously tested (Fields 1999). However, this is *not equivalent* to saying that chronic pain cannot be effectively abolished by selective lesions: while acute pain is necessary for survival, chronic pain is not, and abolition of even focal generators can relieve it. The impression that chronic pain cannot be abolished by focal lesions is due to poor analysis of the relevant literature and misconceptions about the exact generator of a particular chronic pain syndrome, as in the case of CP. On the other hand, the same neural substrates that support the bilateral distribution of nociceptive information processing during acute pain could subserve bilateral spread of chronic pain.

Somatosensation may be served by ipsilateral brain structures (reviewed in Coghill *et al.* 1999), as shown by hemispherectomy cases (Dandy 1933; Muller *et al.* 1991). Noordenbos and Wall (1976) described a patient with spinal cord transection with saving of only a part of one anterolateral quadrant, who could perceive tactile and painful stimuli on both body halves. Patients with corpus callosum transection can report tactile and painful (Stein *et al.* 1989) stimuli from either body half. Contrary to traditional views of spinothalamic transmission of pain, a significant proportion of functional imaging studies (8/20) employing unilateral painful stimuli have detected activation of both the contralateral and ipsilateral thalamus (see references in Coghill *et al.* 1999), which cannot be understood as a generalized arousal in reaction to pain.

Following PNS lesions, there are well-documented events affecting the contra-lateral nonlesioned structures, qualitatively similar to those occurring on the ipsilateral side (although usually smaller in magnitude and with a brief time course): "mirror pains" contralateral to nerve injury in humans have repeatedly been noted, and so bilateral hyperalgesia after unilateral nerve injury (Mohammadian *et al.* 1997, Oaklander *et al.* 1998); a significant percentage of patients with so-called complex regional pain syndrome experience bilateral spread of pain despite an initial, unilateral injury (Veldman and Goris 1996); SCS, like MCS (see Chapter 6) can induce bilateral effects following unilateral stimulation (Lazorthes *et al.* 1978; Garcia-Larrea *et al.* 1989).

This is also the case for CP. Riddoch and Critchley (1937) reported exceptional cases of bilateral pain due to unilateral thalamic lesion. We (Canavero 1996) described a woman with a subparietal cavernoma and contralateral CP who, for about 10 days, complained of the same kind of pain (burning paroxysms to arm and, when severe, the whole hemisoma) on the contralateral arm. Both pains simultaneously responded to propofol. *No sensory deficits were ever observed in involved areas.* Kim (1998) described six patients with unilateral stroke who initially developed painful sensory symptoms on the side contralateral to the lesion. The patient's CPSP progressively worsened for a certain period of time when sensory symptoms also occurred on the side ipsilateral to the lesion. The delayed onset ipsilateral sensory symptom was mild, *unaccompanied by objective sensory deficits* and developed in the body parts mirroring the site of the most severe CPSP. Once developed, they persisted during follow-up (new-onset PNP and strokes were excluded by appropriate exams in some patients). We have already seen examples of bilateral CP elicited by unilateral stimulation in previous sections (Gorecki *et al.* 1989; Chapter 7, Section 2). Kim (1999) also reported on five patients with hemisensory symptoms due to unilateral strokes occurring in the left putamen, left thalamus, right putamen, right lateral medulla and left thalamic-internal capsular area. Sensory symptoms had gradually improved or remained stable after onset. When another stroke occurred on the *contralateral* thalamic-occipital, frontoparietal, lateral medulla, temporoparietal and pontine areas, respectively, previous sensory symptoms significantly worsened and became painful on the previously affected side. Also, two patients with sudden remission of CP following a new stroke in the unaffected hemisphere are on record (see Chapter 7, Section 4). Tasker's group described cases of CP patients with a "silent" thalamus, who most likely engaged the healthy contralateral hemisphere (see Chapter 7, Section 2). Greenspan and colleagues (2004) had 2/13 cases of unilateral CPSP with bilateral cold hypesthesia and other studies described a small number of patients with bilateral cold hypesthesia (Beric *et al.* 1988; Boivie *et al.* 1989; Vestergaard *et al.* 1995). Thus, one fact seems inescapable: *the mechanism that leads to CP engages both hemispheres, so that a corticothalamic pain loop can be activated on either side; importantly, bilateral CP does not depend on structures with bilateral receptive fields (e.g., SII or ACC) or contralateral strokes would not abolish the pain.* CP may likely be shifted contralaterally through the corpus callosum (transfer time: 15 ms; Frot and Mauguière 2003) or through the reticular formation, including spinal and brainstem commissural interneurons (Koltzenburg *et al.* 1999), with its bilateral projections, following loss of GABA tone in SI and reticular formation priming (see previous discussion). Olausson and colleagues (2001) found that cortical areas typically involved in pain processing can be activated by ipsilateral pathways directly from the periphery, but, unlike tactile information, pain activation in the hemisphere contralateral to the stimulation is dependent on transcallosal information processing. In amputees, acute hand deafferentation can elicit a focal increase in excitability in the hand motor MI representation *contralateral* to the deafferented cortex that is influenced by transcallosal interactions; GABA A agonism blocks this increased excitability (Werhahn *et al.* 2002). Meyer and colleagues (1995, and references therein) found that homotopic regions of SI are linked, so that plasticity induced in one hemisphere (in the form of RF expansion brought about by a small peripheral denervation) is immediately mirrored in the other hemisphere: neurons which displayed the plasticity showed no responsiveness to stimulation of the ipsilateral body surface, suggesting a specific role of maintaining integration between corresponding cortical fields. Excitation may be followed by inhibition when the stimulated area is larger or stimulation strength higher (see also Calford and Tweedale 1990). Bilaterality of hand representation in parietal somatosensory areas is under callosal control, since it is lost after callosal section, mostly at BA2 (but much less at BA1 and almost none at BA3b) and BA5/7 levels (Iwamura *et al.* 1994).

Since *facilitatory interhemispheric influences* are possible in patients with agenesis of the corpus callosum, both mechanisms (corpus callosum transfer and reticular formation-processed switch) may play a role.

LESSONS FROM CORD CENTRAL PAIN

For almost 50 years, a dichotomy of response between episodic and constant pains in the setting of spinal injury has been discussed. Botterell and colleagues (1954) stated: "Burning pain has proved a problem difficult of solution...By contrast, jabbing, shooting, crampy, gripping, colicky and vice-like pains, have been regularly relieved by bilateral tractotomy." Porter and colleagues (1966) wrote: "The effectiveness of cordotomy in relieving the symptoms of sharp, lancinating pains in the lower extremities in patients with cauda equina lesions is summarized...The operation had no effect, however, on the frequently encountered burning pain in the lower extremities." White and Sweet (1969), seemingly inferring that intermittent pain is radicular in origin and steady pain of central origin, concluded: "Cordotomy is very useful in paraplegia for relief of pain of radicular origin...Provided the injury involves the cauda equina and does not extend rostrally beyond the conus medullaris to involve the cord, we believe that relief can be obtained in a high proportion of cases by anterolateral cordotomy." Jefferson (1983) noted that cordectomy was differentially effective for discrete pain radiating into the thighs, knees or legs, especially if shooting and episodic, and especially if caused by lower cord lesions. Pain associated with high lesions, particularly if diffuse, steady and in a "bathing trunks" distribution, was relieved poorly. He stated: "One of the very interesting, and perhaps characteristic features of the pain which is likely to respond...is that it is episodic." Tasker and associates (1992) found a statistical correlation between disappearance of intermittent and evoked pain and demolitive procedures, compared to these latter's ineffectiveness for spontaneous pain. They wrote: "destructive surgery is selectively successful in relieving the spontaneous intermittent, often shooting radicular pain that tends to project down the legs ... present in 30% of ... patients with cord central pain...particularly associated with thoracolumbar lesions...evoked pain, present in 47% of...patients, responds similarly to destructive surgery." Intermittent and evoked, but not steady, pains should be dependent upon transmission in somatosensory (probably spinothalamic) pathways, intermittent shooting pain perhaps being the result of ectopic impulses instituted at, or proximal to, injury sites (e.g., through ephapses or peripheral ectopic pacemakers) and then transmitted centrally in these pathways to be perceived as pain. Pagni and Canavero (1995) also noted that the paroxysmal components, often associated with spasms, usually due to lesions at T9–T12 vertebral level, are satisfactorily relieved by cordomyelotomy. On such basis, it has been concluded that evoked pains depend on a local cord generator, whereas diffuse steady pains on more rostrad stations. According to Tasker (2001), intermittent shooting (89%) and allodynia-hyperpathia (84%) respond to cordotomy-cordectomy-DREZ; steady, causalgic, dysesthetic, aching pain only in 26% of the cases.

Another dichotomy has been noted between end-zone or girdle (at-level) pain and diffuse (below-level) pains. On the basis of results of conventional DREZ surgery and cordectomies (Chapter 7), it was concluded that steady burning pain referred to the lower abdomen, and burning or dysesthetic pain diffused to the legs or localized to the retroperitoneal region, buttocks or feet usually are not relieved. Best results were reported for patients complaining of shooting, paroxysmal pain (and spasms), even though referred to apparently totally anesthetic and paralyzed limbs, and girdle pains. Pain worsened by bowel or bladder distension was also likely to be improved by surgery. Results of cordectomies have been less rewarding with lesions and sections at levels higher than T10.

Pain relief in paraplegics after cordectomy appears to be directly related to the extent of the removal, with better results occurring when long rostral segments of the cord are resected, that is, 2–3 cm (three spinal segments) are resected above the site of injury (e.g., Druckman and Lende 1965; Table 7.1). Loeser and colleagues (1968) pointed to the cord segments rostral to injury playing important role in the genesis of pain. Jefferson (1983) noted that, although abnormal tissue was left above the level of his resections, without apparently influencing pain relief, sometimes extension of cordectomy to apparently normal tissue was necessary. Bilateral DREZ lesions that involve two to three spinal cord segments above the spinal injury, and extend into *normal cord*, achieve a better pain relief (coagulation includes laminas I–IV, but may involve up to lamina VI and adjacent white columns), as damage extends for several segments well above injury site (Nashold 1991), whereas extension of DREZ lesions *caudad* into the sacral segments of the cord does not improve the results (only 1 patient with diffuse sacral pain improved in the series of Friedman and Bullitt [1988]; Table 7.1).

Edgar and colleagues (1993) and recently Falci and colleagues (2002) (Table 7.1) found that DREZ surgery can indeed relieve diffuse pains, if lesions are extended sufficiently. In the latter paper, in 62% of patients with below-level pain, spontaneous DREZ hyperactivity was found 3–5 levels cephalad to injury level (7 in the series of Edgar *et al.*). Their findings contradicted traditional dermatomal mapping and thus they hypothesized that below-level pain was mediated significantly by interneuronal pathways, while at-level pain was assumed to be mediated through more traditional pain pathways (e.g., STT) corresponding to the DREZ at injury level. Spinal block studies also (see Chapter 6) found that block above lesion level was necessary for analgesia; failure in two patients (both with below-level pain) despite anesthesia two levels cephalad to injury supports even more rostral mechanisms. Davis and Martin (1947) wrote: "If the distal end of the proximal segment of the injured spinal cord was anesthetized by spinal anesthesia, the pain disappeared" (p. 493), "This suggests that the origin of the pain was the end of the proximal segment of the injured spinal cord...operations upon the sympathetic nervous system [being] ineffective." Studies (Finnerup *et al.* 2003a,b) indicate that changes in somatosensory function in dermatomes rostral to the injury level may be important in the sustenance of CCP, with a significant correlation between intensity of brush-evoked dysesthesia at lesion level and spontaneous below-level pain. The same group (Finnerup *et al.* 2003c) also examined 23 SCI patients above T10 (14 with CP and 9 without CP) in an MRI study. At the level of maximal cord injury,

21 patients had lesions involving the entire cord on axial images, except for a small border of lower signal intensity, whereas 2 patients had central lesions. Rostral to the main injury, the first image with an incomplete lesion showed significantly more involvement of gray matter in pain than in pain-free patients. According to Defrin and colleagues (2001), both a critical level of injury and a state of hyperresponsivity is necessary for CCP to arise. Thus, apparently, above-level hyperactivity may sustain CCP.

This diffuse, likely bilateral, spinal generator involving multisynaptic proprio-spinal systems in and around the lesioned gray matter may feed the thalamocorti-cothalamic loop; a similar generator would be present in the brainstem reticular formation. However, this hyperexcitability is useless without STT-induced changes at corticothalamic levels, which is the first step needed for CP to arise. In thoracolumbar lesions, further excitatory input may derive from peripheral (root/nerve) mechanisms. This "hyperactive core" may have variable extent depending on subject. It is important to remember, though, how previously unreported burning sensations developed after cordectomy (Botterell *et al.* 1954) and even Falci and colleagues, who believed that the higher temperature they used had markedly decreased the development of new "squeezing, pressure" pains, possibly because of a more complete destruction in deeper laminas, triggered new CP sensations; moreover, they could not relieve all their patients of below-level CP, implying even more rostral hyperactivity. Beric (1993) pointed out that the ASAS syndrome is characterized by severe, practically complete interruption of the STT at the spinal level: here, the hypothesis of dorsal horn nociceptive cell hyperactivity at the level of the lesion becomes inconceivable and useless in explaining the painful symptoms of this syndrome. However, propriospinal hyperactivity can still be present and hyperexcitability may have spread more rostrally.

Previously reviewed studies suggest that CP is much more frequent in incomplete cord injuries. Actually, *a majority of seemingly clinically complete transection injuries are subclinically incomplete and retain significant communication between segments above and below the cord injury zone even many years after the original trauma*, as shown both anatomically and electrophysiologically (Dimitrijevic 1987; Beric 1999), so-called *dyscomplete lesions*, i.e., no volitional sensorimotor functions below lesion level, but some residual descending function or control demonstrated by electrophysiology. Also, some sensory cortical evoked responses may still be detected in SCI patients with no clinically appreciable sensory function below the lesion site; prolonged, repeated or continuous application of different stimuli may be transmitted from below lesion level to the brain and produce the awareness that something is happening in seemingly anesthetic areas (this is the case of peripheral or central pathways still transmitting across the traumatic lesion on fast or slow conducting fibers which are, however, functionally useless (Donovan *et al.* 1982)). Finnerup and associates (2004) compared 24 SCI patients (11 with CP and 13 without) with a clinically complete SCI (ASIA grade A), and found that painful or repetitive pinprick stimuli elicited vague localized sensations in 50% of cases. SEPs and MRI found no difference between groups. Thus, sensory communication was retained across injury level (*sensory dyscomplete SCI*).

Kakulas and colleagues (1990, and references therein) observed that out of 197 SCI cases, only 22 reported pain and 5 burning sensations. Of these, 18 had clinically incomplete and 4 a complete cord transection syndrome; in 10 cases the lesion was cervical, in 6 thoracic and in 6 lumbar. They concluded that: "there is a larger proportion of patients with pain and abnormal sensations with anatomically incomplete injuries." They also noted that an extensive regeneration of nerve roots at the level of injury is more frequently observed in patients suffering from pain and that most of seemingly clinically complete cord transection syndromes (63 out of 88) show, on pathological examination, continuity of nervous tracts across the lesion, with a variable residuum of descending and ascending central nervous fibers running in the wall of the lesion. They also noted that *spinal cord lesions are spread over many segments below and above the level of the bony lesion* and lesions may extend well above the injury site (Durward *et al.* 1982). At these levels, loss of myelinated fibers and neurons of the gray substance and gliosis intermingle. Damage of the roots may swing from minor damage to complete or nearly complete loss of nerve fibers. In the chronic stages, nerve root regeneration is a typical feature with formation of neuromas, and is more frequently seen in cases of pain. In traumatic spinal cord damage, the end result is a scar, with collagenous connective tissue and, in the less damaged parts of the cord, demyelination of fibers, intense astrocytic fibrous gliosis (Hughes 1976), involving posterior and anterior horns, plus schwannosis. Surviving axons in injured spinal cord (MS, cervical spondylosis: Hughes 1976; extramedullary tumors: McAlhany and Netsky 1955) have neurophysiological features typical of demyelinated axons (Rasminsky 1980). Then, sensory loss would be due not so much to loss of axons (both during trauma and MS), but to loss of their ability to transmit properly encoded information, conducting slower and ineffectively. Repetitive discharge results in a change of the axon's membrane excitability caused by the propagation of an impulse per se (activity-dependent after-oscillations). Failure of sensation may occur with such activity-dependent changes in axonal excitability, justifying the periodicity of intermittent conduction which occurs in spontaneous discharge in axons with focal demyelination and in spontaneous trains of discharge from axons ending in neuromas (Thalhammer and Raymond 1991). Demyelination may involve cord tracts under the compressing lesion or on the opposite side of the cord.

Pathological afferent discharges may spontaneously originate in the surviving central stumps of divided central nerve fibers and damaged demyelinated fibers of both anterior and posterior cord quadrants, with impulses arising ectopically (Smith and McDonald 1982), both in incomplete and dyscomplete spinal cord traumatic transections. Demyelinated axons may be responsible for pain paroxysms (Pagni and Canavero 1993); minimal mechanical deformation of the cord at the lesion site both increases the level of previous spontaneous activity, inducing spontaneous activity in silent fibers.

Abnormal excitability is likely a general attribute of any demyelinated central nerve fiber, including dorsal columns. These may be at the basis of *Lhermitte's sign* — which would then be a typical mechanical irritative phenomenon of the posterior columns at cervical level — and other electric shock-like pain paroxysms with lesions inside the cord or compressing it from outside. Interestingly, such painful fits may depend on lesions of the dorsal columns, where visceral pain fibers are found (Pagni and Canavero 1993; Willis and Westlund 2004). Here, cordotomies would be ineffective. That scarring-induced irritation of sensory pathways might play a role in CP was surmised by earlier authors: constant bombardment by subliminal impulses from the periphery that under normal conditions are not felt produces painful sensations (Garcin 1937). Traumatic lesions of the spinal cord and cerebral cortex give rise to acute terrible aching pain which fades away in a few hours, days or weeks (Garcin 1937). However, lesions that interrupt central pathways will result in wallerian degeneration of the axons, and thus "there is no way for interrupted central axons to became a source of ectopic nerve impulses, as can happen with peripheral axons, for example, in neuromas" (Willis 1991).

In traumatic lesions at the thoracolumbar passage (T10–L1), which generally involve both the cord lumbar enlargement and caudal roots, neuromas form in the chronic stage (Kakulas 1990; Pagni and Canavero 1995). Nerve root lesion or compression may add to denervation and ectopic impulse generation inducing and maintaining a hyperexcitability of central multimodal neurons. From neuromas, which are powerful ectopic pacemakers (though the amount of spontaneous electrical activity of neuromas may have been overestimated; Burchiel and Russel 1987), and dorsal root ganglion cells of damaged roots, abnormal spontaneous, paroxysmal discharges may sustain the activity of partially deafferented multimodal neurons in the dorsal horns of not completely destroyed cord segments and in the nearby less damaged rostral cord segments, at- and above-level and not necessarily from a change in the excitability of the spinal neuron itself (Pagni and Canavero 1995).

A role of Lissauer's tracts, which lie outside the area included in anterolateral cordotomies, must also be envisioned in the rostral spread of hyperactivity. Denny-Brown and colleagues (1973) found that the medial division of Lissauer's tract seems to exert a facilitatory effect, and the lateral division a suppressor effect on transmission of afferent impulses at the first synapse. Lesion of the lateral part gives rise to hyperesthesia extending both above and below the lesion level on the section side, while "section of the whole Lissauer's tract at any one level had prolonged release effect on the next headward dermatome." Involvement of Lissauer's tract might justify the at-level hyperesthesia on the lesion side after cord hemisection, Lissauer's tract section, section of the posterior columns impinging on the dorsal horn, and girdle pains in spinal tumors.

Roughly half or more of patients with syringomyelia suffer from a blend of at-level and below-level pains. The onset of pain associated with traumatic syringomyelia usually occurs in those dermatomes just above the level of the trauma, but may sometimes be referred to distant dermatomes as the cyst encroaches on high spinal cord segments.

In contrast to other types of pain that usually respond well to surgical treatment of syrinx, dysesthetic CP can persist or even increase postoperatively, despite collapse of the syrinx, and actually new CP can appear ex novo after surgical treatment (Tator and Agbi 1991). In the series of Milhorat and colleagues (1996), surgical treatment of syrinx resulted in total relief in only 7 of 37 patients (19%), with other 15 improved of their dysesthetic pain; 15 patients (41%) reported no improvement or even worsening of pain, despite MR-confirmed collapse of syrinx. Postoperative dysesthetic pain was often disabling and poorly responsive to drugs. One year after surgery, all these 15 patients continued to complain of dysesthesias and pain, although at a lesser level in 9, and most even at 2–6 years postoperatively. Syrinxes often encroached on the dorsolateral quadrant of the cord, but no comparison between pain and non-pain patients was attempted in order to define a possible role of the descending dorsolateral funiculus; similar arguments apply to increase of substance P staining in the dorsal horns below-level and marked reduction or absence at-level (references in Milhorat *et al.* 1997). However, Hida and associates (1994) found that the syrinx cavity in posttraumatic syrinx patients was more central at the caudal than at the rostral end. Sudden onset of pain immediately above the original injury level is the most common presenting complaint from patients with syrinx and often occurs in conjunction with a sudden increase in thoracic pressure (e.g., during a sneeze). Milhorat and associates (1997) noted that patients with syrinx pressures greater than 7.7 cmH_2O tended to have more rapidly progressive symptoms, exhibited greater improvement after shunting and a higher incidence of postoperative dysesthetic pain than patients with normal or almost normal pressures (*30% versus 0%*). Postoperative dysesthetic pain was not found to be due to injury of dorsal roots or posterior columns during myelotomy and chronic irritation of cord by shunt catheter, but only to sudden decompression of hypertensive syrinxes. Such pains resolved spontaneously in two, were less severe in another two, but persisted in a fifth at 1 year: these may have been segmental dysesthetic pains, though. In 75% of patients with pre-drainage SSEPs abnormalities, decompression produced a consistent reduction of N20 latencies and a similar, but less consistent, increase in N20 amplitude. However, all comparisons between high- and low-pressure groups were not statistically significant.

Attal and associates (2004) found that shunting of syrinx significantly improved proprioceptive deficits, but not the magnitude of thermoalgesic deficits in 15 patients, despite collapse of the cavity in 80% of the cases: only pain evoked by effort–cough–movement, *but not pain at rest*, was reduced at 2 years. Moreover, only patients operated within less than 2 years of symptoms onset were improved or stabilized, including 3 patients whose spontaneous pain improved by at least 70%. Not finding a correlation between pain and thermoalgesic deficits, they suggested that pain may result from irritation of the cord at the rostral end of the cyst. A similar conclusion was reached in a study of subjects whose syrinxes were drained and filled with fetal neural grafts (Wirth *et al.* 2002). Despite clear MRI evidence of at least partial cyst obliteration in 7 subjects, complete disappearance of one or more pain symptoms was noted only if collapse of the most rostral portion of the cyst was achieved and no previous or new shunt tube was present in the cyst, suggesting that *syringomyelia pain may result from or be exacerbated by irritation of the cord levels immediately rostral to the cyst*. Irritation may be due to either a mass effect secondary to increased cyst pressure and/or inflammation from tissue damage. In one patient, reopening of a collapsed cyst seemed to cause return of pain. One subject noted a delayed increase of pain after surgery, due to a delayed expansion of a second cyst distant from the transplant site. Pain intensity reports often varied substantially in time, with distribution of dysesthesias more stable. However, *complete disappearance of a dysesthesia was seen in only 2 of 8 subjects.* In one patient, the burning sensation in the dermatomes associated with an upper C6–T3 cyst *disappeared immediately after grafting without shunting* (follow-up 2 years), with complete collapse of cyst. Nonetheless, he developed stabbing pain in the T6–9 dermatomes 3 months after surgery due to expansion of the lower T6–9 cyst, both gradually increasing over 18 months; 27 months after the first surgery, a second graft was placed in this lower cyst, with unsatisfactory results at 1 year, despite 50% collapse of the cyst. Subject 5 had her previous stabbing pain in her legs limited to below knees at 6 weeks and complete disappearance at 9 months (complete obliteration of cyst at 9 months), but full relapse at 18 months (slight reopening at 12 months and persistence through 2 years). In the other 6 unrelieved patients, 5 had substantial collapse of the cyst at the graft site, but also a persistent cyst above the graft site or shunt tubes at or above the graft site. In the ninth, no collapse was seen.

However, Durward and colleagues (1982) reported that, although the syrinx continued upward for many segments above the level of cordectomy and the upper ends of the specimens of the cord showed pathological changes in three of their patients, they were all relieved of their arm pain, indicating that this type of abnormality may not be a generator of pain. On the other hand, in none of other three cases where cordectomy failed was the rostral incision into histologically normal cord. In two of them with a post-traumatic syringomyelia, earlier drainage of the cyst had improved the syndrome, with the exception of the continuing pain. *The pain in these latter three failures was all referred well below the level of the lesion in the cord, and these lesions were all at levels at which Jefferson's cordectomies had also failed.*

In patients with dysesthetic CP due to intramedullary tumors, symptoms tend to persist in many after removal (Epstein *et al.* 1993; McCormick *et al.* 1990). Surgical removal of intramedullary cavernomas may relieve CP initially, but many relapse at follow-up (Kim *et al.* 2006). Also, new CP can appear after excision of the mass (Canavero *et al.* 1994).

In sum, STT damage is the primary event in both BCP and CCP. While segmental pains engage local processes, below-level diffuse pains, even in the best series, are not uniformly relieved (unlike end-zone pains), so that we may conclude that cord foci of hyperactivity play a boosting role only.

THE GENESIS OF ALLODYNIA

That allodynia is not pivotal to CP is proved by the simple observation that not all patients complain of it, unlike steady spontaneous pain. As observed in exceptional patients, allodynia may follow a different time course than spontaneous pain. Greenspan and colleagues (1997) reported a woman with a thalamic lesion observed over 4 years who had CP only during 3 months. Prior to spontaneous pain, there was transient, but intense thermal allodynia several months before. Attal and colleagues (1998) described a patient who presented uniquely with very intense brush-induced allodynia (dynamic mechanical) strictly confined to the left C2/3 dermatomes for several months. Thereafter, spontaneous pain and sensory deficits appeared and a new MRI showed an intraspinal lesion involving the C2/5 segments.

Greenspan and associates (2004), on the basis of a study of 13 CPSP patients, concluded that *sparing of a submodality by lesions causing CP is associated with the occurrence of allodynia in that modality*, i.e., both tactile and cold/heat allodynia, even striking, were significantly associated with the presence, rather than the absence or reduction, of normal tactile and thermal sensibility. Similar observations have been reported in syringomyelia (Ducreux *et al.* 2006). It was also noted how all four patients with insular (posterior) lesions had tactile allodynia, but only one had tactile sensory loss. However, both patients with insular lesions and noninsular lesions had tactile allodynia, cold allodynia and thermotactile sensory deficits without significant differences. Also on the basis of microstimulation studies (Chapter 7, Section 2), Greenspan and associates have suggested that the termination of the STT in the thalamus is reorganized to signal pain instead of cold in CP patients. Cold allodynia would be due to input from an intact cold pathway driving Vc (and not from loss of such input, disinhibiting these regions; see also Garcia-Larrea *et al.* 2002). Tactile allodynia would be due to disinhibition of Vc from loss of insula or SI/SII input. In this context, Beric's focus on a dissociation between STT and (spared) DC-ML conduction would be redirected to explain tactile allodynia.

Tasker (2001, and references therein) observed how the induction of burning and pain appears to be peculiar to patients with pain. Since all those in whom pain was induced and half those in whom burning occurred suffered from evoked pain, the phenomenon may be unrelated to the spontaneous pain ("central allodynia"). He also noted that allodynia and hyperpathia in CPSP appear to be suppressed by PVG DBS, as if depending on spinothalamic transmission. This central allodynia occurs at sites where normally non-painful sensations are evoked, as well at sites where normally no sensations are evoked, being unrelated spatially to the presence of bursting or thalamic reorganization: he ascribed it to third-order neuron sensitization. He also observed how evoked pains in SCI patients may be due to conduction through spinothalamic pathways, and thus differing from steady pain (Tasker *et al.* 1992). Sang and colleagues (1999) also concluded that SCI results in central sensitization, accounting for cephalad spread of cold allodynia and of augmented temporal summation.

Quantitative sensory studies and differential responses to drugs seem to indicate that not all evoked pains have the same genesis, with a difference between thermal evoked pain (amitriptyline responsive) and mechanical evoked pains (lidocaine-morphine responsive). This would argue against a generalized hyper-excitability of nociceptive neurons to any type of stimuli (Attal *et al.* 2000, 2002). Also, the effects of morphine on static mechanical allodynia suggest that static and dynamic (brush evoked) mechano-allodynia associated with CP are sustained by different mechanisms (brush-evoked allodynia having a similar genesis as in PNP). In this regard, it should be noted that some opioids are weak NMDA, but not AMPA, blockers: being hyperalgesia a supposedly NMDA-mediated phenomenon (but see above), this might explain opioid action on hyperalgesia. However, our own studies (Canavero and Bonicalzi 2004) show that both spontaneous pain and allodynia can be abolished simultaneously, although the latter to a greater extent – or even exclusively – in some cases. GABA agonism may thus affect the whole spectrum of CP.

Data suggest that some patients with cold allodynia tend to have more dorsally placed thalamic lesions than those without, and those with movement allodynia more anteriorly placed lesions (Bowsher 2005b).

Thus, sensitization at cord, brainstem and thalamic levels may play a role in the genesis of allodynia only, but not spontaneous pain, with inappropriate activation of the STT through stimulation of receptors and fibers that normally are not involved in nociception. In other words, allodynia could be the result of exaggerated spinal input processed by an arrhythmic thalamus. As we have seen in reviewing neurometabolic studies, allodynia is subserved by additional, widespread activity particularly in frontal areas, perhaps justifying its high unpleasantness. However, sudden disappearances as reviewed above strongly suggest that, once the loop sustaining spontaneous pain has been switched off, allodynia is abolished simultaneously.

Finally, there is no direct proof that expanded receptive fields play a role in human patients.

REFERENCES

Ackermann RF, Finch DM, Babb TL, Engel J Jr. (1984) Increased metabolism during long-duration recurrent inhibition of hippocampal pyramidal cells. *J Neurosci* **4**, 251–264.

Ackerman LL, Follett KA, Rosenquist RW (2003) Long-term outcomes during treatment of chronic pain with intracisternal clonidine or clonidine/opioid combinations. *J Pain Symptom Manage* **26**, 668–677.

Agnew DA, Goldberg VD (1976) A brief trial of phenytoin for thalamic pain. *Bull Los Angeles Neurol Soc* **41**, 9–12.

Ahn SH, Park HW, Lee BS, Moon HW, Jang SH, Sakong J, Bae JH (2003) Gabapentin effect on neuropathic pain compared among patients with spinal cord injury and different durations of symptoms. *Spine* **28**, 341–346.

Akil H, Richardson DE, Hughes DE, Barchas JD (1978) Enkephalin-like material elevated in ventricular cerebrospinal fluid of pain patients after analgesic focal stimulation. *Science* **201**, 463–465.

Alajouanine T (1957) *La douleur et les douleurs.* Paris: Masson.

Alajouanine T, Brunelli A (1935) Les douleurs alterneés dans les lésions bulbo-protubérantielles. Contribution à l'étude de la physiopathologie des douleurs centrales. *Revue Neurol* **63**, 828–837.

Albe-Fessard D (1973) Electrophysiological methods for the identification of thalamic nuclei. *Z Neurol* **205**, 15–28.

Albert ML (1969) Treatment of pain in multiple sclerosis: preliminary report. *N Engl J Med* **280**, 1395.

Amancio EJ, Peluso CM, Santos AC, Pena-Dias AP, Debs FA (2002) [Central pain due to parietal cortex compression by cerebral tumor: report of 2 cases.] *Arq Neuropsiquiatr* **60**, 487–489.

Amano K *et al.* (1976) [in Japanese] cited from Amano 1998.

Amano K, Iseki H, Notani M *et al.* (1980) Rostral mesencephalic reticulotomy for pain relief. Report of 15 cases. *Acta Neurochir Suppl* **30**, 391–393.

Amano K, Tanikawa H, Hiroshi I *et al.* (1982) Endorphins and pain relief. Further observations on electrical stimulation of the lateral part of the periaqueductal gray matter during rostral mesencephalic reticulotomy for pain relief. *Appl Neurophysiol* **45**, 123–135.

Amano K, Kawamura H, Tanikawa T *et al.* (1986) Long-term follow-up study of rostral mesencephalic reticulotomy for pain relief. Report of 34 cases. *Appl Neurophysiol* **49**, 105–111.

Amano K, Kawamura H, Tanikawa T, Kawabatake H, Iseki H, Taira T (1992) Stereotactic mesencephalotomy for pain relief. A plea for stereotactic surgery. *Stereotact Funct Neurosurg* **59**, 25–32.

Amano K (1998) Destructive central lesions for persistent pain: II. Outcome. In Gildenberg PL, Tasker RR, eds., *Textbook of Stereotactic and Functional Neurosurgery.* New York: McGraw-Hill, pp. 1425–1429.

Ameri D (1967) Sindrome talamico de Dejerine–Roussy en una meningitis tuberculosa de la infancia. *Arch Argent Pediatria* **65**, 173–178.

Andersen G, Vestergaard K, Lauritzen L (1994) Effective treatment of post-stroke depression with the selective serotonin re-uptake inhibitor citalopram. *Stroke* **25**, 1099–1104.

Andersen G, Vestergaard K, Ingeman-Nielsen M, Jensen TS (1995) Incidence of central post-stroke pain. *Pain* **61**, 187–193.

Anderson VC, Burchiel KJ (1999) A prospective study of long-term intrathecal morphine in the management of chronic nonmalignant pain. *Neurosurgery* **44**, 289–301.

Andy OJ (1983) Thalamic stimulation for chronic pain. *Appl Neurophysiol* **46**, 116–123.

Angel IF, Gould HJ Jr., Carey ME (1998) Intrathecal morphine pump as a treatment option in chronic pain of nonmalignant origin. *Surg Neurol* **49**, 92–98.

Antonucci O (1938) Chordotomia posterior medialis (dei cordoni di Goll) nelle paraplegie spastiche (tipo Little). *Policlinico (Sez Prat)* **39**, 1761–1768.

Apkarian AV, Stea RA, Mangios SH, Szeverenyi NM, King RB, Thomas FD (1992) Persistent pain inhibits controlateral somatosensory cortical activity in humans. *Neurosci Lett* **140**, 141–147.

Apkarian AV, Stea RA, Bolanowski SJ (1994) Heat-induced pain diminishes vibrotactile perception: a touch gate. *Somatosens Mot Res* **11**, 259–267.

Apkarian AV, Bushnell MC, Treede R-D, Zubieta J-K (2005) Human brain mechanisms of pain perception and regulation in health and disease. *Eur J Pain* **9**, 463–484.

Armour D (1927) Lettsonian lecture on the surgery of the spinal cord and its membranes. *Lancet* **1**, 691–697.

Arnér S, Meyerson BA (1988) Lack of analgesic effect of opioids on neuropathic and idiopathic forms of pain. *Pain* **33**, 11–23.

Arseni G, Boetz MI (1971) *Tulburari viscero-vegetative si trofice in leziunile encefalice.* Bucharest: Editura Academiei Republicii Socialiste Romania.

Ashby P, Rothwell JC (2000) Neurophysiologic aspects of deep brain stimulation. *Neurology* **55**(Suppl. 6), S17–S20.

Attal N, Brasseur B, Parker F, Chauvin M, Bouhassira D (1998a) Effects of gabapentin on the different components of peripheral and central neuropathic pain syndromes: pathophysiological considerations. *Eur Neurol* **40**, 191–200.

Attal N, Brasseur L, Chauvin M, Bouhassira D (1998b) A case of 'pure' dynamic mechano-allodynia due to a lesion of the spinal cord: pathophysiological considerations. *Pain* **75**, 399–404.

Attal N, Gaudè V, Brasseur L *et al.* (2000) Intravenous lidocaine in central pain. A double-blind, placebo-controlled, psychophysical study. *Neurology* **54**, 564–574.

Attal N, Guirimand F, Brasseur L *et al.* (2002) Effects of IV morphine in central pain. A randomized placebo-controlled study. *Neurology* **58**, 554–563.

Attal N, Brasseur L, Guirimand D *et al.* (2004) Are oral cannabinoids safe and effective in refractory neuropathic pain? *Eur J Pain* **8**, 173–177.

Attal N, Parker F, Tadiè M, Bouhassira D (2004) Effects of surgery on central pain and sensory deficits associated with syringomyelia: a long-term prospective psychophysical study. *J Neurol Neurosurg Psych* **75**, 1025–1030.

Awerbuch GI, Sandyk R (1990) Mexiletine for thalamic pain syndrome. *Int J Neurosci* **55**, 129–133.

Babtchine IS (1936) Les résultats immediats et lontains de la cordotomie. *J Chir (Par)* **47**, 26–39.

Backonja M, Gombar K (1992) Response of central pain syndromes to intravenous lidocaine. *J Pain Symptom Manage* **7**, 172–178.

Backonja M, Howland EW, Wang J *et al.* (1991) Tonic changes in alpha power during immersion of the hand in cold water. *Electroenceph Clin Neurophysiol* **79**, 192–203.

Backonja M, Arndt G, Gombar KA, Check B, Zimmermann M (1994) Response of chronic neuropathic pain syndromes to ketamine: a preliminary study. *Pain* **56**, 51–57.

Bailey RA, Glees P, Oppenheimer DR (1954) Midbrain tractotomy. A surgical and clinical report, with observations on ascending and descending tract degeneration. *Mschr Psychiat Neurol* **127**, 316–335.

Bainton T, Fox M, Bowsher D, Wells C (1992) A double-blind trial of naloxone in central post-stroke pain. *Pain* **48**, 159–162.

Ballantine HT Jr., Giriunas IE (1988) Treatment of intractable psychiatric illness and chronic pain by stereotactic cingulotomy. In Schmideck W, Sweet WH, eds., *Operative Neurosurgical Techniques*, 2nd edn. New York: Grune-Stratton, pp. 1069–1075.

Ballantyne JC, Mao J (2003) Opioid therapy for chronic pain. *New Engl J Med* **349**, 1943–1953.

Banerjee T (1974) Transcutaneous nerve stimulation for pain after spinal injury. *New Engl J Med* **291**, 796.

Bang OY, Lee JS, Lee PH, Lee G (2005) Autologous mesenchymal stem cell transplantation in stroke patients. *Ann Neurol* **57**, 874–882.

Baranauskas G, Nistri A (1998) Sensitization of pain pathways in the spinal cord: cellular mechanisms. *Progr Neurobiol* **54**, 349–365.

Barcia-Salorio JL, Roldan P, Lopez-Gomez L (1987) Radiosurgery of central pain. *Acta Neurochir (Wien) Suppl* **39**, 159–162.

Barolat G (1995) Current status of epidural spinal cord stimulation. *Neurosurg Quart* **5**, 98–124.

Barolat G, Ketcik B, He J (1998) Long-term outcome of spinal cord stimulation for chronic pain management. *Neuromodulation* 1, 19–25.

Baron JC, D'Antona R, Pantano R et al. (1986) Effects of thalamic stroke on energy metabolism of the cerebral cortex. *Brain* 109, 1243–1259.

Baron R, Baron Y, Disbrow E, Roberts TP (1999) Brain processing of capsaicin-induced secondary hyperalgesia. A functional MRI study. *Neurology* 53, 548–557.

Barraquer-Bordas L, Molet J, Pascual-sedano B, Català H (1999) Dolor central retardado asociado a hematoma subinsular seguido por tumor parietooccipital. Efecto favorable de la estimulacion cronica del nucleo VPL talamico. *Rev Neurologia* 29, 1044–1048.

Bassetti C, Bogousslavsky J, Mattle H, Bernasconi A (1997) Medial medullary stroke: report of seven patients and review of the literature. *Neurology* 48, 882–890.

Bassetti RD, Bogousslavsky J, Regli F (1993) Sensory syndromes in parietal stroke. *Neurology* 43, 1942–1949.

Bates J, Nathan PW (1980) Transcutaneous electrical nerve stimulation for chronic pain. *Anesthesia* 35, 817–822.

Baudoin A, Puech P (1949) Premiers essais d'intervention directe sur le thalamus (injection, électrocoagulation). *Rev Neurol* 81, 78–81.

Beatty RA (1970) Cold dysesthesia. A symptom of extramedullary tumors of the spinal cord. *J Neurosurg* 33, 75–78.

Becker R, Uhle EI, Alberti O, Bertalanffy H (2000) Continuous intrathecal baclofen infusion in the management of central deafferentation pain. *J Pain Symptom Manage* 20, 313–315.

Behan RJ (1914) *Pain: Its Origin, Conduction, Perception and Diagnostic Significance.* New York: Appleton.

Bejjani B-P, Arnulf I, Houeto J-L et al. (2002) Concurrent excitatory and inhibitory effects of high frequency stimulation: an oculomotor study. *J Neurol Neurosurg Psych* 72, 517–522.

Bejjani GK, Cockerham KP (2001) Adult Chiari malformation. *Contemp Neurosurg* 23.

Belfrage M, Segerdahl M, Arner S, Sollevi A (1999) The safety and efficacy of intrathecal adenosine in patients with chronic neuropathic pain. *Anesth Analg* 89, 136–142.

Bell E, Karnosh LJ (1949) Cerebral hemispherectomy. *J Neurosurg* 6, 285–293.

Bender MB, Jaffe R (1958) Pain of central origin. *Med Clin North Am* 49, 691–700.

Bendok B, Levy RM (1998) Brain stimulation for persistent pain management. In Gildenberg PL, Tasker RR, eds., *Textbook of Stereotactic and Functional Neurosurgery.* New York: McGraw-Hill, pp. 1539–1546.

Berglund B, Harju E-L, Lindblom U (2001) Central and peripheral neuropathic pain characterized by perceived intensity and quality of touch, cold, and warmth. *Arch Center Sensory Res* 6, 31–53.

Beric A, Dimitrijevi'c MR, Lindblom U (1988) Central dysesthesia syndrome in spinal cord injury patients. *Pain* 34, 109–116.

Beric A (1993) Central pain: "new" syndromes and their evaluation. *Muscle Nerve* 16, 1017–1024.

Beric A (1999) Spinal cord damage: injury. In Wall PD, Melzack R, eds., *Textbook of Pain,* 4th edn. Edinburgh: Churchill Livingstone, pp. 915–927.

Berthier M, Starkstein S, Leiguarda R (1988) Asymbolia for pain: a sensory-limbic disconnection syndrome. *Ann Neurol* 24, 41–49.

Bettag W (1966) Results of treatment of pain by interruption of the medial pain tract of the brain stem. *Excerpta Med Int Cong Ser* 110, 771–775.

Bettag W, Yoshida T (1960) Über stereotaktischen schmerzoperationen. *Acta Neurochir* 8, 299–317.

Biella G, Salvadori G, Sotgiu ML (1999) Multifractal analysis of wide dynamic range neuron discharge profiles in normal rats and in rats with sciatic nerve constriction. *Somatosens Motor Res* 16, 89–102.

Biemond A (1956) The conduction of pain above the level of the thalamus opticus. *Arch Neurol Psych* 75, 231–244.

Binder A, Schattschneider J, Wolff S et al. (2002) Inhibition of human motor cortex by tonic cutaneous pain. A fMRI study. In *Abstracts, 10th World Congress on Pain.* Seattle, WA: IASP Press, Abst. 1125-P41.

Bittar RG, Ptito A, Reutens DC (2000) Somatosensory representation in patients who have undergone hemispherectomy: a functional magnetic resonance imaging study. *J Neurosurg* 92, 45–51.

Blond S, Touzet G, Reyns N et al. (2000) Les techniques de neurostimulation dans le traitement de la douleur chronique. *Neurochirurgie* 46, 466–482.

Blumberg H (1988) Zur Entstehung und Therapie des Schmerzsyndroms bei der sympathischen Reflexdystrophie. *Der Schmerz* 2, 125–143.

Boas RA, Corvino BG, Shahnarian A (1982) Analgesic responses to i.v. lignocaine. *Br J Anaesth* 54, 501–505.

Bogousslavsky J, Regli F, Uske A (1988) Thalamic infarcts: clinical syndromes, etiology, and prognosis. *Neurology* **38**, 837–48. Erratum in *Neurology* 1988, **38**, 1335.

Bohm E (1960) Chordotomy for intractable pain due to malignant disease. *Acta Psych Neurol Scand* **35**, 145–155.

Boivie J, Leijon G, Johansson I (1989) Central post-stroke pain. A study of the mechanisms through analyses of the sensory abnormalities. *Pain* **37**, 173–185.

Boivie J, Leijon G (1991) Clinical findings in patients with central poststroke pain. In Casey KL, ed., *Pain and Central Nervous System Disease. The Central Pain Syndromes*. New York: Raven Press, pp. 65–75.

Bonica JJ (1953) *The Management of Pain*. Philadelphia, PA: Lea and Febiger.

Bonica JJ (1991) Introduction: semantic, epidemiologic, and educational issues. In Casey KL, ed., *Pain and Central Nervous System Disease*. New York: Raven Press, pp. 13–30.

Bonicalzi V, Canavero S, Cerutti F *et al.* (1997) Lamotrigine reduces total postoperative analgesic requirement: a randomized double-blind, placebo-controlled pilot study. *Surgery* **122**, 567–570.

Bonicalzi V, Canavero S (1999a) CRPS: are guidelines possible? *Clin J Pain* **15**, 159–169.

Bonicalzi V, Canavero S (1999b) Comments on Kingery. *Pain* **73**, (1997) 123–139. *Pain* **79**, 317–323.

Bonicalzi V, Canavero S (2000) Sympathetic pain again? *Lancet* **360**, 1426–1427.

Bonicalzi V, Canavero S (2004) Intrathecal ziconotide for chronic pain. *JAMA* **292**, 1681–1682.

Bornstein B (1949) Sur le phénomène du membre fantôme. *Encéphale* **38**, 32–46.

Bors E (1951) Phantom limbs of patients with spinal cord injury. *Arch Neurol Psych* **66**, 610–631.

Bosch DA (1991) Stereotactic rostral mesencephalotomy in cancer pain and deafferentation pain. A series of 40 cases with follow-up results. *J Neurosurg* **75**, 747–751.

Botterell EH, Callaghan JC, Jousse T (1954) Pain in paraplegia. Clinical management and surgical treatment. *Proc R Soc Med* **47**, 281–288.

Bouchard G, Mayanagi Y, Martins LF (1977) Advantages and limits of intracerebral stereotactic operations for pain. In Sweet DH, Obradors, Martin-Rodriguez JC, eds., *Neurosurgical Treatment in Psychiatry, Pain and Epilepsy*. Baltimore, MD: University Park Press, pp. 693–696

Bouckoms AF (1989) Psychosurgery for pain. In Wall PD, Melzack R, eds., *Textbook of Pain*. Edinburgh: Churchill Livingstone, pp. 868–881.

Bouhassira D, Attal N, Brasseur L, Parker F (2000) Quantitative sensory testing in patients with painful or painless syringomyelia. In Devor M, Rowbotham MC, Wiesenfeld-Hallin Z, eds., *Proceedings of the 9th World Congress on Pain*. Seattle, WA: IASP Press, pp. 401–409.

Bowsher D, Lahuerta J (1987) A case of tabes dorsalis with tonic pupils and lightning pains relieved by sodium valproate. *J Neurol Neurosurg Psychiatry* **50**, 239–241.

Bowsher D, Foy PM, Shaw MDM (1989) Central pain complicating infarction following subarachnoid hemorrhage. *Br J Neurosurg* **3**, 435–442.

Bowsher D (1989) Contralateral mirror-image pain following anterolateral cordotomy. *Pain* **33**, 63–65.

Bowsher D (1993) Sensory consequences of stroke. *Lancet* **34**, 156.

Bowsher D (1994) La douleur neurogene. *Doul et Analg* **2**, 65–69.

Bowsher D (1995) The management of central poststroke pain. *Postgrad Med J* **71**, 599–604.

Bowsher D (1996) Central pain: clinical and physiological characteristics. *J Neurol Neurosurg Psych* **61**, 62–69.

Bowsher D, Leijon G, Thomas KA (1998) Central poststroke pain: correlation of MRI with clinical pain characteristics and sensory abnormalities. *Neurology* **51**, 1352–1358.

Bowsher D (2001) Stroke and central poststroke pain in an elderly population. *J Pain* **2**, 258–261.

Bowsher D (2002) The time factor in tricyclic treatment of postherpetic neuralgia (PHN) and central post-stroke pain (CPSP). In *10th World Congress on Pain, Book of Abstracts*. Seattle, WA: IASP Press, A890–P160.

Bowsher D (2005a) Dynamic mechanical allodynia in neuropathic pain. *Pain* **116**, 164–165.

Bowsher D (2005b) Allodynia in relation to lesion site in central post-stroke pain. *J Pain* **6**, 736–740.

Bowsher D, Haggett C (2005) Paradoxical burning sensation produced by cold stimulation in patients with neuropathic pain. *Pain* **117**, 230.

Breuer A, Cuervo H, Selkoe DJ (1981) Hyperpathia and sensory level due to parietal lobe arteriovenous malformation. *Arch Neurol* **38**, 722–724.

Brihaye J, Rétif J (1961) Comparaison des résultats obtenus par la cordotomie antéro-latérale au niveau dorsal et au niveau cervical. A propos de 109 observations personnelles. *Neurochirurgie* **7**, 258–277.

Broager B (1974) Commissural myelotomy. *Surg Neurol* **2**, 71–74.

Broggi G, Franzini A, Giorgi C, Servello D, Spreafico R (1984) Preliminary results of specific thalamic stimulation for deafferentation pain. *Acta Neurochir Suppl* **33**, 497–500.

Broggi G, Servello D, Dones I, Carbone G (1994) Italian multicentric study on pain treatment with epidural spinal cord stimulation (SCS). *Stereotact Funct Neurosurg* **62**, 273–278.

Brooks J, Nurmikko TJ, Bimson B (2002) FMRI studies of thermosensation and nociception using graded thermal stimuli. In *10th World Congress on Pain, Book of Abstracts.* Seattle, WA: IASP Press, A1113–P29.

Brooks-Kayal AR, Shumate MD, Jin H, Rikhter TY, Coulter DA (1998) Selective changes in single cell GABA(A) receptor subunit expression and function in temporal lobe epilepsy. *Nature Med* **4**, 1166–72. Erratum in: *Nature Med* 1999, **5**, 590.

Browder J, Gallagher JP (1948) Dorsal cordotomy for painful phantom limbs. *Ann Surg* **128**, 456–469.

Brown JA, Pilitsis JG (2005) Motor cortex stimulation for central and neuropathic facial pain: a prospective study of 10 patients and observations of enhanced sensory and motor function during stimulation. *Neurosurgery* **56**, 290–297.

Buchanan M (2002) *Nexus. Small Worlds and the Groundbreaking Science of Networks.* WW Norton.

Buchhaas U, Koulousakis A, Nittner K (1989) Experience with spinal cord stimulation (SCS) in the management of chronic pain in a traumatic transverse lesion syndrome. *Neurosurg Rev* **12**(Suppl. 1), 582–587.

Budd K (1985) The use of the opiate antagonist naloxone in the treatment of intractable pain. *Neuropeptides* **5**, 419–422.

Bullit E (1991) Abnormal anatomy of deafferentation: regeneration and sprouting within the central nervous system. *Adv Pain Res Ther* **19**.

Burchiel KJ, Russel LC (1987) Has the amount of spontaneous electrical activity in experimental neuromas been overestimated? In Pubols LM, Sessle BJ, eds., *Effects of Injury on Trigeminal and Spinal Somatosensory Systems.* New York: Liss, pp. 77–83.

Burke DC (1973) Pain in paraplegia. *Paraplegia* **10**, 297–313.

Bushnell MC, Duncan GH, Hofbauer RK *et al.* (1999) Pain perception: is there a role for primary somatosensory cortex? *Proc Natl Acad Sci USA* **96**, 7705–7709.

Cahana A, Carota A, Montadon ML, Annoni JM (2004) The long-term effect of repeated intravenous lidocaine on central pain and possible correlation in positron emission tomography measurements. *Anesth Analg* **98**, 1581–1584.

Calford MB, Tweedale R (1990) Interhemispheric transfer of plasticity in the cerebral cortex. *Science* **249**, 805–807.

Cameron T (2004) Safety and efficacy of spinal cord stimulation for the treatment of chronic pain: a 20-year literature review. *J Neurosurg* **100** (Suppl. 3), 254–267.

Campanini A, De Risio C (1962) Sul problema del dolore di origine centrale. *Sist Nerv* **14**, 382–386.

Canavero S, Pagni CA, Castellano G *et al.* (1993) The role of cortex in central pain syndromes: preliminary results of a long-term technetium-99 hexamethylpropyleneamineoxime single photon emission computed tomography study. *Neurosurgery* **32**, 185–191.

Canavero S (1994) Dynamic reverberation. A unified mechanism for central and phantom pain. *Med Hypotheses* **42**, 203–207.

Canavero S, Pagni CA, Duca S, Bradac GB (1994) Spinal intramedullary cavernous angiomas: a literature metaanalysis. *Surg Neurol* **41**, 381–388.

Canavero S, Bonicalzi V, Pagni CA *et al.* (1995a) Propofol analgesia in central pain: preliminary clinical observations. *J Neurol* **242**, 561–567.

Canavero S, Pagni CA, Bonicalzi V (1995b) Transient hyperacute allodynia in Schneider's syndrome: an irritative genesis? *Ital J Neurol Sci* **16**, 555–557.

Canavero S, Bonicalzi V (1995) Cortical stimulation for central pain. *J Neurosurg* **83**, 1117.

Canavero S, Bonicalzi V, Castellano G (1996) Two in one: the genesis of central pain. *Pain* **64**, 394–395.

Canavero S (1996) Bilateral central pain. *Acta Neurol Belg* **96**, 135–136.

Canavero S, Bonicalzi V (1996) Lamotrigine control of central pain. *Pain* **68**, 179–181.

Canavero S, Bonicalzi V, Massa-Micon B (1997) Central neurogenic pruritus: a literature review. *Acta Neurol Belg* **97**, 244–247.

Canavero S, Bonicalzi V (1998a) Review article. The neurochemistry of central pain: evidence from clinical studies, hypothesis and therapeutic implications. *Pain* **74**, 109–114.

Canavero S, Bonicalzi V (1998b) Pain after thalamic stroke: right diencephalic predominance and clinical features in 180 patients. *Neurology* **51**, 927–928.

Canavero S, Bonicalzi V, Castellano G, Perozzo P, Massa-Micon B (1999) Painful supernumerary phantom arm following motor cortex stimulation for central post-stroke pain. *J Neurosurg* **91**, 121–123.

Canavero S, Bonicalzi V, Lacerenza M *et al.* (2001) Disappearance of central pain following iatrogenic stroke. *Acta Neurol Belg* **101**, 221–223.

Canavero S, Bonicalzi V (2001a) Reversible central pain. *Neurol Sci* **22**, 271–273.

Canavero S, Bonicalzi V (2001b) Electroconvulsive therapy and pain. *Pain* **89**, 301–302.

Canavero S, Bonicalzi V, Paolotti R (2002a) Lack of effect of topiramate for central pain. *Neurology* **58**, 831–832.

Canavero S, Bonicalzi V, Paolotti R (2002b) Reboxetine for central pain: a single-blind prospective study. *Clin Neuropharmacol* **25**, 238–239.

Canavero S, Bonicalzi V (2002) Therapeutic extradural cortical stimulation for central and neuropathic pain: a review. *Clin J Pain* **18**, 48–55.

Canavero S, Bonicalzi V (2003a) Chronic neuropathic pain. *New Engl J Med* **348**, 2688–2689.

Canavero S, Bonicalzi V (2003b) Neuromodulation for central pain. *Expert Rev Neurotherapeutics* **3**, 591–607.

Canavero S, Bonicalzi V, Dotta M, Vighetti S, Asteggiano G (2003a) Low-rate repetitive TMS allays central pain. *Neurol Res* **25**, 151–152.

Canavero S, Bonicalzi V, Narcisi P (2003b) Safety of magnesium-lidocaine combination for severe head injury: the Turin Lidomag pilot study. *Surg Neurol* **60**, 165–169.

Canavero S, Bonicalzi V (2004a) Intravenous subhypnotic propofol in central pain. A double-blind, placebo-controlled, crossover study. *Clin Neuropharmacol* **27**, 182–186.

Canavero S, Bonicalzi V (2004b) Motor cortex stimulation for central and neuropathic pain. *Pain* **108**, 199–200.

Canavero S, Bonicalzi V (2005a) Transcranial magnetic stimulation for central pain. *Curr Pain Headache Rep* **9**, 87–89.

Canavero S, Bonicalzi V (2005b) Mexiletine-gabapentin for central pain: an efficacy and long-term study. In *11th World Congress on Pain, Book of Abstracts*. Seattle, WA: IASP Press. P218 A596 P202.

Canavero S, Bonicalzi V (2006) Extradural cortical stimulation for central pain. In Sakas DE, Simpson B, Krames E, eds., *Operative Neuromodulation*. Vienna: Springer Verlag (in press).

Cannon WB, Rosenblueth A (1949) *The Supersensitivity of Denervated Structures, a Law of Denervation*. New York: Macmillan.

Cantor F (1972) Phenytoin treatment of thalamic pain. *Br Med J* **2**, 590.

Cardenas DD, Warms CA, Turner JA *et al.* (2002) Efficacy of amitriptyline for relief of pain in spinal cord injury: results of a randomised controlled trial. *Pain* **96**, 365–373.

Carlsson KC, Hoem NO, Moberg ER, Mathisen LC (2004) Analgesic effect of dextromethorphan in neuropathic pain. *Acta Anaesthesiol Scand* **48**, 328–336.

Carrieri PB, Provitera VV, Lavorgna L, Bruno R (1998) Response of thalamic pain syndrome to lamotrigine. *Eur J Neurol* **5**, 625–626.

Carter ML (2004) Spinal cord stimulation in chronic pain: a review of evidence. *Anaesth Intensive Care* **32**, 11–21.

Casey KL, ed. (1991) *Pain and Central Nervous System Disease. The Central Pain Syndromes*. New York: Raven Press.

Casey KL, Beydoun A, Boivie J *et al.* (1996) Laser-evoked cerebral potentials and sensory function in patients with central pain. *Pain* **64**, 485–491.

Casey KL, Morrow TJ, Lorenz J, Minoshima S (2001) Temporal and spatial dynamics of human forebrain activity during heat pain: analysis by PET. *J Neurophysiol* **85**, 951–959.

Cassinari V, Pagni CA, Infuso L, Marossero F (1964) La chirurgia stereotassica dei dolori incoercibili (esperienza personale a proposito di 20 casi). *Sist Nerv* **16**, 17–28.

Cassinari V, Pagni CA (1969) *Central Pain: A Neurosurgical Survey*. Cambridge, MA: Harvard University Press, pp. 1–192.

Castro-Alamancos MA, Connors BW (1997) Thalamocortical synapses. *Progr Neurobiol* **51**, 581–606.

Cepeda MS, Africano JM, Polo R, Alcala R, Carr DB (2003) What decline in pain intensity is meaningful to patients with acute pain? *Pain* **105**, 151–157.

Cesaro P, Mann MW, Moretti JL *et al.* (1991) Central pain and thalamic hyperactivity: a single photon emission computerized tomographic study. *Pain* **47**, 329–336.

Chatterjee A, Almahrezi A, Ware M, Fitzcharles MA (2002) A dramatic response to inhaled cannabis in a woman with central thalamic pain and dystonia. *J Pain Symptom Manage* **24**, 4–6.

Chen B, Stitik TP, Foyc PM, Nadler SF, DeLisa JA (2002) Central post-stroke pain syndrome: yet another use for gabapentin? *Am J Phys Med Rehab* **81**, 718–720.

Chiou-Tan FY, Tuel SM, Johnson JC *et al.* (1996) Effect of mexiletine on spinal cord injury dysesthetic pain. *Am J Phys Med Rehab* **75**, 84–87.

Chung CS, Caplan LR, Han W et al. (1996) Thalamic haemorrhage. *Brain* **119**, 1873–1886.

Cianchetti C, Zuddas A, Randazzo AP, Perra L, Marrosu MG (1999) Lamotrigine adjunctive therapy in painful phenomena in MS: preliminary observations. *Neurology* **53**, 433.

Cioni B, Meglio M, Pentimalli L, Visocchi M (1995) Spinal cord stimulation in the treatment of paraplegic pain. *J Neurosurg* **82**, 35–39.

Cioni B et al. (1996) cited from Canavero S, Bonicalzi V (2002).

Clifford DB, Trotter JL (1984) Pain in multiple sclerosis. *Arch Neurol* **41**, 1270–1272.

Coghill RC, Sang CN, Maisog JM, Iadarola MJ (1999) Pain intensity processing within the human brain: a bilateral, distributed mechanism. *J Neurophysiol* **82**, 1934–1943.

Coghill RC, McHaffie JG, Yen YF (2003) Neural correlates of interindividual differences in the subjective experience of pain. *Proc Natl Acad Sci USA* **100**, 8538–8542.

Cohen SP, Abdi J (2002) Venous malformations associated with central pain: report of a case. *Anesth Analg* **95**, 1358–1360.

Cohen SP, DeJesus M (2004) Ketamine patient-controlled analgesia for dysesthetic central pain. *Spinal Cord* **42**, 425–428.

Cole JD, Illis LS, Sedgwick EM (1987) Pain produced by spinal cord stimulation in a patient with allodynia and pseudo-tabes. *J Neurol Neurosurg Psych* **50**, 1083–1084.

Cole JD, Illis LS, Sedgwick EM (1991) Intractable central pain in spinal cord injury is not relieved by spinal cord stimulation. *Paraplegia* **29**, 167–172.

Condouris GA (1976) Local anesthetics as modulators of neural information. In Bonica JJ, Albe-Fessard DG, eds., *Advances in Pain Research and Therapy*, vol. 1. New York: Raven Press, pp. 663–667.

Constans JP (1960) Chirurgie frontale de la douleur. *Acta Neurochir(Wien)* **8**, 251–281.

Cook AW, Kawakami Y (1977) Commissural myelotomy. *J Neurosurg* **47**, 1–6.

Cook AW, Nathan PW, Smith MC (1984) Sensory consequences of commissural myelotomy: a challenge to traditional anatomical concepts. *Brain* **107**, 547–568.

Cooper IS (1965) Clinical and physiologic implications of thalamic surgery for disorders of sensory communication: 1. Thalamic surgery for intractable pain. *J Neurol Sci* **2**, 493–519.

Cooper IS, Amin I, Candra R, Waltz JM (1973) A surgical investigation of the clinical physiology of the LP-pulvinar complex in man. *J Neurol Sci* **18**, 89–110.

Cossart R, Bernard C, Ben-Ari Y (2005) Multiple facets of GABAergic neurons and synapses: multiple fates of GABA signalling in epilepsies. *TINS* **28**, 108–113.

Cowie RA, Hitchcoch ER (1982) The late results of antero-lateral cordotomy for pain relief. *Acta Neurochir* **64**, 39–50.

Crabtree JW, Collingridge GL, Isaac JT (1998) A new intrathalamic pathway linking modality-related nuclei in the dorsal thalamus. *Nature Neurosci* **1**, 389–394.

Craig AD (1998) A new version of the thalamic disinhibition hypothesis of central pain. *Pain Forum* **7**, 1–14.

Crawford AS, Knighton RS (1953) Further observations on medullary spino-thalamic tractotomy. *J Neurosurg* **10**, 113–121.

Crawford AS (1960) Medullary spinothalamic tractotomy for high intractable pain. *J Maine Med Assoc* **51**, 233–235.

Crisologo PA, Neal B, Brown R, McDanal J, Kissin I (1991) Lidocaine-induced spinal block can relieve central poststroke pain: role of the block in chronic pain diagnosis. *Anesthesiology* **74**, 184–185.

D'Aleo G, Sessa E, Di Bella P et al. (2001) Topiramate modulation of R3 nociceptive reflex in multiple sclerosis patients suffering paroxysmal symptoms. *J Neurol* **248**, 996–999.

Dandy et al. (1933) cited from Müller et al. (1991).

Daniele O, Fierro B, Brighina F, Magaudda A, Natalè E (2003) Disappearance of haemorrhagic stroke-induced thalamic (central) pain following a further (contralateral ischaemic) stroke. *Funct Neurol* **18**, 95–96.

Dario A et al. (1999) cited from Canavero S, Bonicalzi V (2002).

David M, Talairach J, Hécaen H (1947) Etude critique des interventions neurochirurgicales actuellement pratiquées dans le traitement de la douleur. *Semaine des Hopitaux de Paris* **234**, 1651–1665.

Davidoff G, Roth EJ (1991) Clinical characteristics of central (dysesthetic) pain in spinal cord injury patients. In Casey KL, ed., *Pain and Central Nervous System Disease*. New York: Raven Press, pp. 77–83.

Davidoff G, Guarracini M, Roth E, Sliwa J, Yarkony G (1987a) Trazodone hydrochloride in the treatment of dysesthetic pain in traumatic myelopathy: a randomized, double-blind, placebo-controlled study. *Pain* **29**, 151–161.

Davidoff G, Roth E, Guarracini M, Sliwa J, Yarkony G (1987b) Function-limiting dysesthetic pain syndrome among traumatic spinal cord injury patients: a cross-sectional study. *Pain* **29**, 39–48.

Davis KD, Hutchison WD, Lozano AM, Dostrovsky JO (1994) Altered pain and temperature perception following cingulotomy and capsulotomy in a patient with schizoaffective disorder. *Pain* **59**, 189–199.

Davis KD, Kiss ZHT, Tasker RR, Dostrovsky JO (1996) Thalamic stimulation-evoked sensations in chronic pain patients and in nonpain (movement disorder) patients. *J Neurophysiol* **75**, 1026–1037.

Davis KD, Kiss ZH, Luo L *et al.* (1998) Phantom sensations generated by thalamic microstimulation. *Nature* **391**, 385–387.

Davis KD, Taub E, Duffner F *et al.* (2000) Activation of the anterior cingulate cortex by thalamic stimulation in patients with chronic pain: a positron emission tomography study. *J Neurosurg* **92**, 64–69.

Davis L, Martin J (1947) Studies upon spinal cord injuries: II. The nature and treatment of pain. *J Neurosurg* **4**, 483–491.

Davis L (1954) Treatment of spinal cord injuries. *AMA Arch Surg* **69**, 488–495.

Davis R, Lentini R (1975) Transcutaneous nerve stimulation for treatment of pain in patients with spinal cord injury. *Surg Neurol* **4**, 100–101.

Davis RA, Stokes JW (1966) Neurosurgical attempts to relieve thalamic pain. *Surg Gynecol Obster* **123**, 371–384.

Davison C, Schick W (1935) Spontaneous pain and other subjective sensory disturbances. A clinicopathologic study. *Arch Neur Psych* **34**, 1204–1237.

De Ajuriaguerra J (1937) *La douleur dans les affections du systéme nerveux central.* Paris: Doin.

DeCharms RC, Maeda F, Glover GH *et al.* (2005) Control over brain activation and pain learned by using real-time functional MRI. *Proc Natl Acad Sci USA* **102**, 18626–18631.

Deckers CLP, Czuczwar SJ, Hekster YA *et al.* (2000) Selection of antiepileptic drug polytherapy based on mechanisms of action: the evidence reviewed. *Epilepsia* **41**, 1364–1374.

DeFelipe J, Farinas I (1992) The pyramidal neuron of the cerebral cortex: morphological and chemical characteristics of the synaptic inputs. *Progr Neurobiol* **39**, 563–607.

Defrin R, Ohry A, Blumen N, Urca G (2001) Characterization of chronic pain and somatosensory function in spinal cord injury subjects. *Pain* **89**, 253–263.

Dehen H, Willer JC, Cambier J (1983) Pain in thalamic syndrome: electrophysiological findings in man. *Adv Pain Res Ther* **5**, 936–940.

Dejerine J, Egger M (1903) Contribution à l'étude de la physiologie pathologique de l'incoordination motrice. *Rev Neurol* **11**, 397.

Dejerine J, Roussy G (1906) Le syndrome thalamique. *Rev Neurol* **14**, 521–532.

Dellemijn PL, Vanneste JA (1997) Randomised double-blind active-placebo-controlled crossover trial of intravenous fentanyl in neuropathic pain. *Lancet* **349**, 753–758.

Demirel T, Braun W, Reimers CD (1984) Results of spinal cord stimulation in patients suffering from chronic pain after a two year observation period. *Neurochirurgia (Stuttg)* **27**, 47–50.

Denny-Brown D, Kirk EJ, Yanagisawa N (1973) The tract of Lissauer in relation to sensory transmission in the dorsal horn of the spinal cord in the macaque monkey. *J Comp Neurol* **151**, 175–200.

Derbyshire SW, Jones AK, Gyulai F *et al.* (1997) Pain processing during three levels of noxious stimulation produces differential patterns of central activity. *Pain* **73**, 431–445.

De Salles AF, Bittar GT Jr. (1994) Thalamic pain syndrome: anatomic and metabolic correlations. *Surg Neurol* **41**, 147–151.

Devor M, Basbaum AL, Bennett GJ *et al.* (1991) Group report: mechanisms of neuropathic pain following peripheral injury. In Basbaum I, Besson JM, eds., *Towards a New Pharmacotherapy of Pain.* Chichester: Wiley, pp. 417–440.

Dey DD, Landrum O, Oaklander AL (2005) Central neuropathic itch from spinal-cord cavernous hemangioma: a human case, a possible animal model, and hypotheses about pathogenesis. *Pain* **113**, 233–237.

Diamond ME, Huang W, Ebner FF (1994) Laminar comparison of somatosensory cortical plasticity. *Science* **265**, 1885–1888.

Diaz JM, Slagle DC (1992) Abscesses and thalamic pain. *Neurology* **42**, 2306–2307.

Di Biagio F (1959) Dolore centrale da lesione sopratalamica regredito con atophanyl. *Riv Neurol* **29**, 476–481.

Dieckmann G, Witzmann A (1982) Initial and long-term results of deep brain stimulation for chronic intractable pain. *Appl Neurophysiol* **45**, 167–172.

Dieckmann G, Veras G II (1984) Plexus avulsion pain (neurogenic pain). High frequency coagulation of the dorsal root entry zone in patients with deafferentation pain. *Acta Neurochir (Wien) Suppl* **33**, 445–450.

Diemath EE, Heppner F, Walker AE (1961) Anterolateral chordotomy for relief of pain. *Postgrad Med* **29**, 485–495.

Dierssen G, Odoriz B, Hernando C (1969) Sensory and motor response to stimulation of the posterior cingulate cortex in man. *J Neurosurg* **31**, 435–440.

Dimitrijevic MR (1987) Neurophysiology in spinal cord injury. *Paraplegia* **25**, 205–208.

Di Piero V, Jones AKP, Iannotti F *et al.* (1991) Chronic pain: a PET study of the central effects of percutaneous high cervical cordotomy. *Pain* **46**, 9–12.

Djaldetti R, Shifrin A, Rogowski Z *et al.* (2004) Quantitative measurement of pain sensation in patients with Parkinson disease. *Neurology* **62**, 2171–2175.

Dogliotti AM (1937) Trattamento del dolore nei tumori, *Minerva Med* **28**, 455–461.

Dogliotti AM (1938) First surgical sections in man, of the lemniscus lateralis (pain-temperature paths) at the brainstem, for the treatment of diffused rebellious pain. *Anesth Analg* **17**, 143–145.

Doi N, Nakamura M, Isse K *et al.* (1999) Electroconvulsive therapy for central post-stroke pain. In *9th World Congress on Pain, Book of Abstracts*, A203 P436.

Donovan WH, Dimitrijevic MR, Dahm L, Dimitrijevic M (1982) Neurophysiological approaches to chronic pain following spinal cord injury. *Paraplegia* **20**, 135–146.

Dotson RM (1997) Clinical neurophysiology laboratory tests to assess the nociceptive axis in humans. *J Clin Neurophysiol* **14**, 32–45.

Dowman R (2002) Pain-evoked anterior cingulate activity generating the negative difference potential may reflect response selection processes. *Psychophysiology* **39**, 369–379.

Drake CG, McKenzie KG (1953) Mesencephalic tractotomy for pain. Experience with six cases. *J Neurosurg* **10**, 457–462.

Drevets WC, Burton H, Videen TO *et al.* (1995) Blood flow changes in human somatosensory cortex during anticipated stimulation. *Nature* **373**, 249–252.

Drewes AM, Andreasen A, Poulsen LH (1994) Valproate for treatment of chronic central pain after spinal cord injury. A double-blind cross-over study. *Paraplegia* **32**, 565–569.

Driver J, Mattingley JB (1998) Parietal neglect and visual awareness. *Nature Neurosci* **1**, 17–22.

Drouot X, Nguyen J-P, Peschanski M, Lefaucheur J-P (2002) The antalgic efficacy of chronic motor cortex stimulation is related to sensory changes in the painful area. *Brain* **125**, 1660–1664.

Druckman R, Lende R (1965) Central pain of spinal cord origin. Pathogenesis and surgical relief in one patient. *Neurology* **15**, 518–522.

Druckman R (1966) Personal communication to White and Sweet (1969).

Drury WL, Clarke LC (1970) Ketamine failure in acute brain injury: a case report. *Anaesth Analg* **49**, 859–861.

Ducreux D, Attal N, Parker F, Bouhassira D (2006) Mechanisms of central neuropathic pain: a combined psychophysical and fMRI study in syringomyelia. *Brain* **129**, 963–976.

Duncan GH, Bushnell CM, Marchand S (1991) Deep brain stimulation: a review of basic research and clinical studies. *Pain* **45**, 49–59.

Duncan GH, Kupers RC, Marchand S *et al.* (1998) Stimulation of human thalamus for pain relief: possible modulatory circuits revealed by positron emission tomography. *J Neurophysiol* **80**, 3326–3330.

Durward QJ, Rice GP, Ball MJ, Gilbert JJ, Kaufmann JCE (1982) Selective spinal cordectomy: clinicopathological correlation. *J Neurosurg* **56**, 359–367.

Dworkin GF, Staats WE (1985) Posttraumatic syringomyelia. *Arch Phys Medic Rehab* **66**, 329–331.

Edgar RE, Best LG, Quail PA, Obert AD (1993) Computer-assisted DREZ microcoagulation: posttraumatic spinal deafferentation pain. *J Spinal Dis* **6**, 48–56.

Edinger L (1891) Giebt es central entstehende Schmerzen? *Dtsch Z Nervenheilk* **1**, 262–282.

Edmondson EA, Simpson RK, Stubler DK, Beric A (1993) Systemic lidocaine therapy for poststroke pain. *South Med J* **86**, 1093–1096.

Edwards CL, Sudhakar S, Scales MT *et al.* (2000) Electromyographic (EMG) biofeedback in the comprehensive treatment of central pain and ataxic tremor following thalamic stroke. *Appl Psychophysiol Biofeedback* **25**, 229–240.

Edwards WT, Habib F, Burney RG, Begin G (1985) Intravenous lidoacine in the management of various chronic pain states. *Reg Anaesth* **10**, 1–6.

Eide PK, Stubhaug A, Stenehjem AE (1995) Central dysesthesia pain after traumatic spinal cord injury is dependent on N-methyl-D-aspartate receptor activation. *Neurosurgery* **37**, 1080–1087.

Eide PK, Jorum E, Stenehjem AE (1996) Somatosensory findings in patients with spinal cord injury and central dysesthesia pain. *J Neurol Neurosurg Psych* **60**, 411–415.

Eisenach JC, Rauck RL, Curry R (2003) Intrathecal, but not intravenous adenosine reduces allodynia in patients with neuropathic pain. *Pain* **105**, 65–70.

Eisenberg E, Brecker C (2002) Lumbar spinal cord stimulation for cervical-originated central pain: a case report. *Pain* **100**, 299–301.

Eisenberg E, McNicol ED, Carr DB (2005) Efficacy and safety of opioid agonists in the treatment of neuropathic pain of nonmalignant origin. Systematic review and meta-analysis of randomized controlled trials. *JAMA* **293**, 3043–3052.

Ekbom KA (1966) Tegretol, a new therapy of tabetic lightning pains. *Acta Med Scand* **179**, 251–252.

Ekbom KA, Westerberg CE, Osterman P (1968) Focal sensory motor seizures of spinal origin. *Lancet* **1**, 67

Elliott AM, Smith BH, Chambers WA (2003) Measuring the severity of chronic pain: a research perspective. *Exp Rev Neurotherapeut* **3**, 581–590.

Emmers R (1981) *Pain: A Spike-Interval Coded Message in the Brain.* New York: Raven Press.

Enarson MC, Hays H, Woodroffe MA (1999) Clinical experience with oral ketamine. *J Pain Symptom Manage* **17**, 384–386.

Epstein FJ, Farmer JP, Freed D (1993) Adult intramedullary spinal cord ependymomas. The result of surgery in 38 patients. *J Neurosurg* **79**, 204–209.

Ergenzinger ER, Glasier MM, Hahm JO, Pons TP (1998) Cortically induced thalamic plasticity in the primate somatosensory system. *Nature Neurosci* **1**, 226–229.

Erickson TC, Bleckwenn WJ, Woolsey CN (1952) Observations on the post central gyrus in relation to pain. *Trans Am Neurol Assoc* **77**, 57–59.

Eriksson MBE, Sjolund BH, Nielzen S (1979) Long term results of peripheral conditioning stimulation as an analgesic measure in chronic pain. *Pain* **6**, 335–347.

Eriksson MBE, Sjolund BH, Sundbarg G (1984) Pain relief from peripheral conditioning stimulation in patients with chronic facial pain. *J Neurosurg* **61**, 149–155.

Ervin FR, Brown CE, Mark VH (1966) Striatal influence on facial pain. *Confinia Neurologica* **27**, 75–86.

Espir ML, Millac P (1970) Treatment of paroxysmal disorders in multiple sclerosis with carbamazepine (Tegretol). *J Neurol Neurosurg Psych* **33**, 528–531.

Eysel UT (2003) Illusions and perceived images in the primate brain. *Science* **302**, 789–790.

Fabritius H (1907) *Studien über die sensible Leitung in menschlichen Rückenmark auf grund klinischer und pathologisch-anatomischer Tatsachen.* Berlin: Karger.

Falci S, Best L, Bayles R, Lammertse D, Starnes C (2002) Dorsal root entry zone microcoagulation for spinal cord injury-related central pain: operative intramedullary electrophysiological guidance and clinical outcome. *J Neurosurg* **97**, 193–200.

Falconer MA (1949) Intramedullary trigeminal tractotomy and its place in the treatment of facial pain. *J Neurol Neurosurg Psych* **12**, 297–311.

Falconer MA (1953) Surgical treatment of intractable phantom-limb pain. *Br Med J* **1**, 299–304.

Farmer S (2002) Neural rhythms in Parkinson's disease. *Brain* **125**, 1175–1176.

Favre J, Taha JM, Burchiel KJ (2002) An analysis of the respective risks of hematoma formation in 361 consecutive morphological and functional stereotactic procedures. *Neurosurgery* **50**, 48–56.

Fenollosa P, Pallares J, Cervera J et al. (1993) Chronic pain in the spinal cord injured: statistical approach and pharmacological treatment. *Paraplegia* **31**, 722–729.

Fields HL, Adams JE (1974) Pain after cortical injury relieved by electrical stimulation of the internal capsule. *Brain* **97**, 169–178.

Fields HL (1999) Pain: an unpleasant topic. *Pain* (Suppl. 6), S61–S69.

Fine W (1967) Post-hemiplegic epilepsy in the elderly. *Br Med J* **1**, 199–201.

Finnerty GT, Connors BW (2000) Sensory deprivation without competition yields modest alterations of short-term synaptic dynamics. *Proc Natl Acad Sci USA* **97**, 12864–12868.

Finnerup NB, Yezierski RP, Sang CN, Burchiel KJ, Jensen TS (2001) Treatment of spinal cord injury pain. *Pain Clin Updates* **IX**.

Finnerup NB, Sindrup SH, Bach FW, Johannesen IL, Jensen TS (2002) Lamotrigine in spinal cord injury pain: a randomized controlled trial. *Pain* **96**, 375–383.

Finnerup NB, Gottrup H, Jensen TS (2002) Anticonvulsants in central pain. *Expert Opin Pharmacother* **3**, 1411–1420.

Finnerup NB, Johannesen IL, Bach FW, Jensen TS (2003a) Sensory function above lesion level in spinal cord injury patients with and without pain. *Somatosens Mot Res* **20**, 71–76.

Finnerup NB, Johannesen IL, Fuglsang-Frederiksen A, Bach FW, Jensen TS (2003b) Sensory function in spinal cord injury patients with and without central pain. *Brain* **126**, 57–70.

Finnerup NB, Gyldensted C, Nielsen E et al. (2003c) MRI in chronic spinal cord injury patients with and without central pain. *Neurology* **61**, 1569–1575.

Finnerup NB, Gyldensted C, Fuglsang-Frederiksen A, Bach FW, Jensen TS (2004) Sensory perception in complete spinal cord injury. *Acta Neurol Scand* **109**, 194–199.

Finnerup NB, Biering-Sorensen F, Johannesen IL *et al.* (2005) Intravenous lidocaine relieves spinal cord injury pain. A randomized controlled trial. *Anesthesiology* **102**, 1023–1030.

Fisher K, Hagen NA (1999) Analgesic effect of oral ketamine in chronic neuropathic pain of spinal origin: a case report. *J Pain Symptom Manage* **18**, 61–66.

Fitzek S, Baumgärtner U, Fitzek C *et al.* (2001) Mechanisms and predictors of chronic facial pain in lateral medullary infarction. *Ann Neurol* **49**, 493–500.

Flor H (2003) Cortical reorganisation and chronic pain: implications for rehabilitation. *J Rehab Med* **41**(Suppl.), 66–72.

Foix C, Thevenard A, Nicolesco (1922) Algie faciale d'origine bulbo-trigeminale au cours de la Syringomyelie-Troubles Sympathiques concomitants-Douleur a type cellulaire. *Rev Neurol* **29**, 990–999.

Foltz EL, White LE Jr. (1966) Rostral cingulotomy and pain 'relief'. In Knighton RS, Dumke PR, eds., *Pain. Henry Ford Hospital International Symposium*. Boston, MA: Little Brown, pp. 469–491.

Förster O (1927) *Die Leitungsbahnen des Schmerzgefühls und die chirurgische Behandlung der Schmerzzustände*. Berlin: Urban and Schwarzenberg.

Förster O (1936) Symptomatologie der Erkrankungen des Rückenmarks und seiner Wurzeln. In Bumke O, Förster O, eds., *Handbuch der Neurologie*, vol. 5. Berlin: Springer, pp. 1–403.

Fouad K, Pearson K (2004) Restoring walking after spinal cord injury. *Progr Neurobiol* **73**, 107–126.

Frank F, Tognetti F, Gaist G *et al.* (1982) Stereotaxic rostral mesencephalotomy in treatment of malignant faciothoracobrachial pain syndromes. *J Neurosurg* **56**, 807–811.

Frank F, Frank G, Gaist G, Fabrizi A, Sturiale C (1984) Deep brain stimulation in chronic pain syndromes. *Acta Neurochir (Wien) Suppl* **33**, 491–495.

Franzini A, Ferroli P, Dones I, Marras C, Broggi G (2003) Chronic motor cortex stimulation for movement disorders: a promising perspective. *Neurol Res* **25**, 123–126.

Frazier CH, Lewy FH, Rowe SN (1937) The origin and mechanism of paroxysmal neuralgic pain and the surgical treatment of central pain. *Brain* **610**, 44–51.

Freeman LW, Heimburger RF (1947) Surgical relief of pain in paraplegic patients. *Arch Surg* **55**, 433–440.

Freeman W, Watts JW (1950) *Psychosurgery in the Treatment of Mental Disorders and Intractable Pain*, 2nd edn. Springfield, IL: Thomas.

Fregni F, Boggio PS, Lima MC *et al.* (2006) A sham-controlled, phase II trial of transcranial direct current stimulation for the treatment of central pain in traumatic spinal cord injury. *Pain* **122**, 197–209.

Friedman AH, Nashold BS (1986) DREZ lesions for relief of pain related to spinal cord injury. *J Neurosurg* **65**, 465–469.

Friedman AH, Bullitt E (1988) Dorsal root entry zone lesions in the treatment of pain following brachial plexus avulsion, spinal cord injury and herpes zoster. *Appl Neurophysiol* **51**, 164–169.

Friedman AH (1991) Treatment of deafferentation pains following peripheral nerve injuries. In Nashold BS Jr, Ovelmen-Levitt J, eds., *Deafferentation Pain Syndromes. Pathophysiology and Treatment*. New York: Raven Press.

Friehs GM, Schroettner O, Pendl G (1995) Evidence for segregated pain and temperature conduction within the spinothalamic tract. *J Neurosurg* **83**, 8–12.

Frighetto L, De Salles A, Wallace R *et al.* (2004) Linear accelerator thalamotomy. *Surg Neurol* **62**, 106–113.

Frot M, Mauguiere F (2003) Dual representation of pain in the operculo-insular cortex in humans. *Brain* **126**, 438–450.

Fujii M, Ohmoto Y, Kitahara T *et al.* (1997) Motor cortex stimulation therapy in patients with thalamic pain. *No Shinkei Geka* **25**, 315–319.

Fujita T, Kitani Y (1992) Pituitary adenolysis by electrocoagulation. In *The Pain Clinic IV*. VSP, pp. 25–31.

Fujiwara N, Imai M, Nagamine T *et al.* (2002) Second somatosensory area (SII) plays a significant role in selective somatosensory attention. *Cogn Brain Res* **14**, 389–397.

Fukaya C, Katayama Y, Yamamoto T *et al.* (2003) Motor cortex stimulation in patients with post-stroke pain: conscious somatosensory response and pain control. *Neurol Res* **25**, 153–156.

Fukuhara T, McKhann GM II, Santiago P *et al.* (1999) Resolution of central pain after embolization of an arteriovenous malformation. Case report. *J Neurosurg* **90**, 575–579.

Fukui S, Shigemori S, Nosaka S (2002a) Central pain associated with low thalamic blood flow treated by electroconvulsive therapy. *J Anaesth* **16**, 255–257.

Fukui S, Shigemori S, Nosaka S (2002b) A case of central post-stroke pain with beneficial response to electroconvulsive therapy: a proton magnetic resonance spectroscopy study. *Pain Clinic* **14**, 173–178.

Fukumoto M, Ushida T, Zinchuk VS, Yamamoto H, Yoshida S (1999) Contralateral thalamic perfusion in patients with reflex sympathetic dystrophy syndrome. *Lancet* **354**, 1790–1791.

Gaches J (1952) Résultat thérapeutique des interventions corticales prefrontales limitées dans les traitment de certains syndromes douloureux dit irreductibles. *Semaine des Hopitaux de Paris* **28**, 3667–3675.

Galaretta M, Hestrin S (1998) Frequency-dependent synaptic depression and the balance of excitation and inhibition in the neocortex. *Nature Neurosci* **1**, 587–594.

Gale K (1992) GABA and epilepsy: basic concepts from preclinical research. *Epilepsia* **33**(Suppl. 5), S3–S12.

Galer BS, Miller KV, Rowbotham MC (1993) Response to intravenous lidocaine infusion differs based on clinical diagnosis and site of nervous system injury. *Neurology* **43**, 1233–1235.

Gamble GE, Barberan E, Bowsher D, Tyrrell PJ, Jones AK (2000) Post stroke shoulder pain: more common than previously realized. *Eur J Pain* **4**, 313–315.

Ganz E, Mullan S (1977) Percutaneous cordotomy. In Lipton S, ed., *Persistent Pain*, vol. 1. London: Academic Press, p. 31.

Garcia-Larrea L, Sindou M, Mauguiere F (1989) Nociceptive flexion reflexes during analgesic neurostimulation in man. *Pain* **39**, 145–156.

Garcia-Larrea L, Peyron R, Mertens P *et al.* (1997) Positron emission tomography during motor cortex stimulation for pain control. *Stereotact Funct Neurosurg* **68**, 141–148.

Garcia-Larrea L, Peyron R, Mertens P *et al.* (1999) Electrical stimulation of motor cortex for pain control: a combined PET-scan and electrophysiological study. *Pain* **83**, 259–273.

Garcia-Larrea L, Convers P, Magnin M *et al.* (2000) Laser-evoked potential abnormalities in central pain patients: the influence of spontaneous and provoked pain. *Brain* **125**, 2766–2781.

Garcin R (1937) La douleur dans les affections organiques du système nerveux central. *Rev Neurol* **68**, 105–153.

Garcin R, Lepresle J (1954) Syndrome sensitif de type thalamique et á topographie cheiro-orale par lesion localisée du thalamus. *Rev Neurol* **90**, 124–129.

Garcin R (1957) La douleur dans les affections du système nerveux central (thalamus, region bulbo-protuberantielle). In Alajouanine Th, ed., *La douleur et les douleurs*. Paris: Masson, pp. 199–213.

Garcin R (1968) Thalamic syndrome and pain of central origin. In Soulairac A, Cahn J, Charpentier J, eds., *Pain*. London: Academic Press, pp. 521–539.

Gardner WJ, Karnosh LJ, McLure CC (1955) Residual function following hemispherectomy for tumour and for infantile hemiplegia. *Brain* **78**, 487–502.

Gatscher S, Becker R, Uhle E, Bertalanffy H (2001) Combined intrathecal baclofen and morphine infusion for the treatment of spasticity related pain and central deafferentation pain. *Acta Neurochir* **79**(Suppl.), 75–76.

Gazzaniga MS (1998) The split brain revisited. *Sci Am* **279**, 50–55.

Getting PA (1989) Emerging principles governing the operation of neural networks. *Annu Rev Neurosci* **12**, 185–204.

Gharabaghi A, Hellwig D, Rosahl SK *et al.* (2005) Volumetric image guidance for motor cortex stimulation: integration of three-dimensional cortical anatomy and functional imaging. *Neurosurgery* **57**(ONS Suppl. 1), 114–120.

Gibson JC, White LC (1971) Denervation hyperpathia: a convulsive syndrome of the spinal cord responsive to carbamazepine therapy. *J Neurosurg* **35**, 287–290.

Gimenez-Roldan S, Martin M (1981) Tabetic lightning pains: high-dosage intravenous penicillin versus carbamazepine therapy. *Eur Neurol* **20**, 424–428.

Gioia DF, Wallace PB, Fuste FJ, Greene M (1967) A stereotaxic method of surgery for the relief of intractable pain. *Int Surg* **48**, 409–416.

Glees P, Bailey EA (1951) Schichtung und Fasergroesse des tractus spinothalamicus des Menschen. *Mschr Psychiatr Neurol* **122**, 129–141.

Glynn CJ, Jamous MA, Teddy PJ, Moore RA, Lloyd JW (1986) Role of spinal noradrenergic system in transmission of pain in patients with spinal cord injury. *Lancet* **ii**, 1249–1250.

Glynn CJ, Jamous MA, Teddy PJ (1992) Cerebrospinal fluid kinetics of epidural clonidine in man. *Pain* **49**, 361–367.

Gold L, Lauritzen M (2002) Neuronal deactivation explains decreased cerebellar blood flow in response to focal cerebral ischemia or suppressed neocortical function. *Proc Natl Acad Sci USA* **99**, 7699–7704.

Goldman-Rakic PS (1995) Cellular basis of working memory. *Neuron* **14**, 477–485.

Gonzales GR, Herskovitz S, Rosenblum M *et al.* (1992) Central pain from cerebral abscess: thalamic syndrome in AIDS patients with toxoplasmosis. *Neurology* **42**, 1107–1109.

Gonzales GR, Lewis SA, Weaver AL (2001) Tactile illusion perception in patients with central pain. *Mayo Clin Proc* **76**, 267–274.

Gonzales GR, Tuttle SL, Thaler HT, Manfredi PL (2003) Central pain in cancer patients. *J Pain* **4**, 351–354.

Gorecki J, Hirayama T, Dostrovsky JO, Tasker RR, Lenz FA (1989) Thalamic stimulation and recording in patients with deafferentation and central pain. *Stereotact Funct Neurosurg* **52**, 219–226.

Gorecki JP, Nashold BS (1995) The Duke experience with the nucleus caudalis DREZ operation. *Acta Neurochir (Wien) Suppl* **64**, 128–131.

Graf C (1960) Consideration in loss of sensory level after bilateral cervical cordotomy. *Arch Neurol* **3**, 410–415.

Graff-Radford NR, Damasio H, Yamada T, Eslinger PJ, Damasio AR (1985) Nonhaemorrhagic thalamic infarction. Clinical, neuropsychological and electrophysiological findings in four anatomical groups defined by computerized tomography. *Brain* **108**, 485–516.

Grant FC (1948) Complications accompanying surgical relief of pain in trigeminal neuralgia. *Am J Surg* **75**, 42–47.

Grant FC, Weinberger LH (1941) Experiences with intramedullary tractotomy: IV. Surgery of the brain-stem and its operative complications. *Surg Gyn Obst* **72**, 747–754.

Grant FC, Wood FA (1958) Experiences with cordotomy. *Clin Neurosurg* **5**, 38–65.

Greenspan JD, Joy SE, McGillis SLB, Checkosky CM, Bolanowski SJ (1997) A longitudinal study of somesthetic perceptual disorders in an individual with a unilateral thalamic lesion. *Pain* **72**, 13–25.

Greenspan JD, Ohara S, Sarlani E, Lenz FA (2004) Allodynia in patients with post-stroke central pain (CPSP) studied by statistical quantitative sensory testing within individuals. *Pain* **109**, 357–366.

Greiff F (1883) Zur localisation der Hemichorea. *Arch Psychol Nervenkrankheit* **14**, 598

Guecer G, Niedermeyer E, Long MD (1978) Thalamic recordings in patients with chronic pain. *J Neurol* **219**, 47–61.

Guillaume J, De Seze S, Mazars G (1949) *Chirurgie cerebro-spinale de la douleur*. Paris: Presses Univ France.

Guillery RW, Feig SL, Lozsadi DA (1998) Paying attention to the thalamic reticular nucleus. *TINS* **21**, 28–32.

Gupta A, Wang Y, Markram H (2000) Organizing principles for a diversity of GABAergic interneurons and synapses in the neocortex. *Science* **287**, 273–278.

Gybels JM, Sweet WH (1989) Neurosurgical treatment of persistent pain. In Gildenberg PL, ed., *Pain and Headache*. Basel: Karger, pp. 1–253.

Gybels J, Kupers R, Nuttin B (1993) Therapeutic stereotactic procedures on the thalamus for pain. *Acta Neurochir* **124**, 19–22.

Gybels JM, Kupers RC (1995) Brain stimulation in the management of persistent pain. In Schmideck HH, Sweet WH, eds., *Operative Neurosurgical Techniques. Indications, Methods and Results*, 3rd edn. Philadelphia, PA: WB Saunders, pp. 1389–1398.

Haber SN, Gdowski MJ (2004) The basal ganglia. In Paxinos G, Mai JK, eds., *The Human Nervous System*, 2nd edn. Amsterdam: Elsevier Academic Press, pp. 677–738.

Hachen HJ (1978) Psychological, neurophysiological and therapeutic aspects of chronic pain: preliminary results with transcutaneous electrical stimulation. *Paraplegia* **15**, 353–367.

Hagelberg N, Martikainen IK, Mansikka H *et al.* (2002) Dopamine D2 receptor binding in the human brain is associated with the response to painful stimulation and pain modulatory capacity. *Pain* **99**, 273–279.

Haines DR, Gaines SP (1999) N-of-1 randomised controlled trials of oral ketamine in patients with chronic pain. *Pain* **83**, 283–287.

Hallin RG, Wiesenfeld-Hallin Z (1983) Does sympathetic activity modify afferent inflow at the receptor level in man? *J Auton Nerv Syst* **7**, 391–397.

Hamamci N, Dursun E, Ural C, Cakci A (1996) Calcitonin treatment in reflex sympathetic dystrophy: a preliminary study. *Br J Clin Pract* **50**, 373–375.

Hamby WB, Shinners BM, Marsh IA (1948) Trigeminal tractotomy. Observations on forty-eight cases. *Arch Surg (Lond)* **57**, 171–177.

Hamby WB (1961) Reversible central pain. *Arch Neurol* **5**, 528–532.

Hampf G, Bowsher D (1989) Distigmine and amitriptyline in the treatment of chronic pain. *Anesth Progr* **36**, 58–62.

Hanajima R, Ashby P, Lang AE, Lozano AM (2002) Effects of acute stimulation through contacts placed on the motor cortex for chronic stimulation. *Clin Neurophysiol* **113**, 635–641.

Hankinson J (1962) Neurosurgical aspects of relief of pain at the cerebral level. In Keele CA, Smith R, eds., *The Assessment of Pain in Man and Animals*. Edinburgh: Livingston, pp. 135–143.

Hannington-Kiff LG (1974) Intravenous regional sympathetic block with guanethidine. *Lancet* **1**, 1019–1020.

Hansebout RR, Blight AR, Fawcett S, Reddy K (1993) 4-Aminopyridine in chronic spinal cord injury: a controlled, double-blind, cross-over study in eight patients. *J Neurotrauma* **10**, 1–18.

Hansson P (2004) Post-stroke pain case study: clinical characteristics, therapeutic options and long-term follow-up. *Eur J Neurol* **11**(Suppl. 1), 22–30.

Harbison J, Dennehy F, Keating D (1997) Lamotrigine for pain with hyperalgesia. *Ir Med J* **90**, 56

Harano K, Koga A, Takasaki M, Totoki T (1999) Intracisternal methylprednisolone administration for thalamic and other intractable pains. In *9th World Congress on Pain, Book of Abstracts*. Seattle, WA: IASP Press, A234, p. 445.

Harden RN, Brenman E, Saltz S, Houle T (2002) Topiramate in the management of spinal cord injury pain: a double-blind, randomised, placebo-controlled pilot study. *Progr Pain Res Manage* **23**, 393–407.

Harrington M, Bone I (1981) Spinal meningioma presenting as focal epilepsy; a case report. *Br Med J* **282**, 1984–1985.

Hariz MI, Bergenheim AT (1995) Thalamic stereotaxic for chronic pain: ablative lesion or stimulation? *Stereotact Funct Neurosurg* **64**, 47–55.

Hassenbusch SJ, Stanton-Hicks M, Covington EC, Walsh JG, Guthrey DS (1995) Long-term intraspinal infusions of opioids in the treatment of neuropathic pain. *J Pain Symptom Manage* **10**, 527–543.

Hassler R, Riechert T (1959) Klinische und anatomische Befunde bei sterotaktischen Schmerz-operationen im Thalamus. *Arch Psychiat* **200**, 93–122.

Hassler R (1960) Die zentrale Systeme des Schmerzes. *Acta Neurochir* **8**, 365–423.

Hassler R (1970) Dichotomy of facial pain conduction in the diencephalon. In Hassler R, Walker AE, eds., *Trigeminal Neuralgia*. Philadelphia, PA: WB Saunders, pp. 123–138.

Hawking S (1988) *A Brief History of Time*. London: Bantam.

Hayashi M, Taira T, Ochiai T et al. (2005) Gamma knife surgery of the pituitary: new treatment for thalamic pain syndrome. *J Neurosurg* **102**(Suppl.), 38–41 (includes Hayashi et al. (2003) *Stereotact Funct Neurosurg* **81**, 75–83).

Hayes KC, Potter PJ, Wolfe DL et al. (1994) 4-Aminopyridine-sensitive neurologic deficits in patients with spinal cord injury. *J Neurotrauma* **11**, 433–446.

Head H, Holmes G (1911) Researches into sensory disturbances from cerebral lesions. *Brain* **34**, 102–254.

Hecaen H, Talairach J, David M, Dell MB (1949) Coagulations limitées du thalamus dans les algies du syndrome thalamique. Résultats thérapeutiques et physiopathologiques. *Rev Neurol* **81**, 917–931.

Heilporn A (1978) Two therapeutic experiments on stubborn pain in spinal cord lesions: coupling melitracen-flupenthixol and the transcutaneous nerve stimulation. *Paraplegia* **15**, 368–372.

Heiskanen T, Hartel B, Dahl ML, Seppala T, Kalso E (2002) Analgesic effects of dextromethorphan and morphine in patients with chronic pain. *Pain* **96**, 261–267.

Heiss WD, Pawlik G, Herholz K et al. (1986) Remote metabolic disturbances in lesions of brain stem and diencephalons: a PET study. In Samii M, ed., *Surgery In and Around the Brain Stem and the Third Ventricle*. Berlin: Springer Verlag, pp. 207–212.

Helfant MH, Leksell L, Strang RR (1965) Experiences with intractable pain treated by sterotaxic mesencephalotomy. *Acta Chir Scand* **129**, 573–580.

Helmchen C, Lindig M, Petersen D, Tronnier V (2002) Disappearance of central thalamic pain syndrome after contralateral parietal lobe lesion: implications for therapeutic brain stimulation. *Pain* **98**, 325–330.

Henderson JM, Boongird A, Rosenow JM, LaPresto E, Rezai AR (2004) Recovery of pain control by intensive reprogramming after loss of benefit from motor cortex stimulation for neuropathic pain. *Stereotact Funct Neurosurg* **82**, 207–213.

Henkel K, Bengel D (2005) Gekreuztes zentral-neuropatisches Schmerzsyndrom nach bakterieller Meningoenzephalitis. *Der Schmerz* **19**, 55–58.

Herman RM, D'Luzansky SC, Ippolito R (1992) Intrathecal baclofen suppresses central pain in patients with spinal lesions. A pilot study. *Clin J Pain* **8**, 338–345.

Herregodts P, Stadnik T, Deridder F, D'Haens J (1995) Cortical stimulation for central neuropathic pain: 3-D surface MIZI for easy determination of the motor cortex. *Acta Neurochir (Wien) Suppl* **64**, 132–135.

Hida K, Iwasaki Y, Imamura H, Abe H (1994) Postraumatic syringomyelia: its characteristics, magnetic resonance imaging findings and surgical management. *Neurosurgery* **36**, 886–891.

Hirato M, Kawashima Y, Shibasaki T, Ohye C (1991) Pathophysiology of central (thalamic) pain: a possible role of the intralaminar nuclei in superficial pain. *Acta Neurochir (Wien) Suppl* **52**, 133–136.

Hirato M, Horikoshi S, Kawashima Y et al. (1993) The possible role of the cerebral cortex adjacent to the central sulcus for the genesis of central (thalamic) pain: a metabolic study. *Acta Neurochir (Wien) Suppl* **58**, 141–144.

Hirato M, Ohye C, Shibazaki T et al. (1995) Gamma knife thalamotomy for the treatment of functional disorders. *Stereotact Funct Neurosurg* **64**(Suppl. 1), 164–171.

Hirayama T, Dostrovsky JO, Gorecki J, Tasker RR, Lenz FA (1989) Recordings of abnormal activity in patients with deafferentation and central pain. *Stereotact Funct Neurosurg* **52**, 120–126.

Hitchcock ER, Teixeira MJ (1981) A comparison of results from center-median and basal thalamotomies for pain. *Surg Neurol* **15**, 341–351.

Hodge CJ Jr., King RB (1976) Medical modification of sensation. *J Neurosurg* **44**, 21–28.

Hofbauer RK, Fiset P, Plourde G, Backman SB, Bushnell MC (2004) Dose-dependent effects of propofol on the central processing of thermal pain. *Anesthesiology* **100**, 386–394.

Hoffmann W (1933) Thalamussyndrom auf grund einer kleinen Lesion. *Psychol Neurol* **54**, 362–374.

Holden C (2004) Imaging studies show how brain thinks about pain. *Science* **303**, 1121.

Holland CT, Charles JA, Smith SH, Cortaville PE (2000) Hemihyperaesthesia and hyperresponsiveness resembling central pain syndrome in a dog with a forebrain oligodendroglioma. *Aust Vet J* **78**, 676–680.

Holmes G (1919) Pain of central origin. In Osler W, ed., *Contributions to Medical and Biological Research.* New York: Paul B Hoeber, pp. 235–246.

Holmgren J, Leijon G, Boivie J, Johansson I, Ilievska L (1990) Central post-stroke pain: somatosensory evoked potentials in relation to location of the lesion and sensory signs. *Pain* **40**, 43–52.

Honey CR, Stoessl J, Tsui JK, Schulzer M, Calne DB (1999) Unilateral pallidotomy for reduction of parkinsonian pain. *J Neurosurg* **91**, 198–201.

Hoogenraad TU, Ramos LMP, Van Gijn J (1994) Visually induced central pain and arm withdrawal after right parietal lobe infarction. *J Neurol Neurosurg Psych* **57**, 850–852.

Horrax G (1946) Experiences with cortical excisions for the relief of intractable pain in the extremities. *Surgery* **20**, 593–602.

Horrax G, Lang E (1957) Complications of chordotomy. *Surg Clin N Am* **37**, 849–854.

Hosobuchi Y (1986) Subcortical electrical stimulation for control of intractable pain in humans. Report of 122 cases (1970–1984). *J Neurosurg* **64**, 543–553.

Hosobuchi Y (1990) Alpha-methyldopa blocks the analgesic effect of sensory thalamic stimulation in humans. *Pain* **5**(Suppl.), S274.

Hosobuchi Y (1993) Motor cortical stimulation for control of central deafferentation pain. In Devinsky O, Beric A, Dogari M, eds., *Electrical and Magnetic Stimulation of the Brain and Spinal Cord,* Advances in Neurology Series. New York: Raven Press, pp. 215–217.

Houtchens MK, Richert JR, Sami A, Rose JW (1997) Open label gabapentin treatment for pain in multiple sclerosis. *Mult Scler* **3**, 250–253.

Hsieh J-C, Belfrage M, Stone-Elander S, Hansson P, Ingvar M (1995) Central representation of chronic ongoing neuropathic pain studies by positron emission tomography. *Pain* **63**, 225–236.

Hua SE, Garonzik IM, Lee JI, Lenz FA (2000) Microelectrode studies of normal organization and plasticity of human somatosensory thalamus. *J Clin Neurophysiol* **17**, 559–574.

Hughes JT (1976) Diseases of the spine and spinal cord. In Blackwood W, Corsellis J, eds., *Greenfield's Neuropathology.* London: Arnold, pp. 652–687.

Huguenard JR, Prince DA (1997) Basic mechanisms of epileptic discharges in the thalamus. In Steriade M, Jones EG, McCormick DA, eds., *Thalamus: II. Experimental and Clinical Aspects.* Amsterdam: Elsevier, pp. 295–330.

Hunt WE, Goodman JH, Bingham WG (1975) Stimulation of the dorsal spinal cord for treatment of intractable pain: a preliminary report. *Surg Neurol* **4**, 153–156.

Hutcheon B, Yarom Y (2000) Resonance, oscillation and the intrinsic preference of neurons. *TINS* **23**, 216–222.

Hutchison WD, Davis KD, Lozano AM, Tasker RR, Dostrovsky JO (1999) Pain-related neurons in the human cingulate cortex. *Nature Neurosci* **2**, 403–405.

Hyndman OR (1942) Lissauer's tract section. A contribution to chordotomy for the relief of pain. Preliminary report. *J Int Coll Surg* **5**, 394–400.

Iacono RP, Nashold BS Jr. (1982) Mental and behavioral effects of brain stem and hypothalamic stimulation in man. *Human Neurobiol* **1**, 273–279.

Iannetti GD, Truini A, Romaniello A *et al.* (2003) Evidence of a specific spinal pathway for the sense of warmth in humans. *J Neurophysiol* **89**, 562–570.

Iwamura Y (1998) Hierarchical somatosensory processing. *Curr Opin Neurobiol* **8**, 522–528.

Iwamura Y, Iriki A, Tanaka M (1994) Bilateral hand representation in the postcentral somatosensory cortex. *Nature* **369**, 554–556.

Izhikevich EM, Desai NS, Walcott EC, Hoppensteadt FC (2003) Bursts as a unit of neural information: selective communication via resonance. *TINS* **26**, 161–167.

Jacobs KM, Donoghue JP (1991) Reshaping the cortical motor map by unmasking latent intracortical connections. *Science* **251**, 944–947.

Jänig W, Koltzenburg M (1991) What is the interaction between the sympathetic terminal and the primary afferent fiber? In Basbaum AI, Besson JM, eds., *Towards a New Pharmacotherapy of Pain*. Chichester: John Wiley, pp. 331–335.

Janis KM, Wright W (1972) Failure to produce analgesia with ketamine in two patients with cortical disease. *Anesthesiology* **36**, 405–406.

Jasmin L, Tien D, Janni G, Ohara PT (2003) Is noradrenaline a significant factor in the analgesic effect of antidepressants? *Pain* **106**, 3–8.

Jeanmonod D, Magnin M, Morel A (1996) Low-threshold calcium spike bursts in the human thalamus. Common physiopathology for sensory, motor and limbic positive symptoms. *Brain* **119**, 363–375.

Jeanmonod D, Magnin M, Morel A, Siegemund M (2001) Surgical control of the human thalamocortical dysrhythmia: I Central lateral thalamotomy in neurogenic pain. *Thalam Rel Syst* **1**, 71–79.

Jefferys JGR, Traub RD, Whittington MA (1996) Neuronal networks for induced '40Hz' rhythms. *TINS* **19**, 202–208.

Jefferson A (1983) Cordectomy for intractable pain in paraplegia. In Lipton S, Miles J, eds., *Persistent Pain: Modern Methods for Treatment*, vol. 4. London: Grune and Stratton, pp. 115–132.

Jefferson A (1987) Personal communication to Gybels and Sweet (1989).

Jensen TS, Gottrup H, Johansen P *et al.* (1999) Positron emission tomography (PET) and psychophysical studies in post-stroke pain. In *9th World Congress on Pain, Book of Abstracts*. Seattle, WA: IASP Press, A77.

Jensen TS, Gottrup H, Kristensen AD, Andersen G, Vestergaard K (2002) Cold sensation in central post-stroke pain. In *10th World Congress on Pain, Book of Abstracts*. Seattle, WA: IASP Press, A95-P91.

Johnson RE, Kanigsberg ND, Jimenez CL (2000) Localized pruritus: a presenting symptom of a spinal cord tumor in a child with features of neurofibromatosis. *J Am Acad Dermatol* **43**, 958–961.

Jones AK, Qi LY, Fujirawa T *et al.* (1991) In vivo distribution of opioid receptors in man in relation to the cortical projections of the medial and lateral pain systems measured with positron emission tomography, *Neurosci Lett* **126**, 25–28.

Jones AKP, Watabe H, Cunningham VJ, Jones T (2004) Cerebral decreases in opioid receptor binding in patients with central neuropathic pain measured by [11C] diprenorphine binding and PET. *Eur J Pain* **8**, 479–485.

Jones EG (2001) The thalamic matrix and thalamocortical synchrony. *TINS* **24**, 595–601.

Joyner J, Mealy J Jr., Freeman LW (1966) Cordotomy for intractable pain of non malignant origin. *Arch Surg* **93**, 480–486.

Juliano SL, Ma W, Eslin D (1991) Cholinergic depletion prevents expansion of topographic maps in somatosensory cortex. *Proc Natl Acad Sci USA* **88**, 780–784.

Kaas JH (1999) Is most of neural plasticity in the thalamus cortical? *Proc Natl Acad Sci USA* **96**, 7622–7623.

Kaas JH (2004) Somatosensory system. In Paxinos G, Mai JK, eds., *The Human Nervous System*, 2nd edn. Amsterdam: Elsevier Academic Press, pp. 1061–1093.

Kabirov EI, Staroselseva NG (2002) Transcutaneous electrostimulation in the treatment of dysesthetic pain in syringomyelia. In *10th World Congress on Pain, Book of Abstracts*. Seattle, WA: IASP Press, A1656-P204.

Kakulas BA, Smith E, Gaekwad U, Kaeln C, Jacobsen PF (1990) The neuropathology of pain and abnormal sensation in human spinal cord injury derived from the clinicopathological data base of the Royal Perth Hospital. In Dimitrijevic MR, Wall PD, Lindblom U, eds., *Recent Achievements in Restorative Neurology: 3. Altered Sensation and Pain*. Basel: Karger, p. 38.

Kalman S, Osterberg A, Sorensen J, Boivie J, Bertler A (2002) Morphine responsiveness in a group of well-defined multiple sclerosis patients: a study with i.v. morphine. *Eur J Pain* **6**, 69−80.

Kameda W, Kawanami T, Kurita K *et al.* for the Study Group of the Association of Cerebrovascular Disease in Tohoku (2004) Lateral and medial medullary infarction. A comparative analysis of 214 patients. *Stroke* **35**, 694−699.

Kameyama M (1976−77) Vascular lesions of the thalamus on the dominant and nondominant side. *Appl Neurophysiol* **39**, 171−177.

Kapadia NP, Harden N (2000) Gabapentin for chronic pain in spinal cord injury: a case report. *Arch Phys Med Rehabil* **81**, 1439−1441.

Katayama Y, Fukaya C, Yamamoto T (1998) Poststroke pain control by chronic motor cortex stimulation: neurological characteristics predicting a favorable response. *J Neurosurg* **89**, 585−591.

Katayama Y, Yamamoto T, Kobayashi K *et al.* (2001) Motor cortex stimulation for post-stroke pain: comparison of spinal cord and thalamic stimulation. *Stereotact Funct Neurosurg* **77**, 183−186.

Kawahara N, Sato K, Muraki M *et al.* (1986) CT classification of small thalamic hemorrhages and their clinical implications. *Neurology* **36**, 165−172.

Kendall D (1939) Some observations on central pain. *Brain* **62**, 253−273.

Khedr EM, Kotb H, Kamel NF *et al.* (2005) Long-lasting antalgic effects of daily sessions of repetitive transcranial magnetic stimulation in central and peripheral neuropathic pain. *J Neurol Neurosurg Psych* **76**, 833−838.

Kim D, Park D, Choi S *et al.* (2003) Thalamic control of visceral nociception mediated by T-type Ca^{2+} channels. *Science* **302**, 117−119.

Kim H, Neubert JK, San Miguel A *et al.* (2004) Genetic influence on variability in human acute experimental pain sensitivity associated with gender, ethnicity and psychological temperament. *Pain* **109**, 488−496.

Kim JS, Lee JH, Lee MC (1995) Sensory changes in the ipsilateral extremity. A clinical variant of lateral medullary infarction. *Stroke* **26**, 1956−1958.

Kim JS, Kim HG, Chung CS (1995) Medial medullary syndrome. Report of 18 new patients and a review of the literature. *Stroke* **26**, 1548−1552.

Kim JS, Lee JH, Im JH, Lee MC (1995) Syndromes of pontine base infarction. A clinical-radiological correlation study. *Stroke* **26**, 950−955.

Kim JS (1996a) Bilateral perioral sensory symptom after unilateral stroke: does it have a localizing value? *J Neurol Sci* **140**, 123−128.

Kim JS (1996b) Restricted *nonacral* sensory syndrome. *Stroke* **27**, 988−990.

Kim JS (1998) Delayed-onset ipsilateral sensory symptoms in patients with central post-stroke pain. *Eur Neurol* **40**, 201−206.

Kim JS (1999) Aggravation of poststroke sensory symptoms after a second stroke on the opposite side. *Eur Neurol* **42**, 200−204.

Kim JS (2003) Central post-stroke pain or paresthesia in lenticulocapsular hemorrhages. *Neurology* **61**, 679−682.

Kim JS, Bae YH (1997) Pure or predominant sensory stroke due to brain stem lesion. *Stroke* **28**, 1761−1764.

Kim JS, Choi-Kwon S (1996) Discriminative sensory dysfunction after unilateral stroke. *Stroke* **27**, 677−682.

Kim JS, Choi-Kwon S (1999) Sensory sequelae of medullary infarction: differences between lateral and medial medullary syndrome. *Stroke* **30**, 2697−2703.

Kim SH, Tasker RR, Oh MY (2001) Spinal cord stimulation for nonspecific limb pain versus neuropathic pain and spontaneous versus evoked pain. *Neurosurgery* **48**, 1056−1065.

Kim LJ, Klopfenstein JD, Zabramski JM, Sonntag VK, Spetzler RF (2006) Analysis of pain resolution after surgical resection of intramedullary spinal cord cavernous malformations. *Neurosurgery* **58**, 106−111.

Kimyai-Asadi A, Nousari HC, Kimyai-Asadi T, Dilani F (1999) Poststroke pruritus. *Stroke* **30**, 692.

King CA, Huff FJ, Jorizzo JL (1982) Unilateral neurogenic pruritus: paroxysmal itching associated with central nervous system lesions. *Ann Intern Med* **97**, 222−223.

King RB (1977) Anterior commissurotomy for intractable pain. *J Neurosurg* **47**, 7−11.

Kingery WS (1997) A critical review of controlled clinical trials for peripheral neuropathic pain and complex regional pain syndromes. *Pain* **73**, 123−139.

Kinnier Wilson SA (1927) Dysesthesias and their neural correlates. *Brain* **50**, 428−461.

Kirchner A, Birklein F, Stefan H, Handwerker HO (2001) Vagus nerve stimulation: a new option for the treatment of chronic pain syndromes. *Schmerz* **15**, 272−277.

Kiriakopoulos ET, Tasker RR, Nicosia S, Wood ML, Mikulis DJ (1997) Functional magnetic resonance imaging: a potential tool for the evaluation of spinal cord stimulation. Technical case report. *Neurosurgery* **41**, 501−504.

Kiss ZHT, Dostrovsky JO, Tasker RR (1994) Plasticity in human somatosensory thalamus as a result of deafferentation. *Stereotact Funct Neurosurg* **62**, 153–163.

Kiss ZHT, Davis KD, Tasker RR, Lozano AM, Dostrovsky JO (1995) Human thalamic neurons develop novel receptive fields within minutes of deafferentation. *J Neurosurg* **82**, 373A (A841).

Kittler JT, Moss SJ (2003) Modulation of GABA-A receptor activity by phosphorylation and receptor trafficking: implications for the efficacy of synaptic inhibition. *Curr Opin Neurobiol* **13**, 341–347.

Knecht S, Henningsen H, Elbert T *et al.* (1996) Reorganizational and perceptional changes after amputation. *Brain* **119**, 1214–1219.

Knecht S, Soros P, Guertler S *et al.* (1998) Phantom sensations following acute pain. *Pain* **77**, 209–213.

Kohlhoff H, Lorenz J, Scharein E *et al.* (1999) Cortical disorganization in patients with post-stroke pain studied by MEG. In *9th World Congress on Pain, Book of Abstracts.* Seattle, WA: IASP Press, A27.

Koehling R (2002) GABA becomes exciting. *Science* **298**, 1350–1352.

Koltzenburg M, Wall PD, McMahon SB (1999) Does the right know what the left is doing? *TINS* **22**, 122–127.

Kondziolka D, Wechsler L, Achim C (2002) Neural transplantation for stroke. *J Clin Neurosci* **9**, 225–230.

Kong K-H, Woon V-C, Yang S-Y (2004) Prevalence of chronic pain and its impact on health-related quality of life in stroke survivors. *Arch Phys Med Rehabil* **85**, 35–40.

Koszewski W, Jarosz J, Pernak-De Gast J (2003) Stereotactic posterior capsulo-lentiform deafferentation as an effective treatment in central post-stroke pain. A new surgical method for intractable central pain control? *Pain Clinic* **15**, 115–123.

Koyama T, Arakawa Y, Shibata M, Mashimo T, Yoshiya I (1998) Effect of barbiturate on central pain: difference between intravenous administration and oral administration. *Clin J Pain* **14**, 86–88.

Krainick JU, Thoden U (1989) Spinal cord stimulation. In Wall PD, Melzack R, eds., *Textbook of Pain,* 2nd edn. Edinburgh: Churchill Livingstone, pp. 920–924.

Kramer KM, Levine AM (1997) Posttraumatic syringomyelia. *Clin Orthoped Rel Res* **334**, 190–199.

Krauss JK, Pohle T, Weigel R, Kalbarzcyk A (2001) Somatosensory thalamic stimulation versus center-median-parafascicular complex stimulation in 11 patients with neuropathic pain. *Stereotact Funct Neurosurg* **77**, 194.

Kringelbach ML, Rolls ET (2004) The functional neuroanatomy of the human orbitofrontal cortex: evidence from neuroimaging and neuropsychology. *Progr Neurobiol* **72**, 341–372.

Krueger AG (1960) Management of painful states in injuries of the spinal cord and cauda equina. *Am J Phys Med* **39**, 103–110.

Krupa DJ, Wiest MC, Shuler MG, Laubach M, Nicolelis MAL (2004) Layer-specific somatosensory cortical activation during active tactile discrimination. *Science* **304**, 1989–1992.

Kudo T, Yoshii N, Shimizu S *et al.* (1968) Sterotaxic thalamotomy for pain relief. *Tohoku J Exp Med* **96**, 219–234.

Kuhl DE, Phelps ME, Kowell AP *et al.* (1980) Effects of stroke on local cerebral metabolism and perfusion: mapping by emission computed tomography of 18FDG and 13NH3. *Ann Neurol* **8**, 47–60.

Kuhner A (1981) Percutaneous cordotomy. Actual situation in pain surgery. *Anesth Analg (Paris)* **38**, 357–359.

Kuhn WG (1947) The care and rehabilitation of patients with injuries of the spinal cord and cauda equina. A preliminary report on 133 cases. *J Neurosurg* **4**, 40–68.

Kumagai Y, Taga K, Hokari T *et al.* (1990) The effect of DREZ (dorsal root entry zone) lesions on intractable pain in patients with spinal cord injury. *Masui* **39**, 632–638.

Kumar K, Toth C, Nath RK (1997) Deep brain stimulation for intractable pain: a 15-year experience. *Neurosurgery* **40**, 736–747 (updates *Can J Surg* 1985, **28**, 20–22, *Neurosurgery* 1990, **26**, 774–782).

Kumar K, Hunter G, Demeria D (2006) Spinal cord stimulation in treatment of chronic benign pain: challenges in treatment planning and present status, a 22-year experience. *Neurosurgery* **58**, 481–496 (updates *J Neurosurg* 1991, **75**, 402–407, *Surg Neurol* 1998, **50**, 110–121).

Kumral E, Kocaer T, Ertübey N, Kumral K (1995) Thalamic hemorrhage. A prospective study of 100 patients. *Stroke* **26**, 964–970.

Kumral E, Celebisoy N (1996) Visually evoked hyperpathia due to thalamic hemorrhage: a variant of Dejerine–Roussy syndrome. *Stroke* **27**, 774–775.

Kumral E, Evyapan D, Balkir K, Kutluhan S (2001) Bilateral thalamic infarction. Clinical, etiological and MRI correlates. *Acta Neurol Scand* **103**, 35–42.

Kuong PG (1984) *Practical Neuroanatomy and Neurological Syndromes*. Beijing: People's Army Medical Publishing.

Kupers RC, Konings H, Adriaensen H, Gybels JM (1991) Morphine differentially affects the sensory and affective pain ratings in a neurogenic and idiopathic forms of pain. *Pain* **47**, 5–12.

Kuroda R, Yamada Y, Kondo S *et al.* (2000) Electrical stimulation of the second somatosensory cortex for intractable pain: a case report and experimental study. *Stereotact Funct Neurosurg* **74**, 226.

Kuzniecki R, Pan J, Martin R *et al.* (2002) Modulation of cerebral GABA by *topirate*, lamotrigine and gabapentin in healthy humans. *Neurology* **58**, 368–372.

Kvarnstrom A, Karlsten R, Quiding H, Gordh T (2004) The analgesic effect of intravenous ketamine and lidocaine on pain after spinal cord injury. *Acta Anaesthesiol Scand* **48**, 498–506.

Lahuerta J, Bowsher D, Lipton S, Buxton PH (1994) Percutaneous cervical cordotomy: a review of 181 operations on 146 patients with a study on the location of "pain fibers" in the C-2 spinal cord segment of 29 cases. *J Neurosurg* **80**, 975–985.

Laine E, Gros C (1956) *L'hemispherectomie. Reunion annuelle, Soc Neurochir Langue Franc.* Paris: Masson et Cie.

Laitinen LV (1977) Anterior pulvinotomy in the treatment of intractable pain. In Sweet WH, Obrador S, Martin-Rodriguez JG, eds., *Neurosurgical Treatment in Psychiatry, Pain, and Epilepsy*. Baltimore, MD: University Park Press, pp. 669–672.

Laitinen LV (1988) Mesencephalotomy and thalamotomy for chronic pain. In Lunsford LD, ed., *Modern Sterotactic Neurosurgery*. Boston, MA: Martinus Nijhoff, pp. 269–277.

Lampl Y, Gilad R, Eshel Y, Sarova-Pinhas I (1995) Neurological and functional outcome in patients with supratentorial hemorrhages. A prospective study. *Stroke* **26**, 2249–2253.

Lampl C, Yazdi K, Roeper C (2002) Amitriptyline in the prophylaxis of central post-stroke pain. Preliminary results of 39 patients in a placebo-controlled, long-term study. *Stroke* **33**, 3030–3032.

Lance JW (1996) The red ear syndrome. *Neurology* **47**, 617–620.

Lapresle J, Guiot G (1953) Ètude des résultats éloignés et en particulier des séquelles neurologiques à type de douleur central dans 8 cas de cordotomie antéro-latérale pour coxarthrose. *Semaine des Hopitaux de Paris* **29**, 2189–2198.

Larson SJ, Sances A, Riegel DH *et al.* (1974) Neurophysiological effects of dorsal column stimulation in man and monkey. *J Neurosurg* **41**, 217–223.

Laspiur RD (1956) Estereotaxis. En relacion a dos casos operados de sindrome talamico vascular. *Arch Inst Neurochir* **97**, 113.

La Terre EC, De Volder AG, Goffinet AM (1988) Brain glucose metabolism in thalamic syndrome. *J Neurol Neurosurg Psych* **51**, 427–428.

Laurent B, Peyron R, Garcia-Larrea L *et al.* (1999) Inside the mechanisms of motor cortex stimulation-induced analgesia. In *9th World Congress on Pain, Book of Abstracts*. Seattle, WA: IASP Press, A187.

Lazorthes Y, Verdie JC, Arbus L (1978) Stimulation analgèsique mèdullaire antèrieure et postèrieur par technique d'implantation percutaneè. *Acta Neurochir (Wien)* **40**, 253–276.

Lazorthes Y (1979) European study on deep brain stimulation. *Resumè, Third European Workshop on Electrical Neurostimulation*. Paris: Medtronic.

Lazorthes Y, Siegfried J, Verdie JC, Casaux J (1995) La stimulation mèdullaire chronique dans le traitement des douleurs neurogènes. Etude coopèrative et rètrospective sur 20 ans de suivi. *Neurochirurgie* **41**, 73–88.

Le Beau J, Daum S, Forjaz S (1948) Les tractotomies trigéminales dans les traitement des névralgies faciales. *Brasil Med Chir* **10**, 331–344.

Le Beau J, Choppy M, Gaches J, Rosier M (1954) *Psychochirurgie et fonctions mentales: techniques, résultats, applications physiologiques*. Paris: Masson.

Le Pera D, Svensson P, Valeriani M *et al.* (2000) Long-lasting effect evoked by tonic muscle pain on parietal EEG activity in humans. *Clin Neurophysiol* **111**, 2130–2137.

Lee MS, Choi IS, Chung TS (1989) Thalamic syndrome and cortical hypoperfusion on technetium-99m HM-PAO brain SPECT. *Yonsei Med J* **30**, 151–157.

Leijon G, Boivie J (1989a) Central post-stroke pain: a controlled trial of amitriptyline and carbamazepine. *Pain* **36**, 27–36.

Leijon G, Boivie J (1989b) Central post-stroke pain: the effect of high and low frequency TENS. *Pain* **38**, 187–191.

Leijon G, Boivie J, Johansson I (1989) Central post-stroke pain: neurological symptoms and pain characteristics. *Pain* **36**, 13–25.

Lende RA, Kirsh WM, Druckman R (1971) Relief of facial pain after combined removal of precentral and postcentral cortex. *J Neurosurg* **34**, 537–543.

Lenz FA (1991) The thalamus and central pain syndromes: human and animal studies. In Casey KL, ed., *Pain and Central Nervous System Disease. The Central Pain Syndromes.* New York: Raven Press, pp. 171−182.

Lenz FA, Kwan HC, Martin R *et al.* (1994) Characteristics of somatotopic organization and spontaneous neuronal activity in the region of the thalamic principal sensory nucleus in patients with spinal cord transections. *J Neurophysiol* **72**, 1570−1587.

Lenz FA, Dougherty PM (1997) Pain processing in the human thalamus. In Steriade M, Jones EG, McCormick DA, eds., *Thalamus: II. Experimental and Clinical Aspects.* Amsterdam: Elsevier, pp. 617−652.

Lenz FA, Gracely RH, Baker FH, Richardson RT, Dougherty PM (1998) Reorganization of sensory modalities evoked by stimulation in the region of the principal sensory nucleus (ventral caudal, Vc) in patients with pain secondary to neural injury. *J Comp Neurol* **399**, 125−138.

Leriche R (1937) *La chirurgie de la douleur.* Paris: Masson (3rd edn. 1949).

Levendoglu F, Ogun CO, Ozerbil O, Ogun TC, Ugurlu H (2004) Gabapentin is a first line drug for the treatment of neuropathic pain in spinal cord injury. *Spine* **29**, 743−751.

Levin AB (1988) Stereotactic chemical hypophysectomy. In Lunsford LD, ed., *Modern Stereotactic Neurosurgery.* Boston, MA: M Nijhoff, pp. 365−374 (see also *J Neurosurg* 1983, **59**, 1002−1006).

Levin G (1966) Electrical stimulation of the globus pallidus and thalamus. *J Neurosurg* **24**, 415.

Levy LM, Ziemann U, Chen R, Cohen LG (2002) Rapid modulation of GABA in sensorimotor cortex induced by acute deafferentation. *Ann Neurol* **52**, 755−761.

Levy RM, Lamb S, Adams JE (1987) Treatment of chronic pain by deep brain stimulation: long term follow-up and review of the literature. *Neurosurgery* **21**, 885−893.

Levy R, Lang AE, Dostrovsky JO *et al.* (2001) Lidocaine and muscimol microinjections in subthalamic nucleus reverse Parkinsonian symptoms. *Brain* **124**, 2105−2118.

Lewin W, Philips CG (1952) Observations on partial removal of the post-central gyrus for pain. *J Neurol Neurosurg Psychiat* **15**, 143−147.

Ley A (1957) *Aneurismas arteriovenosos congenitos intracraneales.* Barcelona: Typografia la Académica.

Lhermitte J (1933) Physiologie des ganglions centraux. Les corps stries. La couche optique. Les formations sousthalamiques. In: Binet R, ed., *Traitè de physiologie normale et pathologique*, vol. 9. Paris: Masson, pp. 357−402.

Li J (2000) Clinical analysis and treatment of central pain due to head injury. *Chin J Traumatol* **3**, 126−127.

Libet B (1973) Electrical stimulation of cortex in human subjects and conscious sensory aspects. In Iggo A, ed., *Handbook of Sensory Physiology*, vol. 2. Berlin: Springer, pp. 744−790.

Liepert J, Restemeyer C, Muenchau A, Weiller C (2005) Motor cortex excitability after thalamic infarction. *Clin Neurophysiol* **116**, 1621−1627.

Linazasoro G (2004) Recent failures of new potential symptomatic treatment for Parkinson's disease: causes and solutions. *Mov Disord* **19**, 743−754.

Lind G, Meyerson BA, Winter J, Linderoth B (2004) Intrathecal baclofen as adjuvant therapy to enhance the effect of spinal cord stimulation in neuropathic pain: a pilot study. *Eur J Pain* **8**, 377−383.

Lindblom U, Meyerson BA (1975) Influence on touch, vibration and cutaneous pain of dorsal column stimulation in man. *Pain* **1**, 257−270.

Lindblom U (1991) New directions for basic and clinical research in central pain syndromes. In Casey KL, ed., *Pain and Central Nervous System Disease. The Central Pain Syndromes.* New York: Raven Press, pp. 275−280.

Lippert RS, Hosobuchi Y, Nielsen SL (1974) Spinal commissurotomy. *Surg Neurol* **2**, 373−377.

Lipton S (1989) Percutaneous cordotomy. In Wall PD, Melzack R, eds., *Textbook of Pain*, 2nd edn. Edinburgh: Churchill Livingstone, pp. 832−839.

Lisman J (1997) Bursts as a unit of neural information: making unreliable synapses reliable. *TINS* **20**, 38−43.

Livingstone WK (1943) *Pain Mechanisms: A Physiologic Interpretation of Causalgia and Its Related States.* New York: Macmillan (2nd edn: Plenum, 1946).

Llinas RR, Parè D (1991) Commentary. Of dreaming and wakefulness. *Neuroscience* **44**, 521−535.

Llinas RR, Parè D (1997) Coherent oscillations in specific and nonspecific thalamocortical networks and their role in cognition. In Steriade M, Jones EG, McCormick DA, eds., *Thalamus: II. Experimental and Clinical Aspects.* Amsterdam: Elsevier, pp. 501−516.

Llinas RR, Ribary U, Jeanmonod D, Kronberg E, Mitra PP (1999) Thalamocortical dysrhythmia: a neurological and neuropsychiatric syndrome characterized by magnetoencephalography. *Proc Natl Acad Sci USA* **96**, 15222−15227.

Loeser JD, Ward AA Jr., White LE Jr. (1968) Chronic deafferentation of human spinal cord neurons. *J Neurosurg* **29**, 48–50.

Loh L, Nathan PW (1978) Painful peripheral states and sympathetic blocks. *J Neurol Neurosurg Psych* **41**, 664–671.

Loh L, Nathan PW, Schott GD, Wilson PG (1980) Effects of regional guanethidine infusion in certain painful states. *J Neurol Neurosurg Psych* **43**, 446–451.

Loh L, Nathan PW, Schott GD (1981) Pain due to lesions of central nervous system removed by sympathetic block. *Br Med J* **282**, 1026–1028.

Long DM, Erickson DE (1975) Stimulation of the posterior columns of the spinal cord for relief of intractable pain. *Surg Neurol* **4**, 134–141.

Long DM, Hagfors N (1975) Electrical stimulation in the nervous system: the current status of electrical stimulation of the nervous system for relief of pain. *Pain* **1**, 109–123.

Long DM, Campbell JN, Gucer G (1979) Transcutaneous electrical stimulation for relief of chronic pain. In Bonica JJ, Liebeskind JC, Albe-Fessard DG, eds., *Advances in Pain Research and Therapy.* New York: Raven Press, pp. 593–599.

Lorenz J, Kohlhoff H, Hansen H-C, Kunze, Bromm B (1998) Abeta-fiber mediated activation of cingulate cortex as correlate of central post-stroke pain. *NeuroReport* **9**, 659–663.

Loubser PG, Donovan WH (1991) Diagnostic spinal anaesthesia in chronic spinal cord injury pain. *Paraplegia* **29**, 25–36.

Loubser PG, Clearman RR (1993) Evaluation of central spinal cord injury pain with diagnostic spinal anesthesia. *Anesthesiology* **79**, 376–378.

Loubser PG, Akman NM (1996) Effects of intrathecal baclofen on chronic spinal cord injury pain. *J Pain Symptom Manage* **12**, 241–247.

Lozano AM, Parrent A, Tasker RR (1992) Central pain from thalamic neoplasms. *Stereotact Funct Neurosurg* **59**, 77.

Luessenhop AJ, Dela Cruz T (1969) The surgical excision of spinal intradural vascular malformation. *J Neurosurg* **30**, 552–559.

Magnin M, Jetzer U, Morel A, Jeanmonod D (2001) Microelectrode recording and macrostimulation in thalamic and subthalamic MRI guided stereotactic surgery. *Neurophysiol Clin* **31**, 230–238.

Mailis A, Amani N, Umana M, Basur R, Roe S (1997) Effect of intravenous sodium amytal on cutaneous sensory abnormalities, spontaneous pain and algometric pain pressure thresholds in neuropathic pain patients: a placebo-controlled study. II. *Pain* **70**, 69–81.

Mailis A, Bennett GJ (2002) Dissociation between cutaneous and deep sensibility in central post-stroke pain (CPSP). *Pain* **98**, 331–334.

Maletic-Savatic M, Malinow R, Svoboda K (1999) Rapid dendritic morphogenesis in CA1 hippocampal dendrites induced by synaptic activity. *Science* **283**, 1923–1927.

Mamie C, Morabia A, Bernstein M, Klopfenstein LE, Forster A (2000) Treatment efficacy is not an index of pain intensity. *Can J Anaesth* **47**, 1166–1170.

Manduch M, Davis KD, Lozano AM, Tasker RR, Dostrovsky JO (1999) Thalamic stimulation-evoked pain and temperature sites in pain and non-pain patients. In *9th World Congress on Pain, Book of Abstracts.* Seattle, WA: IASP Press, A70-P151.

Mann L (1892) Kasuisticher Beitrag zur Lehre vom Central entstehenden Schmerze. *Berlin klin Wochenschr* **29**, 244.

Mansuy L, Sindou M, Fischer G, Brunon J (1976) La cordotomie spinothalamique dans les douleurs cancéreuses. Résultats d'une série de 124 malades opérés par abord direct postérieur. *Neurochirurgie* **22**, 437–444.

Marchand S, Bushnell MC, Molina-Negro P, Martinez SN, Duncan GN (1991) The effects of dorsal column stimulation on measures of clinical and experimental pain in man. *Pain* **45**, 249–257.

Marchand S, Kupers RC, Bushnell MC, Duncan GH (2003) Analgesic and placebo effects of thalamic stimulation. *Pain* **105**, 481–488.

Margot-Duclot A, Thiebaut J-B, Simon A *et al.* (2002) Effects of intrathecal baclofen in cauda equina and low spinal cord injury pain. In *10th World Congress on Pain, Book of Abstracts.* Seattle, WA: IASP Press, A221-P217.

Marineo G (2003) Untreatable pain resulting from abdominal cancer: new hope from biophysics? *JOP* **4**, 1–10.

Mark VH, Tsutsumi H (1974) The suppression of pain by intrathalamic lidocaine. *Adv Neurol* **4**, 715–721.

Mark VH, Ervin FR, Hackett TP (1960) Clinical aspects of stereotactic thalamotomy in the human. The treatment of chronic severe pain. *Arch Neurol* **3**, 351–367.

Markram H, Toledo-Rodriguez M, Wang Y *et al.* (2004) Interneurons of the neocortical inhibitory system. *Nature Rev Neurosci* **5**, 793–807.

Marshall J (1951) Sensory disturbances in cortical wounds with special reference to pain. *J Neurol Neurosurg Psych* **14**, 187–204.

Massey EW (1984) Unilateral neurogenic pruritus following stroke. *Stroke* **15**, 901–903.

Masson C, Koskas P, Cambier J, Masson M (1991) Syndrome cortical pseudothalamique gauche et asymbolie à la douleur. *Rev Neurol (Paris)* **147**, 668–670.

Mauguiére F, Desmedt JE (1988) Thalamic pain syndrome of Dejerine–Roussy: differentiation of four subtypes assisted by somatosensory evoked potentials data. *Arch Neurol* **45**, 1312–1320.

Maurer M, Henn V, Dittrich A, Hofmann A (1990) Delta-9-tetrahydrocannabinol shows antispastic and analgesic effects in a single case double-blind trial. *Eur Arch Psychiatry Clin Neurosci* **240**, 1–4.

Max MB, Hagen NA (2000) Do changes in brain sodium channels cause central pain? *Neurology* **54**, 544–545.

Mayanagi Y, Bouchard G (1976–77) Evaluation of stereotactic thalamotomies for pain relief, with reference to pulvinar intervention. *Appl Neurophysiol* **39**, 157–159.

Mayanagi Y, Sano K (1988) Posteromedial hypothalamotomy for behavioral disturbances and intractable pain. In Lunsford LD, ed., *Modern Stereotactic Neurosurgery*. Boston, MA: M Nijhoff, pp. 377–384.

Mayanagi Y, Sano K (1998) Stimulation and coagulation of the posterior hypothalamus for intractable pain. In Gildenberg PL, Tasker RR, eds., *Textbook of Stereotactic and Functional Neurosurgery*. New York: McGraw-Hill, pp. 1453–1454.

Mazars G, Pansini A, Chiarelli J (1960) Coagulation du faisceau spinothalamique et du faiceau quinto-thalamique par stereotaxie. Indications-resultats. *Acta Neurochir* **8**, 324–326 (also includes *J Neurol Neurosurg Psych* 1960, **23**, 352).

Mazars GJ (1975) Intermittent stimulation of nucleus ventralis posterolateralis for intractable pain. *Surg Neurol* **4**, 93–95 (also includes *Neurochirurgie* 1974, **20**, 117–124).

Mazars G (with Merienne L, Cioloca C) (1976) Ètat actuel de la chirurgie de la douleur. *Neurochirurgie* **22**(Suppl.), 1–164.

Mazars GJ, Merienne L, Cioloca C (1979) Comparative study of electrical stimulation of posterior thalamic nuclei, periaqueductal gray, and other midline mesencephalic stuctures in man. *Adv Pain Res Ther* **3**, 541–546.

McAlhany HS, Netsky MG (1955) Compression of the spinal cord by extramedullary neoplasms. *J Neuropath Exp Neurol* **14**, 276–281.

McCance S, Hawton K, Brighouse D, Glynn C (1996) Does electroconvulsive therapy (ECT) have any role in the management of intractable thalamic pain? *Pain* **68**, 129–131.

McCarty GW (1954) The treatment of spastic paraplegia by selective spinal cordectomy. *J Neurosurg* **11**, 539–545.

McCleane G (1998) Lamotrigine can reduce neurogenic pain associated with multiple sclerosis. *Clin J Pain* **14**, 268–270.

McCleane G (1998a) A prospective audit of the use of lamotrigine in 300 chronic pain patients. *The Pain Clinic* **11**, 97–102.

McCormick PC, Torres R, Post KD, Stein BM (1990) Intramedullary ependymoma of the spinal cord. *J Neurosurg* **72**, 523–533.

McCrone J (1999) *Going Inside*. Faber and Faber.

McGowan DJL, Janal MN, Clark WC *et al.* (1997) Central post-stroke pain and Wallenberg's lateral medullary infarction: frequency, character, and determinants in 63 patients. *Neurology* **49**, 120–125.

McQuay HJ, Carroll D, Jadad AR *et al.* (1994) Dextrometorphan for the treatment of neuropathic pain: a double-blind randomised controlled crossover trial with integral n-of-1 design. *Pain* **59**, 127–133.

McQuay HJ, Tramer M, Nye BA *et al.* (1996) A systematic review of antidepressants in neuropathic pain. *Pain* **68**, 217–227.

Meador KJ, Ray PG, Day L, Ghelani H, Loring DW (1998) Physiology of somatosensory perception: cerebral lateralization and extinction. *Neurology* **51**, 721–727.

Meador KJ, Ray PG, Echauz JR, Loring DW, Vachtsevanos GJ (2002) Gamma coherence and conscious perception. *Neurology* **24**, 847–854.

Meadows J, Guarnieri M, Miller K *et al.* (2001) Type I Chiari malformation: a review of the literature. *Neurosurg Quart* **11**, 220–229.

Meglio M (1998) Evaluation and management of central and peripheral deafferentation pain. In Gildenberg PL, Tasker RR, eds., *Textbook of Stereotactic and Functional Neurosurgery*. New York: McGraw-Hill, pp. 1631–1636.

Melzack R, Wall PD (1965) Pain mechanisms: a new theory. *Science* **150**, 971–979.

Melzack R, Loeser JD (1978) Phantom body pain in paraplegics: evidence for a central pattern generating mechanism for pain. *Pain* **4**, 195–210.

Melzack R (1991) Central pain syndromes and theories of pain. In Casey KL, ed., *Pain and Central Nervous System Disease. The Central Pain Syndromes*. New York: Raven Press, pp. 59–64.

Mercadante S (1998) Gabapentin in spinal cord injury pain. *Pain Clinic* **10**, 203–206.

Metzler J, Marks PS (1979) Functional changes in cat somatic sensory-motor cortex short-term during reversible epidural blocks. *Brain Res* **177**, 379–383.

Merren MD (1998) Gabapentin for the treatment of pain and tremor: a large case series. *South Med J* **91**, 739–744.

Merskey H (1994) Classification of chronic pain: descriptions of chronic pain syndromes and definitions of pain terms. *Pain* Suppl. 3, 1986 (with Bogduk N, ed., 2nd edn. Seattle, WA: IASP Press, 1994).

Meyer BU, Roericht S, Graefin von Einsiedel H, Kruggel F, Weindl A (1995) Inhibitory and excitatory interhemispheric transfers between motor cortical areas in normal humans and patients with abnormalities of the corpus callosum. *Brain* **118**, 429–440.

Meyer-Lindenberg A, Ziemann U, Hajak G, Cohen L, Berman KF (2002) Transitions between dynamical states of differing stability in the human brain. *Proc Natl Acad Sci USA* **99**, 10948–10953.

Meyerson BA, Lindblom U, Linderoth B, Lind G, Herregodts P (1993) Motor cortex stimulation as treatment of trigeminal neuropathic pain. *Acta Neurochir* **58**(Suppl.), 150–153.

Meyerson BA, Linderoth B (1999) Electric stimulation of the central nervous system. In Max M, ed., *Pain 1999: An Updated Review*. Seattle, WA: IASP Press, pp. 269–280.

Meyerson BA, Linderoth B (2001) Brain stimulation: intracerebral and motor cortex stimulation. In Loeser JD, ed., *Bonica's Management of Pain*, 3rd edn. Philadelphia, PA: Lippincott Williams & Wilkins, pp. 1877–1889.

Michel D, Laurent B, Convers P et al. (1990), Douleurs corticales. Ètude clinique, électrophysiologique et topographique de 12 cas. *Rev Neurol* **146**, 405–414.

Michelsen JJ (1943) Subjective disturbances of the sense of pain from lesions of the cerebral cortex. *Ass Res Nerv M Dis Proc* **23**, 86–99.

Middleton JW, Siddall PJ, Walker S, Molloy AR, Rutkowski SB (1996) Intrathecal clonidine and baclofen in the management of spasticity and neuropathic pain following spinal cord injury: a case study. *Arch Phys Med Rehabil* **77**, 824–826.

Migita K, Uozumi T, Arita K, Monden S (1995) Transcranial magnetic coil stimulation of motor cortex in patients with central pain. *Neurosurgery* **36**, 1037–1040.

Mikula F, Siroky J, Zapletal B (1959) Le traitement des crises gastralgiques par la tractotomie mésencephalique bilaterale et ses complications auditives inattendues. *Rev oto-neuro oftal (Buenos Aires)* **31**, 456–463.

Milandre L, Brosset C, Khalil R (1993) Infarctus thalamiques lateraux: 22 observations. *Presse Med* **22**, 1865–1869.

Miles J (1998) The pituitary gland and pain relief. In Gildenberg PL, Tasker RR, eds., *Textbook of Stereotactic and Functional Neurosurgery*. New York: McGraw-Hill, pp. 1457–1462.

Milhorat TH, Kotzen RM, Mu HTM, Capocelli AL, Milhorat RH (1996) Dysesthetic pain in patients with syringomyelia. *Neurosurgery* **38**, 940–947.

Milhorat TH, Capocelli AL Jr., Kotzen RM et al. (1997) Intramedullary pressure in syringomyelia: clinical and pathophysiological correlates of syrinx distension. *Neurosurgery* **41**, 1102–1110.

Millan MJ (2002) Descending control of pain. *Prog Neurobiol* **66**, 355–474.

Mirò J, Garcia-Monco C, Leno C, Berciano C (1988) Pelvic pain: an undescribed paroxysmal manifestation of multiple sclerosis. *Pain* **32**, 73–75.

Miserocchi E (1951) Le cordotomie (tractotomie spinali). *Chirurgia* **6**, 519–538.

Mittal B, Thomas DG, Walton P, Calder I (1987) Dorsal column stimulation in chronic pain: report of 31 cases. *Ann R Coll Surg Engl* **69**, 104–109.

Mladinich EK (1974) Diphenylhydantoin in the Wallenberg syndrome. *JAMA* **230**, 372–373.

Modesti LM, Waszak M (1975) Firing pattern of cells in human thalamus during dorsal column stimulation. *Appl Neurophysiol* **38**, 251–258.

Mogil JS (1999) Review. The genetic mediation of individual differences in sensitivity to pain and its inhibition. *Proc Natl Acad Sci USA* **96**, 7745–7751.

Mogilner AY, Rezai AR (2001) Epidural motor cortex stimulation with functional imaging guidance. *Neurosurg Focus* **11**, article 4.

Mohammadian P, Hummel T, Loetsch J, Kobal G (1997) Bilateral hyperalgesia to chemical stimulation of the nasal mucosa following unilateral inflammation. *Pain* **73**, 407–412.

Montes C, Mertens P, Convers P et al. (2002) Cognitive effects of precentral cortical stimulation for pain control: an ERP study. *Neurophysiol Clin* **32**, 313–325.

Montes C, Magnin M, Maarrawi J et al. (2005) Thalamic thermo-algesic transmission: ventral posterior (VP) complex versus Vmpo in the light of a thalamic infarct with central pain. *Pain* **113**, 223–232.

Montgomery BM, King WW (1962) Hemiplegic migraine; a case with paroxysmal shoulder–hand syndrome. *Ann Intern Med* **57**, 450–455.

Moore CEG, Schady W (2000) Investigation of the functional correlates of reorganization within the human somatosensory cortex. *Brain* **123**, 1883–1895.

Moore CI, Nelson SB, Sur M (1999) Dynamics of neuronal processing in rat somatosensory cortex. *TINS* **22**, 513–520.

Moore CI, Stern CE, Dunbar C *et al.* (2000) Referred phantom sensations and cortical reorganization after spinal cord injury in humans. *Proc Natl Acad Sci USA* **97**, 14703–14708.

Morgan M, Loh L, Singer L, Moore PH (1971) Ketamine as the sole anesthetic agent for minor surgical procedures. *Anaesthesia* **26**, 158–159.

Mori S, Sadoshima S, Ibayashi S, Fujishima M, Iino K (1995) Impact of thalamic hematoma on six-month mortality and motor and cognitive functional outcome. *Stroke* **26**, 620–626.

Morin C, Bushnell MC, Luskin MB, Craig AD (2002) Disruption of thermal perception in a multiple sclerosis patient with central pain. *Clin J Pain* **18**, 191–195.

Morley JS, Miles JB, Venn RF, Williams TSC (1991) Dorsal horn enkephalins reduced in human chronic pain. *IASP Congress on Pain*. Seattle, WA: IASP Press, Abstr. 186.

Morley JS, Bridson J, Nash TP *et al.* (2003) Low-dose methadone has an analgesic effect in neuropathic pain: a double-blind randomized controlled cross-over trial. *Palliat Med* **17**, 576–587.

Morrow TJ, Casey KL (2002) Understanding central pain: new insights from forebrain imaging studies of patients and of animals with central lesions. *Progr Pain Res Manage* **23**, 265–279.

Moshè SL (2000) Mechanisms of action of anticonvulsant agents. *Neurology* **55**(Suppl. 1), S32–S40.

Moulin DE, Foley KM, Ebers GC (1988) Pain syndromes in multiple sclerosis. *Neurology* **38**, 1830–1834.

Mukherjee CS, Sarkhel A, Banerjee TK, Sen S (1999) Community survey of central post-stroke pain (CPSP). *9th World Congress on Pain, Book of Abstracts*. Seattle, WA: IASP Press, A338.

Mullan MJ (2002) Descending control of pain. *Progr Neurobiol* **66**, 355–474.

Müller F, Kunesch E, Binkofski F, Frend H-J (1991) Residual sensorimotor functions in a patient after right sided hemispherectomy. *Neuropsychology* **29**, 125–145.

Mundinger F, Becker P (1977) Late results of central stereotactic interventions for pain. *Acta Neurochir Suppl* **24**, 229.

Mundinger F, Salomão JF (1980) Deep brain stimulation in mesencephalic lemniscus medialis for chronic pain. *Acta Neurochir Suppl* **30**, 245–258.

Mundinger F, Neumuller H (1982) Programmed stimulation for control of chronic pain and motor diseases. *Appl Neurophysiol* **45**, 102–111.

Nagaro T, Amakawa K, Kimura S, Arai T (1993) Reference of pain following percutaneous cervical cordotomy. *Pain* **53**, 205–211.

Nagaro T, Shimizu C, Inoue H *et al.* (1995) [The efficacy of intravenous lidocaine on various types of neuropathic pain]. *Masui* **44**, 862–867.

Nair DR, Najm I, Bulacio J, Lueders H (2001) Painful auras in focal epilepsy. *Neurology* **57**, 700–702.

Nakazato Y, Yoshimaru K, Ohkuma A *et al.* (2004) Central post-stroke pain in Wallenberg syndrome. *No To Shinkei* **56**, 385–388.

Namba S, Nakao Y, Matsumoto Y, Ohmoto T, Nishimoto A (1984) Electrical stimulation of the posterior limb of the internal capsule for treatment of thalamic pain. *Appl Neurophysiol* **47**, 137–148 (see also *J Neurosurg* 1985, **63**, 224–234).

Nandi D, Smith H, Owen S *et al.* (2002) Periventricular grey stimulation versus motor cortex stimulation for post-stroke neuropathic pain. *J Clin Neurosci* **9**, 557–561.

Nandi D, Aziz T, Carter H, Stein J (2003) Thalamic field potentials in chronic central pain treated by periventricular gray stimulation – a series of eight cases. *Pain* **101**, 97–107.

Nandi D, Aziz TZ (2004) Deep brain stimulation in the management of neuropathic pain and multiple sclerosis tremor. *J Clin Neurophysiol* **21**, 31–39.

Nashold BS, Wilson WP, Slaughter DG (1969) Stereotactic midbrain lesions for central dysesthesia and phantom pain. Preliminary report. *J Neurosurg* **30**, 116–126.

Nashold BS, Wilson WP (1970) Central pain and irritable midbrain. In Crue B, ed., *Pain and Suffering. Selected Aspects*. Springfield, IL: CC Thomas, pp. 95–118 (also *Conf Neurol* 1966, **27**, 30–34; *Adv Neurol* 1974, 191–196).

Nashold BS, Friedman H Jr. (1972) Dorsal column stimulation for control of pain. Preliminary report on 30 patients. *J Neurosurg* **30**, 590–597.

Nashold BS Jr. (1974) Central pain: its origin and treatment. *Clin Neurosurg* **21**, 311–322.

Nashold BS Jr. (1975) Dorsal column stimulation for control of pain: a three-year follow-up. *Surg Neurol* **4**, 146–147.

Nashold BS Jr., Bullit E (1981) Dorsal root entry zone lesions to control central pain in paraplegics. *J Neurosurg* **55**, 414–419.

Nashold BS Jr. (1982) Brainstem stereotaxic procedures. In Schaltenbrand G, Walker AE, eds., *Stereotaxy of the Human Brain. Anatomical, Physiological and Clinical Applications*, 2nd edn. Stuttgart: Georg Thieme Verlag, pp. 475–483.

Nashold BS (1984) Current status of the DREZ operation. *Neurosurgery* 15, 942–944.

Nashold BS Jr. (1991) Paraplegia and pain. *Adv Pain Res Ther* 19, 301.

Nashold BS, Pearlstein RD, eds. (1996) *The DREZ Operation*. Park Ridge, IL: AANS Publications.

Nasreddine ZS, Saver JL (1997) Pain after thalamic stroke: right diencephalic predominance and clinical features in 180 patients. *Neurology* 48, 1196–1199.

Nasreddine ZS, Saver JL (1998) Pain after thalamic stroke: right diencephalic predominance and clinical features in 180 patients. *Neurology* 51, 927–928.

Nathan PW (1960) Improvement in cutaneous sensibility associated with relief of pain. *J Neurol Neurosurg Psych* 23, 202–206.

Nathan PW, Smith MC (1972) Pain in cancer: comparison of results of cordotomy and chemical rhizotomy. In Fusek I, Kunc Z, eds., *Present Limits of Neurosurgery*. Amsterdam: Excerpta Medica, pp. 513–519.

Nathan PW, Smith MC (1979) Clinico-anatomical correlation in anterolateral cordotomy. In Bonica JJ, Liebeskind JC, Albe-Fessard DG, Jones LE, eds., *Advances in Pain Research and Therapy*. New York: Raven Press, pp. 921–926.

Nathan PW, Smith MC (1984) Dysesthèsie après cordotomie. *Med Hygiene* 42, 1788–1790.

Nathan PW, Smith MC, Cook AW (1986) Sensory effects in man of lesions of the posterior columns and of some other afferent pathways. *Brain* 109, 1003–1041.

Nathanson M (1962) Paroxysmal phenomena resembling seizures related to spinal cord and root pathology. *J Mt Sinai Hosp* 29, 147–151.

Naver H, Blomstrand C, Ekholm S *et al.* (1995) Autonomic and thermal sensory symptoms and dysfunction after stroke. *Stroke* 26, 1379–1385.

Nelson SB, Turrigiano GG (1998) Synaptic depression: a key player in the cortical balancing act. *Nature Neurosci* 1, 539–541.

Nepomuceno C, Fine PR, Richards JS *et al.* (1979) Pain in patients with spinal cord injury. *Arch Phys Med Rehab* 60, 605–609.

Ness TJ, San Pedro EC, Richards JS *et al.* (1998) Clinical note. A case of spinal cord injury-related pain with baseline rCBF brain SPECT imaging and beneficial response to gabapentin. *Pain* 78, 139–143.

Ness TJ, Putzke JD, Liu H-G, Mountz J (2002) Examples of the use of gabapentin in the treatment of spinal cord injury pain. *Progr Pain Res Manage* 23, 379–392.

Nguyen DK, Botez MI (1998) Diaschisis and neurobehavior. *Can J Neurol Sci* 25, 5–12.

Nguyen JP, Keravel Y, Feve A *et al.* (1997) Treatment of deafferentation pain by chronic stimulation of the motor cortex: report of a series of 20 cases. *Acta Neurochir (Wien) Suppl* 68, 54–60.

Nguyen JP, Lefacheur JP, Decq P *et al.* (1999) Chronic motor cortex stimulation in the treatment of central and neuropathic pain: correlations between clinical, electrophysiological and anatomical data. *Pain* 82, 245–251.

Nicholson K, Mailis A, Taylor A (2002) Psychometric correlates of placebo and nocebo responses. In *10th World Congress on Pain, Book of Abstracts*. Seattle, WA: IASP Press, Abst. 317-P596.

Niizuma H, Kwak R, Ikeda S *et al.* (1982) Follow-up results of centromedian thalamotomy for central pain. *Appl Neurophysiol* 45, 324–325.

Nitescu P, Dahm P, Appelgren L, Curelaru I (1998) Continuous infusion of opioid and bupivacaine by externalized intrathecal catheters in long-term treatment of "refractory" nonmalignant pain. *Clin J Pain* 14, 17–28.

Noordenbos W (1959) *Pain, Problems Pertaining to the Transmission of Nerve Impulses Which Give Rise to Pain*. Amsterdam: Elsevier, p. 135.

Noordenbos W, Wall PD (1976) Diverse sensory functions with an almost totally divided spinal cord. A case of spinal cord transection with preservation of part of one anterolateral quadrant. *Pain* 2, 185–195.

North RB, Kidd DH, Zahurak M, James CS, Long DM (1993) Spinal cord stimulation for chronic, intractable pain: experience over two decades. *Neurosurgery* 32, 384–395.

Notcutt W, Price M, Miller R *et al.* (2004) Initial experience with medicinal extracts of cannabis for chronic pain: results from 34 'N of 1' studies. *Anaesthesia* 59, 440.

Nowak LG, Bullier J (1998) Axons, but not cell bodies, are activated by electrical stimulation in cortical gray matter: I. Evidence from chronaxie measurements; II. Evidence from selective inactivation of cell bodies and axon initial segments. *Exp Brain Res* 118, 477–488; 489–500.

Nusser Z, Hajos N, Somogyi P, Mody I (1998) Increased number of synaptic GABA(A) receptors underlies potentiation at hippocampal inhibitory synapses. *Nature* **395**, 172–177.

Nuti C, Peyron R, Garcia-Larrea L *et al.* (2005) Motor cortex stimulation for refractory neuropathic pain: four year outcome and predictors of efficacy. *Pain* **118**, 43–52.

Nyquist JK, Greenhoot JH (1973) Responses evoked from the thalamic centrum medianum by painful input: suppression by dorsal funiculus conditioning. *Exp Neurol* **39**, 215–222.

Oaklander AL, Romans K, Horasek S *et al.* (1998) Unilateral postherpetic neuralgia is associated with bilateral sensory neuron damage. *Ann Neurol* **44**, 789–795.

Obersteiner H (1881) On allochiria. A peculiar sensory disorder. *Brain* **4**, 153–163.

Obeso JA, Rodriguez-Oroz MC, Rodriguez M *et al.* (2000) Pathophysiologic basis of surgery for Parkinson's disease. *Neurology* **55**(Suppl. 6), S7–S12.

Obrador S (1956) Quoted by Laine and Gros (1956).

Obrador S, Dierssen G, Ceballos R (1957) Consideraciones clinicas, neurologicas y anatomicas sobre el llamado dolor talamico. Con motivo de dos casos personales. *Acta Neurol Latinoamer* **3**, 58–77.

Obrador S, Carrascosa R, Sevillano M (1961) Observaciones sobre la estimulacion y lesion talàmica en mano fantasma dolorosa. *Rev esp Oto-Neuro-Oftal* **20**, 149–153.

Ochoa JL (1993) The human sensory unit and pain: new concepts, syndromes, and tests. *Muscle Nerve* **16**, 1009–1016.

Ochoa JL (1999) Truths, errors, and lies around "reflex sympathetic dystrophy" and "complex regional pain syndrome". *J Neurol* **246**, 875–879.

Ohta Y, Akino M, Iwasaki Y, Abe H (1992) Spinal epidural stimulation for central pain caused by a cord lesion. *No Shinkei Geka* **20**, 147–152.

Ohye C, Narabayashi H (1972) Activity of thalamic neurons and their receptive fields in different functional states in man. In Somjen GG, ed., *Neurophysiology Studies in Man*. Amsterdam: Excerpta Medica, pp. 79–84.

Ohye C (1990) Thalamus. In Paxinos G, ed., *The Human Nervous System*. San Diego, CA: Academic Press, pp. 439–468.

Ohye C (1998) Stereotactic treatment of central pain. *Stereotact Funct Neurosurg* **70**, 71–76.

Ojemann JG, Silbergeld DL (1995) Cortical stimulation mapping of phantom limb rolandic cortex. Case report. *J Neurosurg* **82**, 641–644.

Oke A, Keller R, Meffond I, Adams RN (1978) Lateralization of norepinephrine in the human thalamus. *Science* **200**, 1411–1412.

Olausson H, Marchand S, Bittar RG *et al.* (2001a) Central pain in a hemispherectomized patient. *Eur J Pain* **5**, 209–217.

Olausson H, Ha B, Duncan GH *et al.* (2001b) Cortical activation by tactile and painful stimuli in hemispherectomized patients. *Brain* **124**, 916–927.

Olivecrona U (1947) The surgery of pain. *Acta Psych Scand Suppl* **46**, 268–280.

Oliveira RA, Teixeira MJ (2002) Central poststroke pain: clinical–encephalic imaging correlations. In *10th World Congress on Pain, Book of Abstracts*. Seattle, WA: IASP Press, A96-P92.

Olsen RW, Avoli M (1997) GABA and epileptogenesis. *Epilepsia* **38**, 399–407.

Olsen RW, Betz H (2006) GABA and Glycine. In: Siegel GJ, ed., *Basic Neurochemistry*. Amsterdam: Elsevier Academic Press, 291–302.

Orthner H, Roeder F (1966) Further clinical and anatomical experiences with stereotactic operations for relief of pain. *Confin Neurol* **27**, 418–430.

Osterberg A, Boivie J, Holmgren H, Thuomas K, Johansson I (1994) The clinical characteristics and sensory abnormalities of patients with central pain caused by multiple sclerosis. In Gebhart GF, Hammond DL, Jensen TS, eds., *Proceedings of the 7th World Congress on Pain*. Seattle, WA: IASP Press, pp. 789–796.

Osterberg A, Boivie J, Thuomas KA (2005) Central pain in multiple sclerosis: prevalence and clinical characteristics. *Eur J Pain* **9**, 531–542.

Owen SLF, Green AL, Stein JF, Aziz TZ (2006) Deep brain stimulation for the alleviation of poststroke neuropathic pain. *Pain* **120**, 202–206.

Paciaroni M, Bogousslavsky J (1998) Pure sensory syndromes in thalamic stroke. *Eur Neurol* **39**, 211–217.

Pagni CA (1977) Central pain and painful anesthesia. Pathophysiology and treatment of sensory deprivation syndromes due to central and peripheral nervous system lesions. *Progr Neurol Surg* **8**, 132–257.

Pagni CA, Regolo P (1987) Epilessia sensitivo-motoria di origine spinale. Sintomo di esordio raro dei meningiomi spinali. *Minerva Chir* **42**, 2003–2009.

Pagni CA (1989) Central pain due to spinal cord and brain stem damage. In Wall PD, Melzack R, eds., *Textbook of Pain*, 2nd edn. Edinburgh: Churchill Livingstone, pp. 634–655.

Pagni CA, Canavero S (1993) Paroxysmal perineal pain resembling tic douloureux, only symptom of a dorsal meningioma. *Ital J Neurol Sci* **14**, 323–324.

Pagni CA, Lanotte M, Canavero S (1993) How frequent is anesthesia dolorosa following spinal posterior rhizotomy? A retrospective analysis of fifteen patients. *Pain* **54**, 323–327.

Pagni CA, Canavero S (1995a) Functional thalamic depression in a case of reversible central pain due to a spinal intramedullary cyst. Case report. *J Neurosurg* **83**, 163–165.

Pagni CA, Canavero S (1995b) Cordomyelotomy in the treatment of paraplegia pain. Experience in two cases with long-term results. *Acta Neurol Belg* **95**, 33–36.

Panerai AE, Monza G, Movilia P *et al.* (1990) A randomized, within-patient, cross-over, placebo-controlled trial on the efficacy and tolerability of the tricyclic antidepressants chlorimipramine and nortriptyline in central pain. *Acta Neurol Scand* **82**, 34–38.

Pareti G, De Palma A (2004) Does the brain oscillate? The dispute on neuronal synchronization. *Neurol Sci* **25**, 41–47.

Parker HL (1930) Pain of central origin. *Am J Med Sci* **179**, 241–258.

Parrent AG, Tasker RR (1992) Can the ipsilateral hemisphere mediate pain in man? *Acta Neurochir (Wien)* **117**, 89.

Parrent AG, Lozano AM, Dostrovsky JO, Tasker RR (1992) Central pain in the absence of functional sensory thalamus. *Stereotact Funct Neurosurg* **59**, 9–14.

Pattany PM, Widerstroem-Noga EG, Bowen BC *et al.* (2002) Proton magnetic resonance spectroscopy following spinal cord injury: evaluation of patients with chronic neuropathic pain. *Progr Brain Res Manage* **23**, 301–311.

Penfield W, Gage L (1933) Cerebral localization of epileptic manifestations. *Arch Neurol Psychiat* **30**, 709–727.

Penfield W, Welch K (1951) The supplementary motor area of the cerebral cortex: a clinical and experimental study. *Arch Neurol Psych* **66**, 298–317.

Penfield W, Jasper H (1954) *Epilepsy and the Functional Anatomy of the Human Brain*. Boston, MA: Little, Brown.

Penn RD, Paice JA (2000) Adverse effects associated with the intrathecal administration of ziconotide. *Pain* **85**, 291–296.

Percheron G (2004) Thalamus. In Paxinos G, Mai JK, eds., *The Human Nervous System*, 2nd edn. Amsterdam: Elsevier Academic Press, pp. 592–676.

Petit-Dutaillis D, Messimy R, Feld H (1950) Troubles sensitifs et sensorielles apres ablation prefrontal chez l'homme. *Rev Neurol* **83**, 23.

Petit-Dutaillis D, Messimy R, Berges L (1953) La psychochirurgie des algies irreductibles. Étude basée sur 57 cas. *Semaine des Hopitaux de Paris* **29**, 3893–3903.

Petrovic P, Ingvar M (2002) Imaging cognitive modulation of pain processing. *Pain* **95**, 1–5.

Peyron R, Garcia-Larrea L, Deiber MP *et al.* (1995) Electrical stimulation of precentral cortical area in the treatment of central pain: electrophysiological and PET study. *Pain* **62**, 275–286.

Peyron R, Garcia-Larrea L, Gregoire MC *et al.* (1998) Allodynia after lateral-medullary (Wallenberg) infarct. A PET study. *Brain* **121**, 345–356.

Peyron R, Garcia-Larrea L, Costes N *et al.* (1999) The haemodynamic pattern of central pain patients with allodynia. In *9th World Congress on Pain, Book of Abstracts*. Seattle, WA: IASP Press, A78.

Peyron R, Garcia-Larrea L, Gregoire MC *et al.* (2000) Parietal and cingulate processes in central pain. A combined positron emission tomography (PET) and functional magnetic resonance imaging (fMRI) study of an unusual case. *Pain* **84**, 77–87.

Peyron R, Schneider F, Faillenot I *et al.* (2004) An fMRI study of cortical representation of mechanical allodynia in patients with neuropathic pain. *Neurology* **63**, 1838–1846.

Pfeiffer A, Pasi A, Mehraein P, Herz A (1982) Opiate binding sites in human brain. *Brain Res* **248**, 87–96.

Phillips NI, Bhakta BB (2000) Effect of deep brain stimulation on limb paresis after stroke. *Lancet* **356**, 222–223.

Pillay PK, Hassenbusch SJ (1992) Bilateral MRI-guided stereotactic cingulotomy for intractable pain. *Stereotact Funct Neurosurg* **59**, 33–38.

Pioli EY, Gross CE, Meissner W, Bioulac BH, Bezard E (2003) The deafferented nonhuman primate is not a reliable model of intractable pain. *Neurol Res* **25**, 127–129.

Pirotte B, Voordecker P, Neugroschl C *et al.* (2005) Combination of functional magnetic resonance imaging-guided neuronavigation and intraoperative cortical brain mapping improves targeting of motor cortex stimulation in neuropathic pain. *Neurosurgery* **56**(ONS Suppl. 2), 344–359.

Ploner M, Gross J, Timmermann L, Schnitzler A (2002) Cortical representation of first and second pain sensation in humans. *Proc Natl Acad Sci USA* **99**, 12444–12448.

Plotkin R (1982) Results in 60 cases of deep brain stimulation for chronic intractable pain. *Appl Neurophysiol* **45**, 173–178.

Pollo A, Amanzio M, Arslanian A *et al.* (2001) Response expectancies in placebo analgesia and their clinical relevance. *Pain* **93**, 77–84.

Pollock LJ, Boshes B, Finkelmann I *et al.* (1951a) Management of residual injuries to spinal cord and cauda equina. *JAMA* **146**, 1551–1563.

Pollock LJ, Brown M, Boshes B *et al.* (1951b) Pain below the level of injury of the spinal cord. *Arch Neurol Psychiatr* **65**, 319–322.

Pool JL (1946) Posterior cordotomy for relief of phantom limb pain. *Ann Surg* **124**, 386–391.

Porreca F, Ossipov MH, Gebhart GF (2002) Review. Chronic pain and medullary descending facilitation. *TINS* **25**, 319–325.

Portenoy RK, Foley KM (1986) Chronic use of opioid analgesics in non-malignant pain. Report of 38 cases. *Pain* **25**, 171–186.

Portenoy RK, Yang K, Thornton D (1988) Chronic intractable pain: an atypical presentation of multiple sclerosis. *J Neurol* **235**, 226–228.

Portenoy RK, Foley KM, Inturrisi CE (1990) The nature of opioid responsiveness and its implications for neuropathic pain: new hypotheses derived from studies of opioid infusions. *Pain* **43**, 273–286.

Porter RW, Hohmann GW, Bors E, French JD (1966) Cordotomy for pain following cauda equina injury. *Arch Surg* **92**, 765–770.

Potagas C, Avdelidis D, Singounas E, Missir O, Aessopos A (1997) Episodic pain associated with a tumor in the parietal operculum: a case report and literature review. *Pain* **72**, 201–208.

Potter PJ, Hayes KC, Hsieh JT, Delaney GA, Segal JL (1998) Sustained improvements in neurological function in spinal cord injured patients treated with oral 4-aminopyridine: three cases. *Spinal Cord* **36**, 147–155.

Pound P, Ebrahim S, Sandercock P, Bracken MB, Roberts I on behalf of the Reviewing Animal Trials Systematically (RATS) Group (2004) Where is the evidence that animal research benefits humans? *Br Med J* **328**, 514–517.

Powers SK, Barbaro NM, Levy RM (1988) Pain control with laser-produced dorsal root entry zone lesions. *Appl Neurophysiol* **51**, 243–254 (see also *J Neurosurg* 1984, **61**, 841–847).

Preissl H, Flor H, Lutzenberger W *et al.* (2001) Early activation of the primary somatosensory cortex without conscious awareness of somatosensory stimuli in tumor patients. *Neurosci Lett* **308**, 193–196.

Prestor B (2001) Microsurgical junctional DREZ coagulation for treatment of deafferentation pain syndromes. *Surg Neurol* **56**, 259–265.

Procacci P, Maresca M (1991) Central pruritus. Case report. *Pain* **47**, 369–370.

Putzke JD, Richards JS, Kezar L, Hicken BL, Ness TJ (2002) Long-term use of gabapentin for treatment of pain after traumatic spinal cord injury. *Clin J Pain* **18**, 116–121.

Quarti M, Terzian H (1954) L'emisferectomia nel trattamento delle emiplegie infantili. *Chirurgia* **9**, 339–350.

Quigley DG, Arnold J, Eldridge PR *et al.* (2003) Long-term outcome of spinal cord stimulation and hardware complications. *Stereotact Funct Neurosurg* **81**, 50–56.

Rabben T, Skjelbred P, Oye I (1999) Prolonged analgesic effect of ketamine, an *N*-methyl-D-aspartate receptor inhibitor, in patients with chronic pain. *J Pharmacol Exp Ther* **289**, 1060–1066.

Radhakrishnan V, Tsoukatos J, Davis KD *et al.* (1999) A comparison of the burst activity of lateral thalamic neurons in chronic pain and non-pain patients. *Pain* **80**, 567–575.

Raichle ME, McLeod AM, Snyder AZ *et al.* (2001) A default mode of brain function. *Proc Natl Acad Sci USA* **98**, 676–682.

Raij TT, Numminen J, Narvanen S, Hiltunen J, Hari R (2005) Brain correlates of subjective reality of physically and psychologically induced pain. *Proc Natl Acad Sci USA* **102**, 2147–2151.

Ranck JB (1975) Which elements are excited in electrical stimulation of mammalian central nervous system: a review. *Brain Res* **98**, 417–440.

Rasche D, Ruppolt M, Stippich C, Unterberg A, Tronnier VM (2006) Motor cortex stimulation for long-term relief of chronic neuropathic pain: a 10 year experience. *Pain* **121**, 43–52.

Rasmisky M (1980) Physiology of conduction in demyelinated axons. In Waxman, SG ed., *Physiology and Pathobiology of Axons*. New York: Raven Press, pp. 361–376.

Rasmussen PV, Sindrup SH, Jensen TS, Bach FW (2004) Therapeutic outcome in neuropathic pain: relationship to evidence of nervous system lesion. *Eur J Neurol* **11**, 545–553.

Rath SA, Braun V, Soliman N, Antoniadis G, Richter MP (1996) Results of DREZ coagulations for pain related to plexus lesions, spinal cord injuries and postherpetic neuralgia. *Acta Neurochir (Wien)* **138**, 364–369.

Ray CD, Burton CV (1980) Deep brain stimulation for severe chronic pain. *Acta Neurochir (Wien) Suppl* **30**, 289–293.

Reboiledo PE, Gonzalez X, Valenzuela P, Larraguibel F, Mujica A (2002) Study of gabapentin and clomipramine use for chronic pain management in spinal cord injury. In *10th World Congress on Pain, Book of Abstracts*. Seattle, WA: IASP Press, A925-P195.

Regev I, Avrahami A, Bornstein N, Koreczyn AD (1983) Pain and hyperpathia in pontine haemorrhage. *J Neurol* 230, 205–208.

Reig E (1993) *Spinal infusion of morphine for the treatment of neuropathic pain*. Medtronic Conference on Advances in Chronic Pain Treatment, Padova, November 27, 1993.

Remy P, Zilbovicius M, Cesaro P *et al.* (1999) Primary somatosensory cortex activation is not altered in patients with ventroposterior thalamic lesions: a PET study. *Stroke* 30, 2651–2658.

Retif J (1963) Douleur centrale et lesion suprathalamique. Méningiome temporo-pariétal se manifestant par un syndrome algique paroxystique à caractère pseudo-radiculaire du membre inférieur controlateral. *Acta Neurol Psychiat Belg* 63, 955–969.

Rétif J, Brihaye J, Vanderhaegen JJ (1967) Syndrome douloureux "thalamique" et lesion parietale. À propos de trois observations de tumeur à localisation pariétale, s'étant accompagnées de douleurs spontanées de l'hemicorps contralatéral. *Neurochirurgie* 13, 375–384.

Reynolds DV (1969) Surgery in the rat during electrical analgesia induced by focal brain stimulation. *Science* 164, 444–445.

Rezai AR, Lozano AM, Crawley AP *et al.* (1999) Thalamic stimulation and functional magnetic resonance imaging: localization of cortical and subcortical activation with implanted electrodes. Technical note. *J Neurosurg* 90, 583–590.

Richardson DE (1974) Thalamotomy for control of chronic pain. *Acta Neurochir (Wien) Suppl* 21, 77–88.

Richardson DE, Akil H (1977a) Pain reduction by electrical brain stimulation in man: 1. Acute administration in periaqueductal and periventricular sites; 2. Chronic self-administration in the periventricular gray matter. *J Neurosurg* 47, 178–183; 184–194.

Richardson DE, Akil H (1977b) Long-term results of periventricular gray self-stimulation. *Neurosurgery* 1, 199–202.

Richardson RR, Meyer PR, Cerullo LJ (1980) Neurostimulation in the modulation of intractable paraplegic and traumatic neuroma pains. *Pain* 8, 76–84.

Richter HP, Seitz K (1984) Dorsal root entry zone lesions for the control of deafferentation pain: experiences in ten patients. *Neurosurgery* 15, 956–959.

Riddoch G, Critchley McD (1937) La physiopathologie de la douleur d'origine centrale. *Rev Neurol* 68, 77–104.

Riddoch G (1938) The clinical features of central pain. Lumleian lecture. *Lancet* 234, 1093–1098; 1150–1156; 1205–1209.

Ridgeway B, Wallace M, Gerayli A (2000) Ziconotide for the treatment of severe spasticity after spinal cord injury. *Pain* 85, 287–289.

Riechert T (1961) Methodes stéréotaxiques dans la chirurgie de la douleur. *Exc Medica Int Congr Ser* 36, 34–35f.

Rinaldi PC, Young RF, Albe-Fessard D, Chodakiewitz J (1991) Spontaneous neuronal hyperactivity in the medial and intralaminar thalamic nuclei of patients with deafferentation pain. *J Neurosurg* 74, 415–421.

Rodriguez RF, Contreras N (2002) Bilateral motor cortex stimulation for the relief of central dysesthetic pain and intentional tremor secondary to spinal cord surgery: a case report. *Neuromodulation* 5, 189–195.

Roeder F, Orthner H (1961) Erfahrungen mit sterotaktischen Eingriffen. III Mitteilung. Über zerebrale Schmerzoperationen, insbesondere mediale Mesencephalotomie bei thalamischer Hyperpathie und bei Anaesthesia Dolorosa. *Confin Neurol* 21, 51–97.

Rog DJ, Nurmikko TJ, Friede T, Young CA (2005) Randomized, controlled trial of cannabis based medicine in central pain in multiple sclerosis. *Neurology* 65, 812–819.

Rogano L, Teixeira MJ, Lepski G (2003) Chronic pain after spinal cord injury: clinical characteristics. *Stereotact Funct Neurosurg* 81, 65–69.

Rogers R, Painter D, Wise RG, Longe SE, Tracey I (2002) Investigating ketamine analgesia in humans using functional magnetic resonance imaging. In *10th World Congress on Pain, Book of Abstracts*. Seattle, WA: IASP Press, A1123-P39.

Romanelli P, Heit G (2004) Patient-controlled deep brain stimulation can overcome analgesic tolerance. *Stereotact Funct Neurosurg* 82, 77–79.

Rosen JA, Barsoum AH (1979) Failure of chronic dorsal column stimulation in multiple sclerosis. *Ann Neurol* 6, 66–67.

Rosenberg JM, Harrell C, Ristic H, Werner RA, de Rosayro AM (1997) The effect of gabapentin on neuropathic pain. *Clin J Pain* 13, 251–255.

Rosner H, Rubin L, Kestenbaum A (1996) Gaba-pentin adjunctive therapy in neuropathic pain states. *Clin J Pain* 12, 56–58.

Rosomoff HL (1969) Bilateral percutaneous cervical radiofrequency cordotomy. *J Neurosurg* 31, 41–46.

Rossetti AO, Ghika JA, Vingerhoets F, Novy J, Bogousslavsky J (2003) Neurogenic pain and abnormal movements contralateral to an anterior parietal artery stroke. *Arch Neurol* 60, 1004–1006.

Rosso T, Aglioti SM, Zanette G et al. (2003) Functional plasticity in the human primary somatosensory cortex following acute lesion of the anterior lateral spinal cord: neurophysiological evidence of short-term cross-modal plasticity. *Pain* 101, 117–127.

Rousseaux M, Cassim F, Bayle B, Laureau E (1999) Analysis of the perception of and reactivity to pain and heat in patients with Wallenberg syndrome and severe spinothalamic tract dysfunction. *Stroke* 30, 2223–2229.

Roussy G (1906) Les couches optiques: étude anatomique, physiologique et clinique. Thése de Paris.

Roxin A, Riecke H, Solla SA (2004) Self-sustained activity in a small-world network of excitable neurons. *Phys Rev Lett* 92, 198101.

Rowbotham GF (1961) A case of intractable pain in the head and face associated with pathological changes in the optic thalamus. *Acta Neurochir* 9, 1–18.

Rowbotham MC, Twilling L, Davies PS et al. (2003) Oral opioid therapy for chronic peripheral and central neuropathic pain. *New Engl J Med* 348, 1223–1232.

Rudolph U, Antkowiak B (2004) Molecular and neuronal substrates for general anaesthetics. *Nature Rev Neurosci* 5, 709–720.

Sackeim HA, Prudic J, Devanand DP et al. (1993) Effects of stimulus intensity and electrode placement on the efficacy and cognitive effects of electroconvulsive therapy. *New Engl J Med* 328, 839–846.

Sadzot B, Mayberg HS, Frost JJ (1990) Detection and quantification of opiate receptors in man by positron emission tomography: potential applications to the study of pain. *Neurophysiol Clin* 20, 323–334.

Sage JI (2004) Pain in Parkinson's disease. *Curr Treat Options Neurol* 6, 191–200.

Saitoh Y, Kato A, Ninomiya H et al. (2000) Primary motor cortex stimulation within the central sulcus for treating deafferentation pain. *Acta Neurochir Suppl* 87, 149–152.

Saitoh Y, Osaki Y, Nishimura H et al. (2004) Increased regional cerebral blood flow in the contralateral thalamus after successful motor cortex stimulation in a patient with poststroke pain. *J Neurosurg* 100, 935–939.

Sakai T, Tomiyasu S, Ono T, Yamada H, Sumikawa K (2004) Multiple sclerosis with severe pain and allodynia alleviated by oral ketamine. *Clin J Pain* 20, 375–376.

Sakurai M, Kanazawa I (1999) Positive symptoms in multiple sclerosis: their treatment with sodium channel blockers, lidocaine and mexiletine. *J Neurol Sci* 162, 162–168.

Salin PA, Prince DA (1996) I. Spontaneous GABA-a receptor-mediated inhibitory currents in adult rat somatosensory cortex; II. Electrophysiological mapping of GABA-A receptor-mediated inhibition in adult rat somatosensory cortex. *J Neurophysiol* 75, 1573–1588; 1589–1600.

Salmon JB, Hanna MH, Williams M, Toone B, Wheeler M (1988) Thalamic pain: the effect of electroconvulsive therapy. *Pain* 33, 67–71.

Samii M, Moringlane JR (1984) Thermocoagulation of the dorsal root entry zone for the treatment of intractable pain. *Neurosurgery* 15, 953–955.

Sampson JH, Nashold BS Jr. (1992) Facial pain due to vascular lesions of the brain stem relieved by dorsal root entry zone lesions in the nucleus caudalis. Report of two cases. *J Neurosurg* 77, 473–475.

Samuelsson M, Samuelsson L, Lindell D (1994) Sensory symptoms and signs and results of quantitative sensory thermal testing in patients with lacunar infarct syndromes. *Stroke* 25, 2165–2170.

Sanchez-Vives MV, McCormick DA (2000) Cellular and network mechanisms of rhythmic recurrent activity in neocortex. *Nature Neurosci* 3, 1027–1034.

Sandkuehler J (1996) The organization and function of endogenous antinociceptive systems. *Progr Neurobiol* 50, 49–81.

Sandroni P (2002) Central neuropathic itch: a new treatment option? *Neurology* 59, 778–779.

Sandyk R (1985) Spontaneous pain, hyperpathia and wasting of the hand due to parietal lobe haemorrhage. *Eur Neurol* 24, 1–3.

Sanford PR, Lindblom LB, Haddox JD (1992) Amitriptyline and carbamazepine in the treatment of dysesthesia pain in spinal cord injury. *Arch Phys Medic Rehab* 73, 300–301.

Sang CN, Miller VA, Dobosch L, Gracely RH, Hayden D (1999) Temporal summation and reduction of pain thresholds in normal skin in patients with dysesthetic central pain following spinal cord injury. In *9th World Congress on Pain, Book of Abstracts.* Seattle, WA: IASP Press, A114.

Sang CN (2002) Glutamate receptor antagonists in central neuropathic pain following spinal cord injury. *Progr Pain Res Manage* **23**, 365–377.

Sano K, Yoshioka M, Ogashiwa M, Ishijima B, Ohye C (1966) Thalamolaminotomy. A new operation for relief of intractable pain. *Conf Neurol* **27**, 63–66.

Sano K (1977) Intralaminar thalamotomy (thalamolaminotomy), and posteromedial hypothalamotomy in the treatment of intractable pain. In Krayenbühl H, Maspes PE, Sweet WH, eds., *Progress in Neurological Surgery. Pain – Its Neurosurgical Management: II. Central Procedures.* Basel: Karger, pp. 50–103.

Sasaki K (1938) Ueber die Wirkung der Chordotomie auf Spontangangraen. *Arch Klin Chir* **192**, 448–461.

Savas A, Kanpolat Y (2005) Comment to Brown JA and Pilitsis JG. *Neurosurgery* **56**, 296.

Scarff JE (1950) Unilateral prefrontal lobotomy for the relief of intractable pain. Report of 58 cases with special consideration of failures. *J Neurosurg* **7**, 330–336.

Schludermann E, Zubek JP (1962) Effect of age on pain sensitivity. *Percept Skills* **14**, 295–301.

Schmahmann JD, Leifer D (1992) Parietal pseudothalamic pain syndrome. Clinical features and anatomic correlates. *Arch Neurol* **49**, 1032–1037.

Schmahmann JD (2003) Vascular syndromes of the thalamus. *Stroke* **34**, 2264–2278.

Schnitzler A, Ploner M (2000) Neurophysiology and functional neuroanatomy of pain perception. *J Clin Neurophysiol* **17**, 592–603.

Schoenen J, Grant G (2004) Spinal cord: connections. In Paxinos G, Mai JK, eds., *The Human Nervous System*, 2nd edn. Amsterdam: Elsevier Academic Press, pp. 233–250.

Scholz J, Vieregge P, Moser A (1999) Central pain as a manifestation of partial epileptic seizures. *Pain* **80**, 445–450.

Schott B, Laurent B, Mauguire F (1986) Les douleurs thalamiques. Ètude critique de 43 cas. *Rev Neurol* **142**, 308–315.

Schott GD, Loh L (1984) Anticholinesterase drugs in the treatment of chronic pain. *Pain* **20**, 201–206.

Schott GD (1996) From thalamic syndrome to central poststroke pain. *J Neurol Neurosurg Psych* **61**, 560–564.

Schott GD (2001a) Delayed onset and resolution of pain. Some observations and implications. *Brain* **124**, 1067–1076.

Schott GD (2001b) Nosological entities? Reflex sympathetic dystrophy. *J Neurol Neurosurg Psych* **71**, 291–295.

Schvarcz JR (1977) Periaqueductal mesencephalotomy for facial central pain. In Sweet WH, Obrador S, Martin-Rodriguez JG, eds., *Neurosurgical Treatment in Psychiatry, Pain and Epilepsy.* Baltimore, MD: University Park Press, pp. 661–667.

Schvarcz JR (1978) Spinal cord stereotactic techniques for trigeminal nucleotomy and extralemniscal myelotomy. *Appl Neurophysiol* **41**, 99–112.

Schvarcz JR (1980) Chronic self-stimulation of the medial posterior inferior thalamus for the alleviation of deafferentation pain. *Acta Neurochir Suppl* **20**, 295–301.

Schwartz HG (1950) Neurosurgical relief of intractable pain. *Surg Clin N Amer* **30**, 1379–1389.

Schwartz HG (1960) High cervical tractotomy: technique and results. *Clin Neurosurg* **8**, 282–293.

Schwoebel J, Coslett HB, Bradt J, Friedman R, Dileo C (2002) Pain and the body schema: effects of pain severity on mental representations of movement. *Neurology* **59**, 775–777.

Sedan R, Lazorthes Y (1978) La neurostimulation èlectrique thèrapeutique. Soc. Neurochir. Langue Franc. XXVIII Congres Annuel, Neurochirurgie, pp. 1–138.

Seghier ML, Lazeyras F, Vuilleumier P, Schnider A, Carota A (2005) Functional magnetic resonance imaging and diffusion tensor imaging in a case of central poststroke pain. *J Pain* **6**, 208–212.

Selverstone AI, Moulins M (1985) Oscillatory neural networks. *Annu Rev Physiol* **47**, 29–48.

Semyanov A, Walker MC, Kullmann DM, Silver RA (2004) Tonically active GABA A receptors: modulating gain and maintaining the tone. *TINS* **27**, 262–269.

Serpell MG, for the Neuropathic Pain Study Group (2002) Gabapentin in neuropathic pain syndromes: a randomised, double-blind, placebo-controlled trial. *Pain* **99**, 557–566.

Shapiro PE, Braun CW (1987) Unilateral pruritus after a stroke. *Arch Dermatol* **123**, 1527–1530.

Shepherd GM (2004) *The Synaptic Organization of the Brain.* Oxford: Oxford University Press.

Shergill SS, Bays PM, Frith CD, Wolpert DM (2003) Two eyes for an eye: the neuroscience of force escalation. *Science* **301**, 187.

Sherman SM, Guillery RW (2004) Thalamus. In Shepherd GM, ed., *The Synaptic Organization of the Brain.* Oxford: Oxford University Press, pp. 311–360.

Shibasaki H, Kuroiwa Y (1974) Painful tonic seizures in multiple sclerosis. *Arch Neurol* **30**, 47−51.

Shieff C, Nashold BS (1988) Thalamic pain and stereotactic mesencephalotomy. *Acta Neurochir (Wien) Suppl* **42**, 239−242 (same series appearing in *Br J Neurosurg* 1987, **1**, 305−310 and *Neurol Res* 1987, **9**, 101−104).

Shieff C (1991) Treatment of central deafferentation syndromes: thalamic syndrome. In Nashold BS Jr., Ovelmen-Levitt J, eds., *Deafferentation Pain Syndromes. Pathophysiology and Treatment*, New York: Raven Press, pp. 285−290.

Shimodozono M, Kawahira K, Kamishita T *et al.* (2002) Reduction of central poststroke pain with the selective serotonin reuptake inhibitor fluvoxamine. *Int J Neurosci* **112**, 1173−1181.

Shulman R, Turnbull IM, Diewold P (1982) Psychiatric aspects of thalamic stimulation for neuropathic pain. *Pain* **13**, 127−135.

Shulman RG, Rothman DL, Behar KL, Hyder F (2004) Energetic basis of brain activity: implications for neuroimaging. *TINS* **27**, 489−495.

Sicuteri F (1971) Reversible central pain syndrome in man following treatment with P-chlorophenylalanine and reserpine. *Pharmacol Res Commun* **3**, 401.

Siddall PJ, Gray M, Rutkowski S, Cousins MJ (1994) Intrathecal morphine and clonidine in the management of spinal cord injury pain: a case report. *Pain* **59**, 147−148.

Siddall PJ, Taylor DA, McClelland JM, Rutkowski SB, Cousins MJ (1999) Pain report and the relationship of pain to physical factors in the first 6 months following spinal cord injury. *Pain* **81**, 187−197.

Siddall PJ, Molloy AR, Walker S *et al.* (2000) The efficacy of intrathecal morphine and clonidine in the treatment of pain after spinal cord injury. *Anesth Analg* **9**, 1493−1498.

Siddall PJ (2002) Spinal drug administration in the treatment of spinal cord injury pain. *Progr Pain Res Manage* **23**, 353−364.

Siegfried J, Krayenbuhl H (1972) Clinical experience in the treatment of intractable pain. In Janzen R, Keidel WD, Herz A, Steichele C, eds., *Pain: Basic Principles − Pharamacology − Therapy*. Stuttgart: Georg Thieme, pp. 202−204.

Siegfried J (1977) Stereotactic pulvinarotomy in the treatment of intractable pain. *Progr Neurol Surg* **8**, 101−113.

Siegfried J (1991) Therapeutical neurostimulation: indications reconsidered. *Acta Neurochir (Wien) Suppl* **52**, 112−117.

Sillito AM, Jones HE, Gerstein GL, West DC (1994) Feature-linked synchronization of thalamic relay cell firing induced by feedback from the visual cortex. *Nature* **369**, 479−482.

Silver ML (1957) "Central pain" from cerebral arteriovenous aneurysm. *J Neurosurg* **14**, 92−96.

Silverman IE (1998) Central poststroke pain associated with lateral medullary infarction. *Neurology* **50**, 836−837.

Simpson BA (1991) Spinal cord stimulation in 60 cases of intractable pain. *J Neurol Neurosurg Psych* **54**, 196−199.

Simpson BA (1999) Spinal cord stimulation. *Pain Rev* **1**, 199−230.

Sindou M, Keravel Y (1980) Analgesie par la méthode d'electrostimulation transcutanée. Résultats dans les douleurs d'origine neurologique. A propos de 180 cas. *Neurochirurgie* **26**, 153−157.

Sindou MP, Mertens P, Garcia-Larrea L (2001) Surgical procedures for neuropathic pain. *Neurosurg Quart* **11**, 45−65.

Sindou M, Mertens P, Bendavid U, Garcia-Larrea L, Mauguiere F (2003) Predictive value of somatosensory evoked potentials for long-lasting pain relief after spinal cord stimulation: practical use for patient selection. *Neurosurgery* **52**, 1374−1384.

Sindrup SH, Jensen TS (1999) Efficacy of pharmacological treatments of neuropathic pain: an update and effect related to mechanism of drug action. *Pain* **83**, 389−400.

Sist TC, Filadora VA II, Miner M, Lema M (1997) Experience with gabapentin for neuropathic pain in the head and neck: report of ten cases. *Reg Anesth* **22**, 473−478.

Sjölund BH (1991) Role of transcutaneous electrical nerve stimulation, central nervous system stimulation, and ablative procedures in central pain syndromes. In Casey KL, ed., *Pain and Central Nervous System Disease. The Central Pain Syndromes*. New York: Raven Press, pp. 267−275.

Sjölund BH (1993) Transcutaneous electrical stimulation in neuropathic pain. *Pain Digest* **3**, 23−26.

Sjöqvist O (1950) La section chirurgicale des cordons et des voies de la douleur dans la moêlle et le tronc cérébral. *Rev Neurol* **83**, 38−40.

Slaughter RF (1938) Relief of causalgic-like pain in the isolated extremity by sympathectomy. *JMA Georgia* **27**, 253−256.

Slawek J, Reclowicz D, Zielinski P, Sloniewski P, Nguyen JP (2005) [Motor cortex stimulation in the central pain syndrome]. *Neurol Neurochir Pol* **39**, 237−240.

Sleghart W, Sperk G (2002) Subunit composition, distribution and function of GABA A receptor subunits. *Curr Top Med Chem* **2**, 795−816.

Slonimski M, Abram SE, Zuniga RE (2004) Intrathecal baclofen in pain management. *Reg Anesth Pain Med* **29**, 269−276.

Smith AJ, Blumenfeld H, Behar KL *et al.* (2002) Cerebral energetics and spiking frequency: the neurophysiological basis of fMRI. *Proc Natl Acad Sci USA* **99**, 10765−10770.

Smith KJ, McDonald WI (1982) Spontaneous and evoked electrical discharges from a central demyelinating lesion. *J Neurol Sci* **55**, 39−47.

Smolik FA, Nash FP, Machek O (1960) Spinal cordectomy in the management of spastic paraplegia. *Am Surg* **26**, 639−645.

Solaro C, Brichetto G, Amato MP *et al.*, and the PaIMS Study group (2004) The prevalence of pain in multiple sclerosis. A multicenter cross-sectional study. *Neurology* **63**, 919−921.

Soria ED, Fine EJ (1991) Disappearance of thalamic pain after parietal subcortical stroke. *Pain* **44**, 285−288.

Soros P, Imai T, Bantel C *et al.* (1999) Plasticity of the somatosensory cortex during cluster headache attacks. In *9th World Congress on Pain, Book of Abstracts.* Seattle, WA: IASP Press, Abst. 91-P403.

Sourek K (1969) Commissural myelotomy. *J Neurosurg* **31**, 524−527.

Spaic M, Markovic N, Tadic R (2002) Microsurgical DREZotomy for pain of spinal cord and cauda equina injury origin: clinical characteristics of pain and implications for surgery in a series of 26 patients. *Acta Neurochir (Wien)* **144**, 453−462.

Spiegel EA, Wycis HT, Freed H (1952) Stereoencephalotomy. Thalamotomy and related procedures. *JAMA* **148**, 446−451.

Spiegel EA, Kletzkin M, Szekely EG, Wycis HT (1954) Role of hypothalamic mechanisms in thalamic pain. *Neurology* **4**, 735−751.

Spiegel EA, Wycis HT (1962) *Stereoencephalotomy: II. Clinical and Physiological Applications.* New York: Grune & Stratton.

Spiegel EA, Wycis HT, Szekely EG, Gildenberg PL (1966) Medial and basal thalamotomy in so-called intractable pain. In Knighton RS, Dumke PR, eds., *Pain.* Boston, MA: Little Brown, pp. 503−517.

Spiegelmann R, Friedman WA (1991) Spinal cord stimulation: a contemporary series. *Neurosurgery* **28**, 65−71.

Stein BE, Price DD, Gazzaniga MS (1989) Pain perception in a man with total corpus callosum transection. *Pain* **38**, 51−56.

Steinke W, Sacco RL, Mohr JP *et al.* (1992) Thalamic stroke. Presentation and prognosis of infarcts and hemorrhages. *Arch Neurol* **49**, 703−710.

Stenager E, Knudsen L, Jensen K (1991) Acute and chronic pain syndromes in multiple sclerosis. *Acta Neurol Scand* **84**, 197−200.

Steriade M, Jones EG, McCormick DA (1997) *Thalamus.* Amsterdam: Elsevier.

Steriade M (1999) Coherent oscillations and short-term plasticity in corticothalamic networks. *TINS* **22**, 337−345.

Stewart I (1997) *Does God Play Dice? The New Mathematics of Chaos.* London: Penguin Books.

Stewart WA, Stoops WL, Pillone PR, King RB (1964) An electrophysiologic study of ascending pathways from nucleus caudalis of the spinal trigeminal nuclear complex. *J Neurosurg* **21**, 35−48.

Stoermer S, Gerner HJ, Grueninger W *et al.* (1997) Chronic pain/dysaesthesiae in spinal cord injury patients: results of a multicentre study. *Spinal Cord* **35**, 446−455.

Stone TT (1950) Phantom limb pain and central pain. Relief by ablation of portion of posterior central cerebral convolution. *Arch Neurol Psych* **63**, 739−748.

Stoodley MA, Warren JD, Oatey PE (1995) Thalamic syndrome caused by unruptured cerebral aneurysm. Case report. *J Neurosurg* **82**, 291−293.

Strogatz S (2003) Sync: *The Emerging Science of Spontaneous Order.* New York: Hyperion.

Sugita K, Mutsuga N, Rakaoka T, Doi T (1972) Results of stereotaxic thalamotomy for pain. *Conf Neurol* **34**, 265−274.

Sullivan MJ, Drake ME Jr. (1984) Unilateral pruritus and nocardia brain abscess. *Neurology* **34**, 828−829.

Supèr H, Spekreijse H, Lamme VAF (2001) Two distinct modes of sensory processing observed in monkey primary visual cortex (V1). *Nature Neurosci* **4**, 304−310.

Suzuki M, Davis C, Symon L, Gentili F (1985) Syringoperitoneal shunt for treatment of cord cavitation. *J Neurol Neurosurg Psych* **48**, 620−627.

Svendsen KB, Jensen TS, Bach FW (2004) Does the cannabinoid dronabinol reduce central pain in multiple sclerosis? Randomised double blind placebo controlled crossover trial. *Br Med J* **329**, 253.

Svendsen KB, Jensen TS, Hansen HJ, Bach FW (2005) Sensory function and quality of life in patients with multiple sclerosis and pain. *Pain* **114**, 473−481.

Svensson P, Minoshima S, Beydoun A, Morrow TJ, Casey KL (1997) Cerebral processing of acute skin and muscle pain in humans. *J Neurophysiol* **78**, 450−460.

Sweet WH, Wepsic JG (1974) Stimulation of pain suppressor mechanisms. A critique of some current methods. *Adv Neurol* **4**, 734–746.

Sweet WH, Wepsic J (1975) Stimulation of the posterior columns of the spinal cord for pain control. *Surg Neurol* **4**, 133.

Sweet WH, Poletti CE (1989) Operations in the brain stem and cord, with an appendix on open cordotomy. In Wall PD, Melzack R, eds., *Textbook of Pain*, 2nd edn. Edinburgh: Churchill Livingstone, pp. 811–831.

Sweet WH (1991) Deafferentation syndromes in humans: a general discussion. In Nashold BS Jr., Ovelmen-Levitt J, eds., *Deafferentation Pain Syndromes. Pathophysiology and Treatment*, New York: Raven Press, pp. 259–274.

Szentirmai O, Carter BS (2004) Genetic and cellular therapies for cerebral infarction. *Neurosurgery* **55**, 283–297.

Tai Q, Kirschblum S, Chen B *et al.* (2002) Gabapentin in the treatment of neuropathic pain after spinal cord injury: a prospective, randomized, double-blind, crossover trial. *J Spinal Cord Med* **25**, 100–105.

Taira T, Tanikawa T, Kawamura H, Iseki H, Takakura K (1994) Spinal intrathecal baclofen suppresses central pain after a stroke. *J Neurol Neurosurg Psych* **57**, 381–382.

Taira T, Kawamura H, Tanikawa T *et al.* (1995) A new approach to control central deafferentation pain: spinal intrathecal baclofen. *Stereotact Funct Neurosurg* **65**, 101–105.

Taira T (1998) Comments on Eisenberg and Pud, *Pain* 74, 337–339. *Pain* **78**, 221–226.

Takahashi Y, Hashimoto K, Tsuji S (2004) Successful use of zonisamide for central poststroke pain. *J Pain* **5**, 192–194.

Takano M, Takano Y, Sato I (1999) The effect of oral amantadine in chronic pain patients with positive ketamine challenge test. In *9th World Congress on Pain, Book of Abstracts*. Seattle, WA: IASP Press, Abst. 220-P68.

Talbot JD, Villemure JG, Bushnell MC, Duncan GH (1995) Evaluation of pain perception after anterior capsulotomy: a case report. *Somatosens Mot Res* **12**, 115–126.

Talairach J, Hecaen H, David M, Monnier M, De Ajuraguerra J (1949) Recherches sur la coagulation thèrapeutique des structures sous-corticales chez l'homme. *Rev Neurol* **81**, 4–24.

Talairach J (1955) *Chirurgie stéréotaxique du thalamus*. Bases anatomiques et techniques. Indications et résultats thérapeutiques. VI Congr Lat Am Neurocir (Montevideo), pp. 865–925.

Talairach J, Tournoux P, Bancaud J (1960) La chirurgie pariétale de le douleur. *Acta Neurochir (Wien)* **8**, 153–250.

Tasker RR, Organ LW, Hawrylyshyn P (1980) Deafferentation and causalgia. In Bonica JJ, ed., *Pain*. New York: Raven Press, pp. 305–330.

Tasker RR, Tsuda T, Hawrylyshyn P (1983) Clinical neurophysiological investigation of deafferentation pain. *Adv Pain Res Ther* **5**, 713–738.

Tasker RR (1984) Deafferentiation. In Wall PD, Melzack R, eds., *Textbook of Pain*. London: Churchill Livingstone, pp. 119–132.

Tasker RR, Yoshida M, Sima AAF, Deck J (1986) Stimulation mapping of the periventricular-periaqueductal gray (PVG-PAG) in man: an autopsy study. In Samii M, ed., *Surgery In and Around the Brain Stem and the Third Ventricle*. Berlin: Springer Verlag, pp. 161–167.

Tasker RR, Dostrovsky J (1989) Deafferentation and central pain. In: Wall PD, Melzack R, eds., *Textbook of Pain*. London: Churchill Livingstone, pp. 154–180.

Tasker RR (1989) Stereotactic surgery. In Wall PD, Melzack R, eds., *Textbook of Pain*, 2nd edn. Edinburgh: Churchill Livingstone, pp. 840–855.

Tasker RR (1990) Thalamotomy. *Neurosurg Clin N Am* **1**, 84–86.

Tasker RR, DeCarvalho G, Dostrovsky JO (1991) The history of central pain syndromes, with observations concerning pathophysiology and treatment. In Casey KL, ed., *Pain and Central Nervous System Disease: The Central Pain Syndromes*. New York: Raven Press, pp. 31–58.

Tasker RR, DeCarvalho GTC, Dolan EJ (1992) Intractable pain of spinal cord origin: clinical features and implications for surgery. *J Neurosurg* **77**, 373–378.

Tasker RR, Parrent AG, Kiss Z, Davis K, Dostrovsky JO (1994) Surgical treatment of stroke-induced pain. *Stereotact Funct Neurosurg* **62**, 311–312.

Tasker RR, North RB (1997) Cordotomy and myelotomy. In North RB, Levy RM, eds., *Neurosurgical Management of Pain*. New York: Springer, pp. 191–220.

Tasker RR (2001a) Central pain states. In Loeser JD, ed., *Bonica's Management of Pain*, 3rd edn. Philadelphia, PA: Lippincott Williams & Wilkins, pp. 433–457 (see also previous edn., 1990).

Tasker RR (2001b) Microelectrode findings in the thalamus in chronic pain and other conditions. *Stereotact Funct Neurosurg* **77**, 166–168.

Tator CH, Agbi CB (1991) Complications in the management of syringomyelia. *Perspect Neurol Surg* **2**, 143–150.

Taub E, Munz M, Tasker RR (1997) Chronic electrical stimulation of the gasserian ganglion for the relief of pain in a series of 34 patients. *J Neurosurg* **86**, 197–202.

Teixeira MJ (1998) Various functional procedures for pain: II. Facial pain. In Gildenberg PL, Tasker RR, eds., *Textbook of Stereotactic and Functional Neurosurgery.* New York: McGraw-Hill, pp. 1389–1402.

Teixeira MJ, Lepski G, Aguiar PHP *et al.* (2003) Bulbar trigeminal stereotactic nucleotractotomy for treatment of facial pain. *Stereotact Funct Neurosurg* **81**, 37–42.

Thalhammer JG, Raymond SA (1991) Does the axon only ax? IASP newsletter, July–August, pp. 2–4.

Thomas DGT, Jones SJ (1984) Dorsal root entry zone lesions (Nashold's procedure) in brachial plexus avulsion. *Neurosurgery* **15**, 966–968.

Thompson SC (1981) Will it hurt less if I can control it? A complex answer to a simple question. *Psychol Bull* **90**, 89–101.

Thomson AM, Deuchars J (1994) Temporal and spatial properties of local circuits in neocortex. *TINS* **17**, 119–126.

Tirsch WS, Stude P, Scherb H, Keidel M (2004) Temporal order of nonlinear dynamics in human brain. *Brain Res Rev* **45**, 79–95.

Tommerdahl M, Delemos KA, Vierck CJ Jr., Favorov OV, Whitsel BL (1996) Anterior parietal cortical response to tactile and skin-heating stimuli applied to the same skin site. *J Neurophysiol* **75**, 2662–2670.

Tommerdahl M, Delemos KA, Favorov OV *et al.* (1998) Response of anterior parietal cortex to different modes of same-site skin stimulation. *J Neurophysiol* **80**, 3272–3281.

Tommerdahl M, Whitsel BL, Favorov OV, Metz CB, O'Quinn BL (1999) Responses of contralateral SI and SII in cat to same-site cutaneous flutter versus vibration. *J Neurophysiol* **82**, 1982–1992.

Tommerdahl M, Delemos KA, Whitsel BL, Favorov OV, Metz CB (1999) Response of anterior parietal cortex to cutaneous flutter versus vibration. *J Neurophysiol* **82**, 16–33.

Torvik A (1959) Sensory, motor and reflex changes in two cases of intractable pain after stereotactic mesencephalic tractotomy. *J Neurol Neurosurg Psychiat* **22**, 299–305.

Toth S, Sólyom A, Tóth Z (1984) One possible mechanism of central pain. Autokindling phenomenon on the phantom limb or sensory loss oriented patients. *Acta Neurochir (Wien) Suppl* **33**, 459–469.

Tourian AY (1987) Narcotic responsive "thalamic" pain treatment with propranolol and tricyclic antidepressants. *Pain Suppl* **4**, 411.

Tourian AY (1991) Deafferentation syndrome: medical treatment. In: Nashold BS Jr., Ovelmen-Levitt J, eds., *Deafferentation Pain Syndromes. Pathophysiology and Treatment,* New York: Raven Press, pp. 331–340.

Tovi D, Schisano G, Liljequist B (1961) Primary tumors of the region of the thalamus. *J Neurosurg* **18**, 730–740.

Treede R-D, Bromm B (1991) Neurophysiological approaches to the study of spinothalamic tract function in humans. In Casey KL, ed., *Pain and Central Nervous System Disease.* New York: Raven Press, pp. 117–127.

Tremont-Lukats IW, Challapalli V, McNicol ED, Lau J, Carr DB (2005) Systemic administration of local anesthetics to relieve neuropathic pain: a systematic review and meta-analysis. *Anesth Analg* **101**, 1738–1749.

Trentin L, Visentin M (2000) La predittività del test con lidocaina nel trattamento del dolore neuropatico. *Minerva Anestesiol* **66**, 157–161.

Triggs WJ, Beric A (1992) Sensory abnormalities and dysaesthesias in the anterior spinal artery syndrome. *Brain* **115**, 189–198.

Triggs WJ, Beric A (1993) Giant somatosensory evoked potentials in a patient with the anterior spinal artery syndrome. *Muscle Nerve* **16**, 492–497.

Triggs WJ, Beric A (1994) Dysaesthesiae induced by physiological and electrical activation of posterior column afferents after stroke. *J Neurol Neurosurg Psych* **57**, 1077–1080.

Tsai PS, Buerkle H, Huang LT *et al.* (1998) Lidocaine concentrations in plasma and cerebrospinal fluid after systemic bolus administrations in humans. *Anesth Analg* **87**, 601–604.

Tseng SH (2000) Treatment of chronic pain by spinal cord stimulation. *J Formos Med Assoc* **99**, 267–271.

Tsubokawa T, Moriyasu N (1975) Follow-up results of centre median thalamotomy for relief of intractable pain. *Conf Neurol* **37**, 280–284.

Tsubokawa T, Yamamoto T, Katayama T, Hirayama T, Sibuya H (1984) Thalamic relay nucleus stimulation for relief of intractable pain. Clinical results and beta-endorphin immunoreactivity in the cerebrospinal fluid. *Pain* **18**, 115–126.

Tsubokawa T, Katayama Y, Yamamoto T, Hirayama T (1985) Deafferentation pain and stimulation of the thalamic sensory relay nucleus: clinical and experimental study. *Appl Neurophysiol* **48**, 166–171.

Tsubokawa T, Katayama Y, Yamamoto T, Hirayama T, Koyama S (1991) Treatment of thalamic pain by chronic motor cortex stimulation. *PACE* **14**, 131–134.

Tsubokawa T, Katayama Y, Yamamoto T, Hirayama T, Koyama S (1993) Chronic motor cortex stimulation in patients with thalamic pain. *J Neurosurg* **78**, 393–401.

Turnbull F (1939) Cordotomy for thalamic pain. A case report. *Yale J Biol Med* **2**, 411–414.

Turnbull IM (1972) Bilateral cingulumotomy combined with thalamotomy or mesencephalic tractotomy for pain. *Surg Gynecol Obstet* **134**, 958–962.

Turnbull IM (1984) Brain stimulation. In Wall PD, Melzack R, eds., *Textbook of Pain*, Edinburgh: Churchill Livingstone, pp. 706–714.

Turner JA, Lee JS, Schandler SL, Cohen MJ (2003) An fMRI investigation of hand representation in paraplegic humans. *Neurorehab Neural Repair* **17**, 37–47.

Ullman S (1995) Sequence seeking and counter streams: a computational model for bidirectional information flow in the visual cortex. *Cereb Cortex* **5**, 1–11.

Urabe M, Tsubokawa T (1965) Stereotaxic thalamotomy for the relief of intractable pain. *Tohoku J Exp Med* **85**, 286–300.

Urban BJ, Nashold BS Jr. (1978) Percutaneous epidural stimulation of the spinal cord for relief of pain. *J Neurosurg* **48**, 323–328.

Usubiaga J, Moya F, Wikinski J (1967) Relationship between the passage of local anesthetics across the blood brain barrier and their effects on the central nervous system. *Br J Anaesth* **39**, 943–947.

Van Bastelaere M, De Laat M (1999) Lamotrigine: a morphine-sparing drug for central pain. In *9th World Congress on Pain, Book of Abstracts*. Seattle, WA: IASP Press, A211-P65.

Van der Bruggen MA, Huisman HB, Beckermann H et al. (2001) Randomized trial of 4-aminopyridine in patients with chronic incomplete spinal cord injury. *J Neurol* **248**, 665–671.

Vega-Bermudez F, Johnson KO (2002) Spatial acuity after digit amputation. *Brain* **125**, 1256–1264.

Velasco M, Brito F, Jimenez F et al. (1998) Effect of fentanyl and naloxone on a thalamic induced painful response in intractable epileptic patients. *Stereotact Funct Neurosurg* **71**, 90–102.

Veldman PHJM, Goris RJ (1996) Multiple reflex sympathetic dystrophy. Which patients are at risk for developing a recurrence of reflex sympathetic dystrophy in the same or another limb? *Pain* **64**, 463–466.

Verdugo R, Ochoa JL (1991) High incidence of placebo responders among chronic neuropathic pain patients. *Ann Neurol* **30**, 229.

Verhoeff NP, Petroff OA, Hyder F et al. (1999) Effects of vigabatrin on the GABAergic system as determined by [123I] iomazenil SPECT and GABA MRS. *Epilepsia* **40**, 1433–1438.

Vestergaard K, Nielsen J, Andersen G et al. (1995) Sensory abnormalities in consecutive, unselected patients with central post-stroke pain. *Pain* **61**, 177–186.

Vestergaard K, Andersen G, Jensen TS (1996) Treatment of central post-stroke pain with a selective serotonin reuptake inhibitor. *Eur J Neurol* **3**(Suppl. 5), 169.

Vestergaard K, Andersen G, Gottrup H, Kristensen BT, Jensen TS (2000) Lamotrigine for central poststroke pain: a randomized controlled trial. *Neurology* **56**, 184–190.

Vick PG, Lamer TJ (2001) Treatment of central post-stroke pain with oral ketamine. *Pain* **92**, 311–313.

Vierck CJ (1973) Alterations of spatio-tactile discrimination after lesions of primate spinal cord. *Brain Res* **58**, 69–79.

Vilela Filho O, Tasker RR (1994) Pathways involved in thalamic ventrobasal stimulation for pain relief: evidence against the hypothesis VB stimulation-rostroventral medulla excitation-dorsal horn inhibition. *Arq Neuropsiquiatr* **52**, 386–391.

Vilela Filho O (1996) Risk factors for unpleasant paresthesiae induced by paresthesiae-producing deep brain stimulation. *Arq Neuropsiquiatr* **54**, 57–63.

Villemure C, Wassimi S, Bennett GJ, Shir Y, Bushnell MC (2006) Unpleasant odors increase pain processing in a patient with neuropathic pain: psychophysical and fMRI investigation. *Pain* **120**, 213–220.

Vogel HP, Heppner B, Humbs N, Schramm J, Wagner C (1986) Long term effects of spinal cord stimulation in chronic pain syndromes. *J Neurol* **233**, 16–18.

Vogt BA, Berger GR, Derbyshire SW (2003) Structural and functional dichotomy of human mid-cingulate cortex. *Eur J Neurosci* **18**, 3134–3144.

Von Hagen KO (1957) Chronic intolerable pain. Discussion of its mechanism and report of eight cases treated with electroshock. *JAMA* **165**, 773–777.

Voris HC, Whisler WW (1975) Results of stereotaxic surgery for intractable pain. *Conf Neurol* **37**, 86–96.

Vranken JH, Dijkgraaf MG, Kruis MR, van Dasselaar NT, van der Vegt MH (2005) Iontophoretic administration of S(+)-ketamine in patients with intractable central pain: a placebo-controlled trial. *Pain* **118**, 224–231.

Vuadens PH, Regli F, Dolivo M, Uske A (1994) Segmental pruritus and intramedullary vascular formation. *Schw Arch Neurol Psych* **145**, 13–16.

Wade DT, Makela P, Robson P, House H, Bateman C (2004) Do cannabis-based medicinal extracts have general or specific effects on symptoms in multiple sclerosis? A double-blind, randomized, placebo-controlled study on 160 patients. *Mult Scler* **10**, 434–441.

Waijima Z, Shitara T, Inoue T, Ogawa R (2000) Severe lightning pain after subarachnoid block in a patient with neuropathic pain of central origin: which drug is best to treat the pain? *Clin J Pain* **16**, 265–269.

Walker AE (1942a) Relief of pain by mesencephalic tractotomy. *Arch Neurol Psych* **48**, 865–883.

Walker AE (1942b) Mesencephalic tractotomy. A method for the relief of unilateral intractable pain. *Arch Surg* **44**, 953–962.

Walker AE (1950) The neurosurgical treatment of intractable pain. *Lancet* **70**, 279–282.

Walker AE (1955) Pain: the neurosurgeon's viewpoint. *J Chron Dis* **2**, 91–95.

Wall PD (1995) Pain in the brain and lower parts of the anatomy. *Pain* **62**, 389–391.

Walshe TM, Davis KR, Fisher CM (1977) Thalamic hemorrhage: a computed tomographic–clinical correlation. *Neurology* **27**, 217–222.

Waltz TA, Ehni G (1966) The thalamic syndrome and its mechanisms. Report of two cases, one due to arteriovenous malformation in the thalamus. *J Neurosurg* **24**, 735–742.

Wang XJ (2001) Synaptic reverberation underlying mnemonic persistent activity. *Trends Neurosci* **24**, 455–463.

Warms CA, Turner JA, Marshall HM, Cardenas DD (2002) Treatments for chronic pain associated with spinal cord injuries: many are tried, few are helpful. *Clin J Pain* **18**, 154–163.

Waxman SG, Hains BC (2006) Fire and phantoms after spinal cord injury: Na(+) channels and central pain. *Trends Neurosci* **29**, 207–215.

Weigel R, Krauss JK (2004) Center median-parafascicular complex and pain control. *Stereotact Funct Neurosurg* **82**, 115–126.

Weiller C, Chollet F, Friston KJ, Wise RJ, Frackowiak RS (1992) Functional reorganization of the brain in recovery from striatocapsular infarction in man. *Ann Neurol* **3**, 463–472.

Weimar C, Kloke M, Schlott M, Katsarava Z, Diener HC (2002) Central poststroke pain in a consecutive cohort of stroke patients. *Cerebrovasc Dis* **14**, 261–263.

Weisenberg M, Schwarzwald J, Tepper I (1996) The influence of warning signal timing and cognitive preparation on the aversiveness of cold-pressor pain. *Pain* **64**, 379–385.

Werhahn KJ, Mortensen J, Kaelin-Lang A, Boroojerdi B, Cohen LG (2002) Cortical excitability changes induced by deafferentation of the contralateral hemisphere. *Brain* **125**, 1402–1413.

Werner A (1961) Myélectomie dans un cas de paraplégie spastique douloureuse. *Neurochirurgie* **7**, 140–145.

Wertheimer P, Mansuy L (1949) Reflexions sur la topectomie prefrontale. *Rev Neurol* **81**, 866–871. (see also 401–408)

Wertheimer P, Lecuire J (1953) La myélotomie commissurale postérieure: à propos de 107 observations. *Acta Chir Belg* **52**, 568–574.

Wessel K, Vieregge P, Kessler CH, Kömpf D (1994) Thalamic stroke: correlation of clinical symptoms, somatosensory evoked potentials, and CT findings. *Acta Neurol Scand* **90**, 167–173.

Wester K (1987) Dorsal column stimulation in pain treatment. *Acta Neurol Scand* **75**, 151–155.

White JC, Sweet WH (1955) *Pain: Its Mechanisms and Neurosurgical Control.* Springfield, IL: Thomas.

White JC (1962) Modifications of fronto-leukotomy for relief of pain and suffering in terminal malignant diseases. *Ann Surg* **156**, 394–403.

White JC (1963) Anterolateral chordotomy – its effectiveness in relieving pain of non-malignant disease. *Neurochirurgia (Stuttgart)* **6**, 83–102.

White JC, Sweet WH (1969) *Pain and the Neurosurgeon. A Forty-Year Experience.* Springfield, IL: Thomas.

Widar M, Samuelsson L, Karlsson-Tivenius S, Ahlstroem G (2002) Long-term pain conditions after a stroke. *J Rehabil Med* **34**, 165–170.

Widar M, Ek A-C, Ahlstroem G (2004) Coping with long-term pain after a stroke. *J Pain Symptom Manage* **27**, 215–225 (see also *J Clin Nurs* 2004, **13**, 497–505).

Widerstroem-Noga E, Felipe-Cuervo E, Yezierski RP (2001) Chronic pain after spinal injury: interference with sleep and daily activities. *Arch Phys Med Rehabil* **82**, 1571–1577.

Wiegand H, Winkelmuller W (1985) Behandlung des Deafferentierungsschmerzes durch Hochfrequenzläsion der Hinterwurzeleintrittszone. *Deutsche medizinische Wochenschrift* **110**, 216–220.

Wiffen P, Collins S, McQuay H *et al.* (2000) Anticonvulsant drugs for acute and chronic pain. *Cochrane Database Syst Rev* CD001133.

Willis WD (1985) *The Pain System. The Neural Basis of Nociceptive Transmission in the Mammalian Nervous System.* Basel: Karger.

Willis WD (1991) Central neurogenic pain: possible mechanisms. *Adv Pain Res Ther* **19**, 81−102.

Willis WD (2002) Possible mechanisms of central neuropathic pain. *Progr Pain Res Manage* **23**, 85−115.

Willis WD, Westlund KN (2004) Pain system. In Paxinos G, Mai JK, eds., *The Human Nervous System,* 2nd edn. Amsterdam: Elsevier Academic Press, pp. 1137−1170.

Willoch F, Schindler F, Wester HJ *et al.* (2004) Central poststroke pain and reduced opioid receptor binding within pain processing circuitries: a [11C] diprenorphine PET study. *Pain* **108**, 213−220.

Winkelmuller M, Winkelmuller W (1996) Long-term effects of continuous intrathecal opioid treatment in chronic pain of nonmalignant etiology. *J Neurosurg* **85**, 458−467.

Wirth ED III, Vierck CJ Jr., Reier PJ, Fessler RG, Anderson DK (2002) Correlation of MRI findings with spinal cord injury pain following neural tissue grafting into patients with posttraumatic syringomyelia. *Progr Pain Res Manage* **23**, 313−330.

Witting N, Kupers RC, Svensson P *et al.* (2001) Experimental brush-evoked allodynia activates posterior parietal cortex. *Neurology* **57**, 1817−1824.

Wolskee PJ, Gracely RH, Greenberg RP, Dubner R, Lees D (1982) Comparison of effects of morphine and deep brain stimulation on chronic pain. *Am Pain Soc Abst* 36.

Wood T, Sloan R (1997) Successful use of ketamine for central pain. *Palliat Med* **11**, 57.

Woodrow KM, Friedman GD, Siegelaub AB, Collen MF (1972) Pain tolerance: differences according to age, sex and race. *Psychosom Med* **34**, 548−556.

Woolsey CN, Erickson TC, Gilson WE (1979) Localization in somatic sensory and motor areas of human cerebral cortex as determined by direct recording of evoked potentials and electrical stimulation. *J Neurosurg* **51**, 476−506.

Wu Q, Garcia-Larrea L, Mertens P *et al.* (1999) Hyperalgesia with reduced laser evoked potentials in neuropathic pain. *Pain* **80**, 209−214.

Wycis HT, Spiegel EA (1962) Long-range results in the treatment of intractable pain by stereotaxic midbrain surgery. *J Neurosurg* **19**, 101−107.

Yamamoto T, Katayama Y, Hirayama T, Tsubokawa T (1997) Pharmacological classification of central post-stroke pain: comparison with the results of chronic motor cortex stimulation therapy. *Pain* **72**, 5−12.

Yamamoto T, Katayama Y, Fukaya C *et al.* (2000) Thalamotomy caused by cardioversion in a patient treated with deep brain stimulation. *Stereotact Funct Neurosurg* **74**, 73−82.

Yamashiro K, Iwayama K, Karihara M *et al.* (1991) Neurons with epileptiform discharge in the central nervous system and chronic pain. Experimental and clinical investigations. *Acta Neurochir (Wien) Suppl* **52**, 130−132.

Yen HL, Chan W (2003) An East−West approach to the management of central post-stroke pain. *Cerebrovasc Dis* **16**, 27−30.

Yoshii N, Mizokami T, Ushikubo T, Kuramitsu T, Fukuda S (1980) Long-term follow-up study after pulvinotomy for intractable pain. *Appl Neurophysiol* **43**, 128−132.

Young GB, Blume WT (1983) Painful epileptic seizures. *Brain* **106**, 537−554.

Young RF, Goodman SJ (1979) Dorsal spinal cord stimulation in the treatment of multiple sclerosis. *Neurosurgery* **5**, 225−230.

Young RF, Chambi I (1987) Pain relief by electrical stimulation of the periaqueductal and periventricular gray matter. Evidence for a non-opioid mechanism. *J Neurosurg* **66**, 364−371.

Young RF (1989) Brain stimulation. In Wall PD, Melzack R, eds., *Textbook of Pain.* New York: Churchill Livingstone, pp. 925−929.

Young RF (1990) Clinical experience with radiofrequency and laser DREZ lesions. *J Neurosurg* **72**, 715−720.

Young RF, Tronnier V, Rinaldi PC (1992) Chronic stimulation of the Kolliker-Fuse nucleus region for relief of intractable pain in humans. *J Neurosurg* **76**, 979−985.

Young RF, Vermeulen SS, Grimm P *et al.* (1995) Gamma knife thalamotomy for the treatment of persistent pain. *Stereotact Funct Neurosurg* **64**(Suppl. 1), 172−181.

Young RF (1995) Commentary. In Schmideck HH, Sweet WH, eds., *Operative Neurosurgical Techniques. Indications, Methods and Results,* 3rd edn. Philadelphia, PA: WB Saunders, pp. 1399−1401.

Young RF, Rinaldi PC (1997) Brain stimulation. In North RB, Levy RM, eds., *Neurosurgical Management of Pain.* New York: Springer, pp. 283−301.

Young RF (1998) Deep brain stimulation for failed back syndrome. In Gildenberg PL, Tasker RR, eds.,

Textbook of Stereotactic and Functional Neurosurgery. New York: McGraw-Hill, pp. 1621–1626.

Zachariah SB, Borges EF, Varghese R, Cruz AR, Ross GS (1994) Positive response to oral divalproex sodium (Depakote) in patients with spasticity and pain. *Am J Med Sci* **308**, 38–40.

Zeki S, Ffychte DH (1998) The Riddoch syndrome: insights into the neurobiology of conscious vision. *Brain* **121**, 25–45.

Zimmermann M (1979) Peripheral and central nervous mechanisms of nociception, pain, and pain therapy: facts and hypotheses. *Adv Pain Res Ther* **3**, 3–32.

Zimmermann M (1991) Central nervous mechanisms modulating pain-related information: do they become deficient after lesions of the peripheral or central nervous system? In Casey KL, ed., *Pain and Central Nervous System Disease. The Central Pain Syndromes.* New York: Raven Press, pp. 183–200.

Zubieta J-K, Dannals RF, Frost JJ (1999) Gender and age influences on human brain mu-opioid receptor binding measured by PET. *Am J Psychiat* **156**, 842–848.

Zubieta J-K, Smith YR, Bueller JA *et al.* (2001) Regional mu opioid receptor regulation of sensory and affective dimensions of pain. *Science* **293**, 311–315.

Zuelch KJ (1960) Schmerzbefunde nach operativen Eingriffen am Zentralnervensystem. *Acta Neurochir (Wien)* **8**, 282–286.

Zuelch KJ, Schmid EE (1953) Uber die Schmerzarten und den Begriff der Hyperpathie. *Acta Neuroveg* **7**, 147–159.

Zylicz Z (1997) Opioid responsive central pain of cerebrovascular origin: a case report. *Palliat Med* **11**, 495–496.

INDEX